Laughing Your Way To Passing The Neurology Boards

Amy McGregor, M.D.
David Z. Rose, M.D

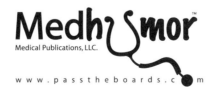

MedHumor Medical Publications, Stamford, Connecticut

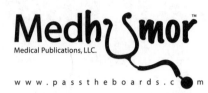

www.passtheboards.com

Published by:
Medhumor Medical Publications, LLC
1127 High Ridge Road, Suite 332
Stamford, CT 06905 U.S.A.

ISBN: 978-1-60743-535-8

Printed in the United States of America

This book is designed to provide information and guidance in regard to the subject matter covered.

It is to be used as a study guide for physicians preparing for the Part I examination for initial certification in Neurology administered by the American Board of Psychiatry and Neurology. It is not meant to be a clinical manual. The reader is advised to consult textbooks and other reference manuals in making clinical decisions. It is not the purpose of this book to reprint all the information that is otherwise available, but rather to assist the Board Candidate in organizing the material to facilitate study and recall on the exam. The reader is encouraged to read other sources of material, in particular picture atlases that are available.

Although every precaution has been taken in the preparation of this book, the publisher, author, and members of the editorial board assume no responsibility for errors, omissions or typographical mistakes. Neither is any liability assumed for damages resulting from the direct and indirect use of the information contained herein. The book contains information that is up-to-date only up to the printing date. Due to the very nature of the medical profession, there will be points out-of-date as soon as the book rolls off the press. The purpose of this book is to educate and entertain.

If you do not wish to be bound by the above, you may return this book to the publisher for a full refund within 30 days from the date of purchase.

Acknowledgments

First, I want to express my deepest gratitude to my husband, Dave McGregor, for his support and for reading the entire first draft of the first edition.

I wish to acknowledge my mom, whose strength and compassion are an inspiration to me, and who is a wonderful listener.

I want to thank Lisa Armitige for years of friendship and for cheering me on every step of the way.

I am indebted to Fred Perkins for writing the Foreword and to Vickie Brewer for writing the Exams are a Fact of Life chapter.

I am grateful to many individuals for reading over chapters of the first edition: Lisa Armitige (Infectious Diseases), Tulio Bertorini (Neuromuscular Diseases), Vickie Brewer (Behavioral Neurology), Linda Buckleair (Neuropathology and Neuro-oncology), Ian Butler (Pediatric Neurology), Mazen Dimachkie (Neurophysiology), Stanley Fisher (Movement Disorders), Bob Foehring (Anatomy), Collin Hovinga (Neurotransmitters), Michael Jacewicz (Toxins), Andrew Lawton (Neuro-ophthalmology), Pedro Mancias (Neurocutaneous Disorders), Brannon Morris (Neuro-oncology), Ronald Pfeiffer (Neurodegenerative diseases), William Pulsinelli (Stroke), Aparajitha Verma (Reflexes and Triads), Jewell Ward (Metabolic Diseases), James Wheless (Epilepsy and Neurophysiology), and Bryan Williams (Toxins).

Jackie Brown created the fantastic drawings, including the sketches for the cover of the first edition, and was delightful to work with. I wish to thank Louise Storey for her help with graphics and for her enthusiasm.

Dave Clarke, Fred Perkins, and Jim Wheless, my terrific (and funny) colleagues, gave me advice and answered numerous questions.

Douglas McGregor, Jeremy Slater, and Milvia Pleitez encouraged me at pivotal times in the development in this book. I am also thankful for the support of my brother Greg and my friends Rebecca Gelber and Appu Verma.

I want to express my appreciation to Ian Butler, Sharon Crandell, James Ferrendelli, Louisa Kalsner, Pedro Mancias, Mya Schiess, John Slopis, and all the other wonderful attendings at The University of Texas-Houston Medical School who trained me.

I am grateful to Stu Silverstein and Medhumor Medical Publications, LLC for their interest in this book. Todd Van Allen provided valuable assistance.

Amy McGregor, M.D.

In memory of my dad, who had a wonderful sense of humor.

Acknowledgments

A million thanks to my terrific parents, Burton A. Rose & Celeste C. Rose for all those years of encouragement, enthusiasm, and enlightenment; my beautiful and intelligent esposa Liz Evora for keeping me on-track; and my sister Dayna C. Rose-Benn and her husband Andrew R. Benn for all the intangibles. My loyal family always supports my ideas with alacrity. Who else could love this punim? Only Goblin, Mamsickle, Boo-boo, Schwayna, and Bunny.

Secondly, thanks to Medhumor Medical Publications, LLC (Stu Silverstein, M.D., Brian Cahn, and Antoinette D'Amore) for this opportunity to expand upon the groundbreaking, hilarious Neurology mnemonic book by Amy McGregor, M.D. I'm honored to have built upon Amy's creative right-brained tome.

Thirdly, thanks to all the wonderful M.D.'s who have trained me over the years, taking the time to "show one, do one, teach one." These compassionate humanoids are:

- At the University of Pennsylvania in Philadelphia: Drs. Kasner, Messe, Mullen, Cucchiara and Detre;

- At the University of Miami in Florida: Drs. Sacco, Rundek, Isaacson, Bradley, McCarthy, Verma, Lopez-Alberola, Sanchez, Thomas, Tornes, Maldonado, Rodriguez and Romano;

- At the Cleveland Clinic in Ohio: Drs. Furlan, Sila, DeGeorgia, Nielsen, Jacobs, Babu, Schaus, Lefferts, and Lowenthal;

- At the University of Virginia in Charlottesville: Drs. Serkin, Smolarz, Gaughen, and Mr. Hershman, Batten and Koussa;

- And at the University of South Florida in Tampa: Drs. Burgin, Decker, Agazzi, VanLovern, Gooch, Muntean, Kan, Frontera, Bozorg, Brock, and Ms.'s Clancy, Moret, Lund, Wilson, Bozeman, Cypress-West, Bisick, Bodiford, Giarratano, McTigue, and all the terrific people at the USF-CAMLS building (Center for Advanced Medical Learning and Simulation) in downtown Tampa Bay who helped put together our Thrombolysis in Acute Ischemic Stroke, Team Practice Approach (TPA) simulation project."

Lastly, thanks to my attorneys Robert L. Achor and Michael H. Leibowitz; my hair stylists Wiz Donato and Georgina Panache; the good folks at Bastion Construction and Barlow's Hardware; the Infomas TV news crew; the foot-stompin' band of "Koblick and the Cartagena Cinco"; and of course, the Greek Goddess Mnemosyne and her jo Zeus – my sincerest "Gracias, Amigos!"

David Z. Rose, M.D.

"I am certain of nothing but the holiness of the heart's affections, and the truth of imagination."
— John Keats

Foreward to the First Edition

Here it is guys, the beginning of the rest of your life. Congratulations! You have worked very, very hard and should be rightfully proud of your accomplishments. No doubt, your spouse/significant other is proud. Your children (if you have had time to make any) are proud. Your parents are proud. Your Aunt Minnie is proud. Heck, my Aunt Minnie is proud but then again my Aunt Minnie is happy if she can make it to the bathroom on time and her 'lumbago isn't actin' up.'

Reality Check: Most of you are in your early thirties. You're in debt up to your eyeballs. Some of you are working in fellowships which is academicalese for "he who works for low pay and high responsibility." Most of you are trying to figure out where you're going to work next year. How much money will you earn? Is there a good sign on bonus? What should you look out for in your contract? Unfortunately, this book won't help you with any of that. Adding insult to injury, the world thinks you are now a rich doctor and even your family is wondering what you are complaining about. Now comes that last niggling little detail: the board exam.

The bad news is that you are about to take one of the hardest medical specialty boards in existence. The good news is that every resident can pass this exam. The other good news is that the Part II Oral Exams have been mothballed in favor of local mock orals conducted by the residency programs themselves. This book CAN help you with the former.

I have a confession to make. I never properly studied (if I studied at all) for any of my exams. I didn't study for the SAT, ACT, or the MCAT. I barely studied for my USMLE part I. For parts II and III, I didn't even crack a book. Don't get me wrong, I'm no genius. Like you, I was a fairly smart person and I simply played the odds. Luckily for me, that had always paid off. When I got to neurology residency, I had a similar attitude (although I took my work very seriously). I didn't study for my first Residency In Training Exam (RITE) and the results were abysmal. It was a wake up call. I knew at that point that I would have to study for the neurology board.

There are always people who say, "I didn't study for this exam or that exam and I did just fine." This might be fine for people passing their Health Board exam prior to an engaging career in body piercing or tattooing but you won't find neurologists making such statements. I've seen colleagues stress so much over the board that they generated enough sphincter tone to convert coal to diamonds. I even saw one or two I thought might rip a temporary hole in the fabric of space-time. I'm telling you now, this is NOT helpful. Although, given the current circumstances of healthcare finance, the diamond making trick might come in handy.

Are these fears founded on reality? Well, the answer is "yes" and "no." It's hard to get any real data from the ABPN because they tend to keep the pass/fail rate numbers fairly closely guarded. When I was in training, not so many moons ago, my program director informed us that we had about a sixty-something percent chance of passing part I, the first time around, and a sixty-something chance of passing part II, the first time around. That didn't sound very good to me especially when they told me there was a study that supported the notion that residents who did very well in the RITE exam also tended to do very well on the boards. The only credible data that I have seen published came from the Journal of Child Neurology (J Child Neurol 2005;20:25-27) which followed graduates of neurology and child neurology residency from 1994. To summarize, the first time pass rate for both neurology and child neurology for part I was 75%. Neurology graduates first time pass rate for part II was a bit higher at 73% compared with child neurology at 57%. Furthermore, the paper goes on to say that the pass rates for all first time takers between 1990-1999 were 68% for part I (neurology and child neurology combined) and 65% for part II child neurology and 67% for part II neurology. Finally, getting back to the class of '94, 82% of those seeking certification ultimately got it. So I suppose my program director was right. Oh and to soothe the concerns of our child neurology brothers and sisters, remember this: There are approximately ten adult neurologists in training for every one child neurologist. Furthermore, the number of child neurologists taking the board in a given year is around two dozen, this is compared with a couple hundred (or more) adult candidates. It's really hard to extrapolate much from the limited data that the ABPN has released and it's even harder to compare the two groups.

So how do you prepare? First of all, you have identified yourself as very motivated because you're reading this book. That alone probably increases your chances of passing – self selection, Heisenberg principle, insert your method of analysis here _____. In addition to this book, a couple other resources may be handy. A good, basic clinical book (not necessarily one of the mega-books) is a great study aide for weak areas. A good functional neuroanatomy text is useful and another helpful method is to review the old RITE exam answers/explanations including the slide sets. Most residency programs keep copies and I strongly recommend you review them. There are only so many academic neurologists in the world, writing only so many questions which cover so many disorders. In other words, the tests are not the same but by my observation, there seems to be some cross pollination. Set yourself a schedule several months in advance of the test. Read this book and review the RITE answers/slides first and use the textbooks to fill in the voids. Finally, attend every local neurology review conference you can reasonably get to. If you are following the steps listed above, then it will only reinforce your knowledge base.

My final advice is to relax a moment, take a step back and breathe. I like to keep a few things in mind. One, the test can only last a few hours, so all pain much like bleeding, does stop. Second, you will see things in the board you have never heard of before. Don't let this throw you off your game. Trust in the quality of your knowledge, the quantity is already there. Don't forget to take care of yourself. Eat properly. Exercise. Spend time with your family. If you are married and/or have children, keep in mind that those people who are supporting you and also enduring this process. Don't forget about them either.

There are no guarantees in life, but if you do these things, then your chances of success are quite good indeed.

Good Luck!

F. Frederick Perkins, Jr., MD

Table of Contents

Copyright 2013 by Medhumor Medical Publications, LLC

Chapter 19: Reflexes, Signs and Other Phenomenon 677

Chapter 20: X-Linked Diseases................................683

Chapter 21: Psychiatry for Neurologists 685

Guideposts Along the Way

As you read the book, you will notice pictures in the margin that emphasize important points. These "Guideposts" will indicate a particular category of information.

DEFINITION	*Definition*	This points to a definition.
PERIL / WARNING	*Perils*	This alerts you to possible big mistakes and traps that can be laid down for you on the exam.
MNEMONIC	*Mnemonic Device*	This indicates a mnemonic that will help you memorize difficult but important information.
HOT TIP	*Hot Tip*	"This draws attention to a "Board Pearl," to help you on potential trouble areas in the exam.
BUZZ WORDS	*Buzz Words*	This describes buzzwords or key phrases that are typical for a given disorder. By learning this, you will often be able to recognize the answer in the wording of the question itself.
EITHER OR CHOICES	*Down to two choices*	This points out minute differences between similar disorders, which are critical to answering many questions correctly.
TAKE HOME MESSAGE	*Take Home Message*	Important take home points to remember.
TREATMENT	*Treatment*	This points to specific treatments for a given diagnosis or disorder.
VERY BORING MATERIAL WARNING!	*Boring*	Warning! Very boring material. Do not handle heavy machinery while reading.

Exams Are A Fact Of Life

Even if you manage to escape the obligatory death and taxes, standardized exams are a fact of life, no matter how desperately you attempt to avoid eye contact with this reality.

If you continue to deny the need to study, eventually reality will make eye contact *with you*: which was eloquently pointed out in the foreward by Dr. Perkins.

Of course you always have the option of taking the exam more than once, but the purpose of this book is to help you avoid this inconvenient fate.

If you have already taken the exam once before, it is important to **remain confident** and *see the first time around as a learning experience.*

What follows is information regarding test preparation and test-taking skills.

BEFORE THE TEST

Begin your preparation early with a **game plan**. Begin by reviewing the material and narrowing in and keeping notes on the key points you are expected to have at your fingertips.

Reinforce with Review

Review should be a part of your regular weekly study schedule.

Reviews are much more than reading and rereading. You need to read over your notes and **focus on the material you don't know well**. The tendency is to review material you know well since that is more gratifying, but it won't take you closer to your goal of passing the exam.

If your notes are relatively complete and well organized, you may find that very little rereading of the textbook for detail is needed.

Once you have consolidated the important information, you need to begin reading for the purpose of memorizing. This will typically be material on cases you have not actually seen during your training.

Lemmings and Lemons

There will be pressure from colleagues to form *study groups* but don't feel you have to do that. Groups are not always beneficial to everyone, and you might just be following lemmings off a cliff. Often studying in groups is inconvenient and may force you to focus on details that are not necessary to the exam or material you have already mastered.

Choose what works best for you. If you do better studying on your own at your convenience, do that.

Avoid talking about the process with egotistic, overly optimistic peers. It will just make you mad. *Sometimes the level of ego is inversely proportional to test performance.* Often you will either gain a false sense of security or insecurity depending on the neurosis of the colleague you happen to be speaking to.

Fun Memory Lane

This book provides several mnemonics to help you remember important facts. In doing so we hope to demonstrate, by example, how you can develop your own. **Mnemonics are the fast lane to making it impossible to forget material.** Mnemonics are a great way to remember material because it helps your brain use multiple modalities and humor to not only help you remember the material, but to make it impossible to forget.

Sprinting and Sleeping to Avoid Marathon Fatigue

Review for several short periods rather than one long period. You will find that you retain information better and get less fatigued.

Review some material at night prior to going to bed. Sleep helps consolidate memories so that information is moved more readily into long term storage. *Research shows that information studied right before going to sleep is more readily remembered.* There is less interference, and some theories suggest that dreams are a way of processing material.

Be a Flasher

It may seem "old-fashioned", but flashcards may be a helpful way to review material that involves details that are more difficult to memorize. Review the cards in random order, removing the cards that become etched in your memory until you have no cards left.

What me Worry? What to do about Test Anxiety?

Anxiety is your worst enemy. If you have reached this point you can and will pass the exam, and you must tell yourself this over and over. Anxiety interferes with your ability to effectively form strategies for retrieving information. *An individual may do poorly on an exam despite knowing the material if anxiety prevented them from developing strategies to learn the material or retrieve it on the exam if they did.*

The following strategies will help you reduce anxiety and gain precious points on the exam:

1. Always **arrive early** and take a moment to relax and reduce your anxiety.

   · This brief time period will boost your confidence.

   · Use this time to focus your mind and think positive thoughts.

2. **Rest well the night before the exam**.

   Don't stay up late reviewing the night before the exam. Any information you might learn in those last hours will be offset by information you will forget due to fatigue.

3. **Have a proper balanced diet.**

   Don't forget to eat a balanced meal before the exam. This is not the time to suffer from fatigue due to low glucose levels. The same goes for lunch.

4. **No time to quit caffeine**.

   If you are a serious coffee drinker, don't take this opportunity to cut back on caffeine intake. You'll just get a headache and feel tired. Drink the usual amount you drink daily

5. **Meds require a trial run**.

   If you are considering medications to help you with anxiety, **don't take the medication for the first time the day before or day of the test**. Use common sense; all medications can have side effects and this is not the time to experiment and find out that body odor and frequent urination is a common side effect.

6. **Do not dwell on the negative**.

   In fact you should focus on positive statements such as "I deserve to and will pass the exam". Maybe even think of an imaginary crowd cheering you on as if this is a sporting event and you are a world class famous athlete.

7. **Do relax. Take a deep breath**.

   Remember from basic physiology that taking a deep breath slows your heart rate and lowers your blood pressure. This can also be achieved through ocular compression but I wouldn't suggest pushing on your eyeballs in the middle of your board exam since it may raise eyebrows.

DURING THE TEST

Arrive Early.

Arriving early will give you time to relax and reduce panic. However, *don't make the mistake of chatting with friends and colleagues.* Use this time to focus and relax. Talking about the test and being around people who are either overly optimistic or pessimistic isn't going to help. *Try to go into the test alert and calm instead of tense and anxious.*

Read Carefully.

Read each question carefully and completely before picking your answer. Re-read if you are at all confused.

Don't worry if you forget something that you would normally know. A lapse in memory is normal and it will likely come back to you later when you need it. Just put a check mark by the item and return later. If you have the opportunity to go back and return to questions do so. Most computerized exams have this option and track unanswered questions for you.

Don't Spend Too Much Time on Any Question.

Figure out how much time you have to spend on each question and as you go through put a check mark by the ones you are uncertain about. Then after completing the test, go back to those with check marks. This will also give you some idea of how you are doing. Don't worry if there are lots of check marks. Statistically, if there are 4 answers to multiple choice questions, you'll get 25% of those correct just by guessing.

A Legal Cheat Sheet

Do a quick dumping of information you don't want to forget. If there is something that you just keep forgetting, review it right before going in and then immediately write it down on the scrap paper you are given at the test center. Sort of a legal cheat sheet.

Watch the Double Negatives

Reread all questions containing negative wording such as "not" or "least". Be especially alert for the use of double or even triple negatives within a sentence, as these must be read very carefully to assure full understanding.

When facing a choice that is a double negative restate the choice as a positive statement and then assess if it is the correct choice.

With such questions you are often looking for the "incorrect choice" and we are trained to look for correct choices. Therefore it is very easy to carelessly pick a "correct choice" which is actually the "incorrect answer".

Eliminate!!!

Instead of looking for the right choices, look for the wrong choices first and eliminate them. You can usually eliminate 2 choices rather quickly. **Question options that are totally unfamiliar to you.**

You might want to note on your scrap paper which choices to focus on for each question to help you focus on this process. Some of the items will be obviously wrong. If you have to guess, at least you have narrowed it down so that your chances are better of getting it right.

True False Questions Dressed in Multiple Choice Clothing

Be alert for multiple choice questions that ask you to pick the one choice that is correct or the one choice that is incorrect.

In this format **all** parts of the statement must be true or the entire statement is false.

Be alert for grammatical inconsistencies between the question stem and the answer choices on multiple-choice questions. **A choice is almost always wrong if it and the stem do not make a grammatically correct sentence.**

First Guess is Best

Be cautious about changing your answer without a good reason. Your first "guess" is more likely to be correct than are subsequent "guesses", so be sure to have a sound reason for changing your answer. Look for the central idea of each question. What is the fact or concept are they testing you on?

Of course if you are sure the original answer is incorrect by all means go ahead and change it. Sometimes an answer may become apparent in a later question.

Always and Never are (Usually) Never Correct

Question options that contain negative or absolute words. Statements that begin with always, never, any, except, most, or least-are probably NOT the answer.
Try substituting a qualified term for an absolute one as follows:

Substitute *frequently* for *always*

Substitute *typical* for *every*

This will help you clarify if the statement is accurate.

GUESSING!

If you have to guess, make it an educated guess and follow some simple rules.

A. Choose the longest choice

B. If two choices are opposites, choose one of them.

C. The most general alternative is usually the right answer.

D. Never be afraid to guess. Remember your statistics. If there are 4 answers you have a 25% chance of getting it right. But narrow it down. There is always at least one that is obviously wrong. If you eliminate even one, you've improved your chances to 33.33% of getting it right.

"All of the Above:"

If you know two of three options seem correct, then "all of the above" is a strong possibility.

"Look Alike Options"

If two choices look alike then one is probably correct.

If two alternatives seem correct, **compare them for differences**, and then **refer to the stem to find your best answer.**

Following the suggestions in this chapter and taking a systematic approach to studying for the exam should put you in a good position to pass the exam.

Exams Are a Fact of Life

was written by:

Dr. Vickie R. Brewer

Chapter 1

Anatomy

Cerebellum

Gross Anatomy of Cerebellum

The cerebellum consists of:

· 2 cerebellar hemispheres
· The vermis
· The flocculonodulus

The cerebellar hemispheres are responsible for appendicular control, and the vermis is responsible for axial control.

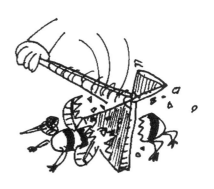

 To remember both, just AX the VERMIN!!!

Lobes of Cerebellum

The flocculonodulus has a role in vestibular function and is discussed below.

The cerebellum has 3 lobes: anterior, posterior, flocculonodular.

Lobe of the Cerebellum Alternative names:

To associate the cerebellar lobes with their more antiquated names, think of an APe'S FAVorite PreNuP.

Anterior = Paleocerebellum = Spinocerebellum
Flocculonodular = Archicerebellum = Vestibulocerebellum
Posterior = Neocerebellum = Pontocerebellum

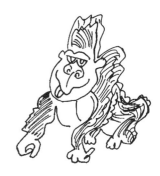

Anterior Lobe/Paleocerebellum/Spinocerebellum

 To remember the **A**nterior lobe is called **P**aleocerebellum or **S**pinocerebellum: Remember **APe'S**

The spinocerebellum receives input from the:

· Dorsal (posterior) spinocerebellar tract
· Ventral (anterior) spinocerebellar tract
· Cuneocerebellar tract

(These tracts are discussed below.)

Lesions of the **A**nterior lobe cause **A**taxic gait.

Posterior Lobe/ Neocerebellum/Pontocerebellum (PreNuP)

The **P**osterior lobe, or **N**eocerebellum, or **P**ontocerebellum is important for precise movement.

The **P**osterior lobe is responsible for **P**recise movement.

Flocculonodular Lobe/ Archicerebellum/ Vestibulocerebellum (FAVorite)

The vestibulocerebellum is important for equilibrium and eye movements. It receives input from the vestibulocerebellar tract.

To remember the **F**locculonodular lobe is also known as the **A**rchicerebellum or **V**estibulocerebellum: Remember FAVorite in APe'S FAVorite PreNuP.

Cerebellar Peduncles

There are 3 peduncles, which connect the cerebellum to the brainstem: superior, middle, inferior.

Cerebellar peduncle	Alternative name for the peduncle	Area of brainstem to which peduncle connects
Superior	Brachium conjunctivum	Midbrain
Middle	Brachium pontis	Pons
Inferior	Restiform body / corpus restiform	Medulla

Just as you would expect based on brainstem neuroanatomy:

Superior cerebellar peduncle ———> midbrain

Middle cerebellar peduncle ———> pons

Inferior cerebellar peduncle ———> medulla

The superior cerebellar peduncle primarily carries outputs from the cerebellum; whereas, the other peduncles mainly carry inputs.

 The **s**uperior cerebellar peduncle **s**ends information from the cerebellum.

Nuclei of the Cerebellum

There are deep cerebellar and vestibular nuclei. **These carry the output of the cerebellum.**

The deep cerebellar nuclei are called dentate, emboliform, fastigial, and globose. Their order from lateral to medial is: dentate, emboliform, globose, fastigial.

 To remember the names of the deep cerebellar nuclei :

    Dentate

    Emboliform

    Globose

    Fastigial

 DENTISTS EMULATE GREAT FRIENDS

This mnemonic is in anatomic order!

Dentate Nucleus

The dentate nucleus is part of the neocerebellum/pontocerebellum.

The dentate nucleus is the most lateral of the deep nuclei, and the lateral hemispheres of the cerebellum project to it.

The dentate nucleus contributes to dexterity.

 The **de**ntate assists with **de**xterity, which you want your dentist to have.

The dentate nucleus is part of the **Triangle of Guillain Mollaret**, which is described below.

The **dentatorubrothalamic tract** is important in planning and synergy of movement. It is a major output from the cerebellum; it travels through the superior cerebellar peduncle.

The dentatorubrothalamic pathway:

Purkinje cells ⇨ dentate nucleus ⇨ contralateral red nucleus ⇨ ventral lateral thalamus ⇨ areas 4,6 motor cortex

Fastigial Nucleus

The fastigial nucleus is associated with the flocculonodular lobe/archicerebellum/vestibulocerebellum.

It has a role in stance and walking.

 The **f**astigial nucleus is associated with the **f**locculonodular lobe.[1] *foot traffic*

Another way to remember that the **fast**igial nucleus is associated with the flocculonodular lobe/archicerebellum/vestibulocerebellum, remember FAST FAVorite.

Emboliform and Globose Nuclei

The emboliform and globose nuclei are also known as the **interposed nuclei**.

 They are associated with the **APeS**: **A**nterior lobe/**P**aleocerebellum/**S**pinocerebellum.

The interposed nuclei have a role in stability and speed of initiation of movement.

---

[1] Mnemonic courtesy of Dr. Foehring.

Lesions of the interposed nuclei result in **T**itubation, **A**ction tremor, abnormal **R**apid alternating movements, and **DY**smetria on finger-nose-finger and heel-knee-shin testing.

DENTISTS EMULATE GREAT FRIENDS... until they INTERPOSE by being TARDY!

> **T**itubation
> **A**ction tremor
> **R**apid alternating movements off
> **DY**smetria

Cerebellar Cortex

Layers of the Cerebellar Cortex - M.P.G. (as in Mile Per Gallon)

The cerebellar cortex has 3 layers:

1. **M**olecular layer
2. **P**urkinje cell layer
3. **G**ranule cell layer

The molecular layer contains:

- Basket cells
- Stellate cells
- Purkinje cell dendrites
- Parallel fibers of the granule cells
- Golgi cell dendrites

The Purkinje cell layer just contains Purkinje cells.

The granule cell layer contains:

- Granule cells
- Golgi cells
- Glomeruli (synapse of granule and Golgi cells)

(handwritten annotations: GLUT, (-) Taurine, (+), (+), GABA, (-), input climbing fibers, output deep cerebellar + vestibular nuclei, (+) aspartate, (-) GABA, input mossy fibers, GLUT)

The **M**olecular layer contains a **Mile** of cells. The **P**urkinje cell layer contains just **Per**-kinje cells, and the **G**ranule cell layer contains cells that have a "G" and "l" like **Gall**on: **Granule, Golgi and Glomeruli.**

Cell type	Neurotransmitter	Role	Cells upon which it acts
Golgi	GABA	Inhibitory	Granule
Granule	Glutamate	Excitatory(+)***	Basket, Golgi, stellate **Note: only Granules are excitatory!!!!!!!!!!!!!!!!**
Purkinje	GABA	Inhibitory (-)	Deep cerebellar nuclei and vestibular nuclei
Stellate	Taurine	Inhibitory (-)	Purkinje

Basket cells use GABA as their neurotransmitter and are inhibitory to Purkinje cells.

Stellate cells, which use taurine as their neurotransmitter, are also inhibitory to Purkinje cells.

Basket cells ——————————→ Purkinje cells ←—————————— Stellate cells
GABA   Taurine

Golgi cells use GABA as their neurotransmitter and are inhibitory to granule cells.

Purkinje cells are GABAergic and are inhibitory to deep cerebellar and vestibular nuclei.

Granule cells are glutamatergic and are excitatory to basket, Golgi, and stellate cells.

Note: only Granules are excitatory!!!!!!!!!!!!!!!!!!!!!

In summary:

· Basket, Golgi, Purkinje, and stellate cells are inhibitory.
- ○ Purkinje cells inhibit intracerebellar and vestibular nuclei.
- ○ Stellate, basket, and Golgi cells act as inhibitory interneurons.
- ○ Basket, Golgi, and Purkinje cells are GABAergic.
    Stellate cells use taurine as their neurotransmitter.

·Granule cells are excitatory and use glutamate as their neurotransmitter.

Granule cells get the basket, Golgi, and stellate cells groovin' with glutamate.

Golgi cells gouge the granule cells. Granule cells excite the Golgi cells, but the Golgi cells inhibit the granule cells.

Inputs to the Cerebellar Cortex

The two main sources of input to the cerebellar cortex are mossy fibers and climbing fibers.

 Mossy fibers mosey and climbing fibers climb into the cerebellar cortex.

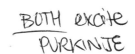

BOTH excite PURKINJE

Mossy Fibers

The mossy fibers provide most of the input to the cerebellum. The neurotransmitter they use is **aspartate**.

Mossy fibers synapse on granule cells, which they excite.

 Let's toast the mossy fibers with diet Coke (with aspartame), someone is finally willing to excite the granule cells.

Axons from the granule cells form **parallel fibers** in the molecular layer.

The parallel fibers excite Purkinje cells, which carry output from the cerebellar cortex.

One mossy fiber may stimulate thousands of Purkinje cells via the granule cells.

The mossy fibers are bossy.

Climbing Fibers

Climbing fibers also provide input to the cerebellum. They come from the contralateral inferior olivary nucleus, through the inferior cerebellar peduncle, to the molecular layer of the cerebellum, where they excite Purkinje cells.

One climbing fiber excites about 10 Purkinje cells. It makes multiple synaptic contacts with each Purkinje cell. This climbing fiber sends a few branches to synapse with stellate and basket cells nearby.

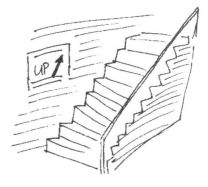

Outputs from the Cerebellar Cortex

Purkinje cells provide output from cerebellar cortex.

Purkinje cells are perky and outgoing (from the cerebellar cortex).

Afferent and Efferent Pathways

Afferent Information

From the Cortex

The cortex provides input to the cerebellum through 3 pathways:

- Corticopontocerebellar pathway
- Cerebro-olivocerebellar pathway
- Cerebroreticulocerebellar pathway

Information from the corticopontocerebellar pathway enters the cerebellum through the middle cerebellar peduncle. (Recall that the pons is connected to the cerebellum by the middle cerebellar peduncle.)

To remember that the cortex sends input to the cerebellum by the corticoPONTOcerebellar, Cerebro-OLIVOcerebellar, and cerebroRETICULOcerebellar pathways: The cortex sent the cerebellum input in the OLIVE RETICULE PRONTO.

Input from the cerebro-olivocerebellar pathway enters the cerebellum as climbing fibers, which are excitatory to Purkinje cells.

To remember that climbing fibers are the fibers of the olivocerebellar tract, think of climbing an olive tree.

The cerebroreticulocerebellar pathway is important for controlling voluntary movement.

From the Spinal Cord

The spinal cord sends information to the cerebellum via 4 tracts:

- Cuneocerebellar tract
- Dorsal (posterior) spinocerebellar tract
- Rostral spinocerebellar tract
- Ventral (anterior) spinocerebellar tract

Cuneocerebellar Tract

The cuneocerebellar tract carries afferent information about movement of the ipsilateral upper extremity and rostral body to the cerebellum.

Dorsal Spinocerebellar Tract

The dorsal spinocerebellar tract carries afferent information about ipsilateral lower extremity limb movement and the trunk to the cerebellum. Fibers in the dorsal spinocerebellar tract give rise to mossy fibers that travel in the inferior cerebellar peduncle to the cerebellum.

Ventral Spinocerebellar Tract

Like the dorsal spinocerebellar tract, the ventral spinocerebellar tract carries unconscious proprioceptive information from the trunk and lower extremities to the cerebellum; however, some fibers cross. Also, information in the ventral spinocerebellar tract travels to the cerebellum via the superior cerebellar peduncle.

Rostral Spinocerebellar Tract

The rostral spinocerebellar tract carries unconscious proprioceptive information from the upper limbs and rostral body, similar to the cuneocerebellar tract.

	Movement	Proprioception
UE & rostral body:	Cuneocerebellar	Rostral spinocerebellar
LE & trunk:	Dorsal spinocerebellar	Ventral spinocerebellar

From the Vestibular Nerve

Information from the vestibular nerve enters the cerebellum through the inferior cerebellar peduncle (ICP). Mossy fibers carry this information to the flocculonodular lobe. (Recall that the flocculonodular lobe is also known as the vestibulocerebellum.)

Other Afferent Fibers

The cerebellum receives information from the red nucleus and tectum.

The cerebellar cortex also receives input from the raphe nuclei (serotonergic) and the locus ceruleus (noradrenergic). These inputs have diffuse actions.

Efferent Information

The Purkinje cells carry output from the cerebellum.

Most of the Purkinje cells synapse on neurons of the deep cerebellar nuclei; some Purkinje cell axons travel directly to the lateral vestibular nucleus.

Efferent Pathways

Efferent pathways from the cerebellum are:
- Globose-emboliform-rubral pathway
- Dentatothalamic and dentatorubral pathways
- Fastigial vestibular pathway
- Fastigial reticular pathway

Globose-Emboliform-Rubral Pathway

Information leaves the globose and emboliform nuclei and travels in the decussation of the superior cerebellar peduncles to the contralateral red nucleus.

Dentatothalamic and Dentatorubral Pathways

The **dentatothalamic pathway** carries information to the contralateral ventral lateral (VL) nucleus of the thalamus.

To remember that the dentatothalamic tract travels from the dentate to the ventral lateral nucleus: Dentists are eViL[2].

The **dentatorubral tract** transmits information to the contralateral red nucleus. These fibers are often branches of the dentatothalamic tract.

---

[2] This is just a mnemonic; it's not meant to be a slur of our dental colleagues.

To remember that the dentate nucleus also sends a tract to the red nucleus: Dentists cause lots of red blood.

The dentatorubrothalamic pathway is how the cerebellum exerts its effect on synergy of movement.

The dentatorubrothalamic pathway:

Purkinje cells → dentate nucleus → contralateral red nucleus → ventral lateral thalamus → areas 4,6 of the motor cortex

One can use the dentist mnemonics to remember that the information travels from the dentate to the red nucleus and then the ventral lateral thalamus.

Fastigial Vestibular Pathway

Information travels from the fastigial nucleus to the lateral vestibular nucleus via the inferior cerebellar peduncle.

The **lateral vestibulospinal tract**, which facilitates ipsilateral extensor muscle tone, is formed from neurons of the lateral vestibular nucleus.

Fastigial Reticular Pathway

Information also travels from the fastigial nucleus to the reticular formation via the inferior cerebellar peduncle.

The **reticulospinal tract**, which affects ipsilateral muscle tone, arises from the reticular formation.

The Cerebellar Peduncles and Afferent and Efferent Information

As mentioned above, the superior cerebellar peduncle connects the cerebellum to the midbrain, the middle cerebellar peduncle connects the cerebellum to the pons, and the inferior cerebellar peduncle connects the cerebellum to the medulla.

Cerebellar Peduncles and Afferent Pathways

Try Real VODCA inferior input

Inferior Cerebellar Peduncle	Middle Cerebellar Peduncle	Superior Cerebellar Peduncle
Arcuatocerebellar tract	Pontocerebellar (corticopontocerebellar) tract	Cerulocerebellar tract
Cuneocerebellar tract		Tectocerebellar tract
Dorsal spinocerebellar tract		Trigeminocerebellar tract
Olivocerebellar tract		Ventral spinocerebellar tract
Reticulocerebellar tract		
Trigeminocerebellar tract		
Vestibulocerebellar tract		

Cerebellar Peduncles and Efferent Pathways

Inferior Cerebellar Peduncle	Middle Cerebellar Peduncle	Superior Cerebellar Peduncle
Fastigial vestibular pathway		Dentatorubral tract
Fastigial reticular pathway		Dentatothalamic tract
		Globose-emboliform-rubral pathway
		Uncinate bundle of Russell

GED, superior, Russell

Inferior Cerebellar Peduncle

 A lot of the **in**put to the cerebellum comes in through the **in**ferior cerebellar peduncle.

To remember the inputs to the inferior cerebellar peduncle: **Try Real VODCA (vodka), because yours is <u>INFERIOR</u>! I won't <u>input</u> it into my mouth!**

This refers to **T**rigeminocerebellar , **R**eticulocerebellar, **V**estibulocerebellar, **O**livocerebellar, **D**orsal spinocerebellar, **C**uneocerebellar, and **A**rcuatocerebellar tracts.

The **Rest**iform body and **Juxt**arestiform body are components of the inferior cerebellar peduncle.
After Trying Real VODCA, you Juxt want to Rest!

The **restiform body** has fibers from spinocerebellar tracts (dorsal spinocerebellar, rostral spinocerebellar, and cuneocerebellar tracts), which project to the spinocerebellum.

The restiform body also contains olivocerebellar fibers.

The **juxtarestiform body** has afferent and efferent fibers related to the vestibular system: vestibulocerebellar and cerebellovestibular fibers.

Cerebellovestibular and cerebelloreticular pathways exit the cerebellum through the inferior cerebellar peduncle.

Middle Cerebellar Peduncle

The middle cerebellar peduncle carries only afferent fibers. Specifically, afferent fibers of the pontocerebellar (corticopontocerebellar) tract travel in the middle cerebellar peduncle, which is also known as the brachium pontis.

Superior Cerebellar Peduncle

The superior cerebellar peduncle primarily carries outputs from the cerebellum; whereas, the other peduncles mainly carry inputs.

The superior cerebellar peduncle is formed by fibers from the globose, emboliform, and dentate nuclei.

Following a GED (globose, emboliform, dentate nuclei) you can get superior (superior cerebellar peduncle) education, like Uncle Russell.

The **uncinate bundle of Russell (Uncle Russell)** transmits information to the vestibular nuclei and reticular formation via the superior cerebellar peduncle.

The Triangle of Guillain Mollaret

The Triangle of Guillain Mollaret is a feedback loop.

Fibers travel from the red nucleus to the ipsilateral inferior olive in the **central tegmental tract**.

Then climbing fibers travel from the inferior olive to the contralateral dentate nucleus in the inferior cerebellar peduncle (ICP).

Next, fibers travel from the dentate nucleus to the contralateral (original) red nucleus in the superior cerebellar peduncle (SCP).

The Triangle of Guillain Mollaret

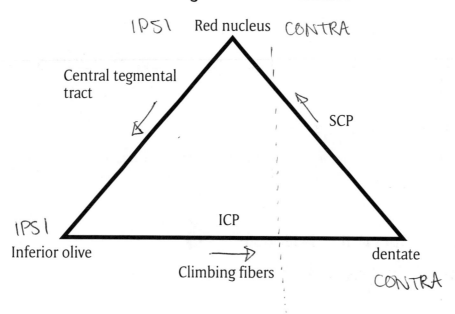

 A lesion in the pathways of the Triangle of Guillain Mollaret causes **palatal myoclonus**.

Cerebral Cortex

Layers of the cerebral cortex:

    I.   Molecular Layer

    II.   External granular layer

    III. External pyramidal layer

    IV. Internal granular layer

    V.   Internal pyramidal / ganglionic layer

    VI. Multiform layer

Layer I is the most superficial.
Layers II and III are responsible for cortical-cortical connections.
Layer IV, receives information from the thalamus.
Layer VI sends information to the thalamus.

For Your Reference (I don't remember being tested on this):

Area of cortex	Brodmann's area	Lobe
Primary somatosensory cortex	3,1,2	Parietal
Premotor cortex	6	Frontal
Primary motor cortex	4	Frontal
Primary olfactory cortex	34	Temporal
Frontal eye fields	8	Frontal
Primary visual cortex	17	Occipital
Visual association cortex	39,19,18	Occipital
Primary auditory cortex	41	Temporal
Auditory association cortex (Wernicke's speech area)	22	Temporal
Broca's speech area	44,45	Frontal

MNEMONIC Primary visual cortex is Brodmann's area 17. At 17 you can take your first (primary) view of a rated-R movie.

Visual association cortex is nearby at Brodmann's areas 18,19, and 39. (Brodmann's area 39 is the angular gyrus.)

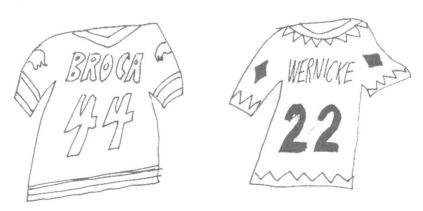

Cranial Nerves

A mnemonic for cranial nerve names (in order) is:

Oh, **O**h, **O**h, **T**o **T**ouch **A**nd **F**eel **V**elvet, **G**ood **V**elvet, **A**h, **H**eaven!

Cranial nerve	Name of cranial nerve
I	**O**lfactory nerve
II	**O**ptic nerve
III	**O**culomotor nerve
IV	**T**rochlear nerve
V	**T**rigeminal nerve
VI	**A**bducens nerve
VII	**F**acial nerve
VIII	**V**estibulocochlear nerve
IX	**G**lossopharyngeal nerve

Cranial nerve	Name of cranial nerve
X	**V**agus nerve
XI	spinal **A**ccessory nerve
XII	**H**ypoglossal nerve

A common-use, well known mnemonic for cranial nerve function (in order) is:

Some **S**ay **M**arry **M**oney, **B**ut **M**y **B**rother **S**ays **B**ig **B**rains **M**atter **M**ost!

Where S, M, and B are:

S = Sensory

M = Motor

B = Both (Sensory + Motor)
the mnemonic for function

Cranial nerve	Function
Olfactory nerve (CN I)	**S**ensory: Olfaction.
Optic nerve (CN II)	**S**ensory: Vision.
Oculomotor nerve (CN III)	**M**otor: eye muscles (except Superior Oblique and Lateral Rectus) and pupillary constrictors.
Trochlear nerve (CN IV)	**M**otor: Superior Oblique muscle (SO_4).
Trigeminal nerve (CN V)	**B**oth: facial sensation and mastication If you try to masticate (muscles of **mastication**) a mile (**mylohyoid**) of food, your "A+" belly (**A**nterior **belly** of digastric) becomes tense (**tensors**).
Abducens (CN VI)	**M**otor: Lateral Rectus muscle (LR_6).
Facial nerve (CN VII)	**B**oth: Facial movement, taste (anterior 2/3 tongue), salivation, lacrimation. **To Zanzibar By Motor Car** – *motor branches of VII* – Temporal – *motor branches of VII* – **T**emporal, **Z**ygomatic, **B**uccal, **M**andibular, **C**ervical.
Vestibulocochlear nerve (CN VIII)	**S**ensory: Hearing.
Glossopharyngeal nerve (CN IX)	**B**oth: stylopharyngeus muscle; taste (posterior 1/3 tongue); sensation to middle and external ear, pharynx, posterior 1/3 tongue; innervates parotid gland and carotid body and sinus.

Cranial nerve	Function
Vagus nerve (CN X)	**B**oth: motor to lift palate, pharynx[3], larynx, and viscera; efferent limb of oculocardiac and carotid sinus reflexes; sensory to taste (pharynx).
Spinal accessory nerve (CN XI)	**M**otor: trapezius, sternocleidomastoid, and laryngeal muscles[4].
Hypoglossal nerve (CN XII)	**M**otor: Tongue movement.

Function	Cranial nerves
Pure **M**otor	3,4,6,11,12
Pure **S**ensory	1,2,8
Both motor and sensory	5,7,9,10
Parasympathetic	3,7,9,10

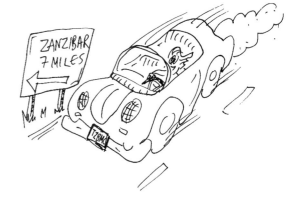

---

[3] Except the stylopharyngeus muscle, which is innervated by CN IX, and the tensor veli palatini muscle, which is innervated by CN V.

[4] Except the cricothyroid, which is supplied by a branch of the vagus nerve.

Mnemonic for foramina, in order:
Cleaners **O**nly **S**praying **S**alty **S**cents **R**ight
Onto **S**melly **I**guanas **I**s **J**ustified, **J**ustified,
Justified, **H**owever!

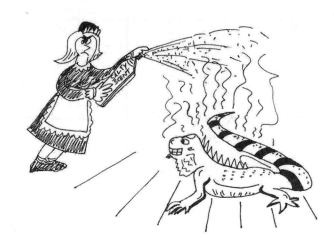

Cranial nerve (CN)	Foramina through which CN exits skull
I	**C**ribriform plate
II	**O**ptic canal
III, IV, V$_1$-*ophthalmic division*	**S**uperior orbital fissure *(S,S,S for III, IV, and V$_1$)*
V$_2$-*maxillary division*	Foramen **R**otundum
V$_3$-*mandibular division*	Foramen **O**vale
VI	**S**uperior orbital fissure
VII	**I**nternal auditory meatus then stylomastoid foramen
VIII	**I**nternal auditory meatus
IX, X, XI	**J**ugular foramen *(J,J,J for IX, X, and XI)*
XII	**H**ypoglossal foramen

The internal carotid artery travels through the foramen lacerum.

Think **rum** on **ic**e to remember that the **ICA** travels through the foramen lace**rum**.

The middle meningeal artery travels through the foramen spinosum.

Recall that epidural hematomas are often due to injury to the middle meningeal artery.

Cranial Nerves in Detail

CN I (Olfactory Nerve)

CN I is a sensory nerve that is responsible for olfaction.

It exits the skull through the cribriform plate of the ethmoid bone.

Olfaction

Olfactory receptor neurons send axons in the olfactory nerves to the olfactory bulbs, where they synapse. Then, the olfactory tracts (lateral striae) carry information from the olfactory bulbs to the olfactory cortex. The **primary olfactory cortex consists of the piriform cortex and the periamygdaloid cortex and is found in the anterior temporal lobe.**

Fibers project from the olfactory cortex to the orbitofrontal cortex, entorhinal cortex, medial dorsal nucleus of the thalamus, and the hippocampus. The entorhinal area of the parahippocampal gyrus is the secondary olfactory cortex.

Fibers from the olfactory tract also project to the amygdala and olfactory tubercle in the anterior perforated substance.

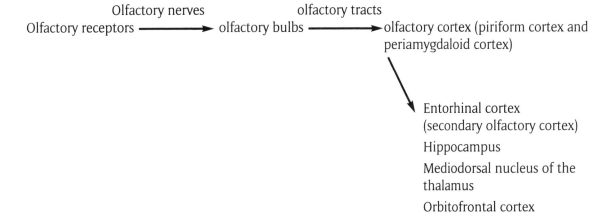

Olfactory nerves   olfactory tracts

Olfactory receptors ⟶ olfactory bulbs ⟶ olfactory cortex (piriform cortex and periamygdaloid cortex)

Entorhinal cortex (secondary olfactory cortex)

Hippocampus

Mediodorsal nucleus of the thalamus

Orbitofrontal cortex

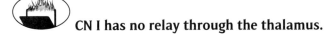 **CN I has no relay through the thalamus.**

The olfactory nerve does not go through the thalamus because it's smelly, and the other cranial nerves don't want it there.

Lesions of CN I

Head trauma can cause loss of smell if the olfactory nerves traveling through the cribriform plate are damaged.

Recall that olfactory groove meningiomas can cause **Foster-Kennedy Syndrome** (ipsilateral optic atrophy, contralateral papilledema, ipsilateral anosmia).

 To remember the details of F̲oster-**Kennedy** Syndrome, think of president John **F. Kennedy**:

> If he couldn't **see (ipsilateral optic atrophy, contralateral papilledema),** and
> he couldn't **smell (ipsilateral anosmia),**
> he'd still be **groovin' man (olfactory groove meningiomas).**

Lesions of the uncus cause olfactory hallucinations.

To remember that the uncus is associated with olfactory hallucinations, think of un̲c̲le Olaf (olfactory) in *Lemony Snicket's A Series of Unfortunate Events.*

CN II (Optic Nerve)

The optic nerve is a sensory nerve that is formed by axons from the ganglion layer of the retina.

Please see the Neuro-ophthalmology chapter.

CN III (Oculomotor Nerve)

The oculomotor nerve is a motor nerve. It innervates the levator palpebrae superior and the extraocular muscles except the superior oblique and lateral rectus.

It also provides parasympathetic innervation to the pupillary constrictor and ciliary muscle of the lens.

CN IV (Trochlear Nerve) (SO$_4$)

The trochlear nerve is a motor nerve that innervates the **S**uperior **O**blique muscle, which causes **depression** and **intorsion** of the eye—People who are SO depressed become introverted!

This is the longest and smallest cranial nerve. It is the only cranial nerve that crosses the midline. It is also the only cranial nerve to leave from the dorsal aspect of the brainstem.[5]

---

[5] For more information on CN IV, please see the Neuro-ophthalmology chapter.

MNEMONIC

The <u>tr</u>ochlear nerve is <u>tr</u>icky. It exits out the back and crosses. As a result, it has a long distance to travel. Maybe it does this because it's the **smallest** nerve, it's **depressed**, and has become S**O** **introverted** that it exits out the back to avoid everyone.

CN V (Trigeminal Nerve)

The trigeminal nerve has both sensory and motor functions, which are described below.

Branches

CN V has 3 branches:
V_1 is the ophthalmic branch.
V_2 is the maxillary branch.
V_3 is the mandibular branch.

As mentioned above, V_1 exits the skull through the **S**uperior orbital fissure; V_2 exits through the foramen **R**otundum, and V_3 exits through the foramen **O**vale.

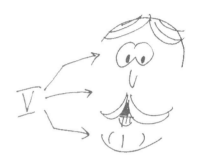

MNEMONIC

To remember that the **mandib**ular division of the trigeminal nerve exits by the foramen **oval**e, remember that you move your **mandib**le to drink **Oval**tine.

V_1 and V_2, which are purely sensory, pass through the cavernous sinus. V_3 has sensory and motor functions; it does not travel through the cavernous sinus.

MNEMONIC

V_3, which has to do both motor and sensory functions, doesn't have time to go into the **cave (cavernous sinus)** with V_1 and V_2 (which are **sensory only**).

Sensory Functions of CN V

The trigeminal nerve provides sensation to the face, mouth, sinuses, and meninges. It also provides sensation (not taste) to the anterior 2/3 of the tongue.

The trigeminal (gasserian) ganglion, which is the sensory ganglion of the trigeminal nerve, is in Meckel's cave. "*semilunar*"

Motor Functions of CN V

V3 innervates the following muscles:

- · Muscles of mastication (temporalis, masseter, pterygoids)
- · Mylohyoid
- · Anterior belly of digastric
- · Tensors (Tensor Tympani, and Tensor Veli Palatini)

 To remember the muscles that the trigeminal nerve innervates remember this phrase: If you try to masticate a mile of food, your belly becomes tense.

 If you try (**trigeminal**) to masticate (muscles of **mastication**) a mile (**mylohyoid**) of food, your "A+" belly (**A**nterior **belly** of digastric) becomes tense (**tensors**).

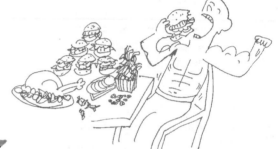

 CN VII supplies the posterior belly of the digastric.

 Contractions of the tensor veli palatini are found in essential palatal tremor.

The tensor tympani dampens movements of the malleus (one of the middle ear ossicles).

Reflexes Involving CN V

The trigeminal nerve is involved in many reflexes.

Corneal Reflex

When the cornea is touched, the corneal reflex causes the eyelids to close.

The afferent limb is the ophthalmic division of the trigeminal nerve (V_1).

The efferent limb is the facial nerve (VII) via the orbicularis oculi muscle.

Jaw Jerk

 The afferent and efferent limbs of the jaw jerk are the mandibular nerve (V_3).

The Tearing (Lacrimal) Reflex

 The afferent limb of the tearing reflex is V_1, and the efferent limb is the facial nerve.

The Oculocardiac Reflex

As a result of the oculocardiac reflex, pressure on the eye results in bradycardia. (Please don't do this at home.)

 The afferent limb is V_1 (ophthalmic nerve), and the efferent limb is the vagus nerve (X).

Nuclei of CN V

 The trigeminal nerve has 4 nuclei:
- Main sensory nucleus
- Mesencephalic nucleus
- Motor nucleus
- Spinal nucleus

Trigeminal Sensory Nuclei

Nucleus	Function
Main sensory nucleus of V	Fine touch
Spinal nucleus of V	Pain and temperature sensation
Mesencephalic nucleus of V	Position sense

The spinal nucleus of V carries spinothalamic information e.g. pain and temperature.

The mesencephalic nucleus is the only example of a primary sensory neuron being located in the central nervous system (CNS) rather than peripheral ganglia.

To remember that the mesencephalic nucleus is in the CNS, think of mesencephalic as Me's in cephalic.

Pain and temperature, fine touch, and position sense for the face first converge in the **ventroposterior medial nucleus (VPM)**. The VPM projects to postcentral gyrus.

The various modalities of CN V meet in the VPM, which could be thought of as VPMeeting.

Tracts of CN V

Ventral Trigeminothalamic Tract

The ventral trigeminothalamic tract is responsible for carrying *pain and temperature* sensation from the face and oral cavity.

To remember that the ventral trigeminothalamic tract is responsible for pain sensation, remember that people vent when they are in pain.

Information is carried to first-order neurons in the trigeminal (gasserian) ganglion. Information is then carried in the spinal trigeminal tract to the spinal trigeminal nucleus, where the second-order neurons are located.

Like the **spin**othalamic tract, the **spin**al nucleus receives pain and temperature information.

The third order neurons are located in the contralateral ventral posteromedial (VPM) nucleus of the thalamus.

Information is then carried through the posterior limb of the internal capsule to the somatosensory cortex responsible for face (Brodmann's areas 3,1,2) in the parietal lobe.

Dorsal Trigeminothalamic Tract

The dorsal trigeminothalamic tract carries information about *touch and pressure* from the face and oral cavity.

The dorsal trigeminothalamic tract is analogous to the dorsal columns.

The first-order neurons are in the trigeminal (gasserian) ganglion.

Second-order neurons are located in the principal sensory nucleus of CN V. These neurons project to the ipsilateral VPM nucleus.

From the VPM nucleus, information is carried through the posterior limb of the internal capsule to the ipsilateral somatosensory cortex (Brodmann's areas 3,1,2) for the face.

Lesions of CN V

Trigeminal Neuralgia

Trigeminal neuralgia is characterized by intermittent lancinating pain in the distribution of a branch or branches of the trigeminal nerve.

It can be triggered by chewing.

CN VI (Abducens Nerve) (LR$_6$)

CN VI innervates the **L**ateral **R**ectus muscle, which abducts the eye.

CN VII (Facial Nerve)

CN VII exits the brainstem in the cerebellopontine angle. It then travels through the internal auditory meatus and the facial canal. It exits the skull through the **stylomastoid foramen**.

The facial nerve has sensory, motor, and parasympathetic functions.

Roles of CN VII:
- Innervates facial muscles (except the muscles of mastication): frontalis, orbicularis oculi, orbicularis oris, buccinator, and platysma.
- Innervates the stapedius, occipitalis, posterior belly of the digastric, stylohyoid, and anterior and superior auricular muscles.
- Innervates the lacrimal, parotid, sublingual, and submandibular glands.
- Provides taste sensation to the anterior 2/3 of the tongue.
- Provides sensation to the external ear.

Motor Functions of CN VII

The main motor nucleus of CN VII is in the pons.

The main portion of the nerve exits the skull through the stylomastoid foramen and divides into 5 branches that control facial movement:

· Buccal

· Cervical

· Mandibular

· Temporal

· Zygomatic

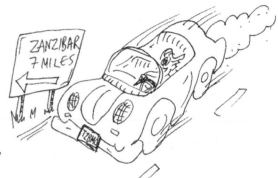

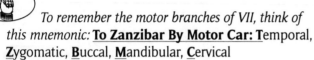 To remember the motor branches of VII, think of this mnemonic: **To Zanzibar By Motor Car: T**emporal, **Z**ygomatic, **B**uccal, **M**andibular, **C**ervical

Branch of facial nerve	Muscle innervated
Buccal	Buccinator
Cervical	Platysma
Mandibular	Orbicularis oris
Temporal	Frontalis
Zygomatic	Orbicularis oculi

The motor neurons to the upper facial muscles receive innervation from both cerebral hemispheres. The motor neurons to the lower facial muscles receive only contralateral cortical input.

Upper motor neuron lesions of CN VII cause *contralateral* facial weakness *sparing the forehead*. **Lower motor neuron lesions** cause *ipsilateral* facial weakness that *affects the upper and lower face*.

CN VII also innervates the stapedius, occipitalis, posterior belly of the digastric, stylohyoid, and anterior and superior auricular muscles.

The stapedius dampens movements of the stapes.

The stapedius is a silencer!

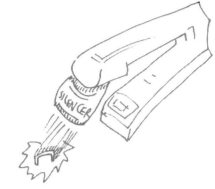

 The muscles of mastication are innervated by the trigeminal nerve, not the facial nerve.

Sensory Functions of CN VII

The first-order sensory neurons for CN VII are located in the **geniculate ganglion**, which is in the temporal bone.

 CN VII provides sensation to the external ear and auditory canal.

It is responsible for taste sensation from the anterior 2/3 of the tongue. The information is carried via the lingual branch of V3 to the **chorda tympani**, which is a branch of CN VII.

The chorda tympani carries taste to the geniculate ganglion. Then information about taste travels to the nucleus tractus solitarius. From there, the **central tegmental tract** carries the information to tertiary sensory neurons in the Ventral Posteromedial (VPM) nucleus of the thalamus. Then taste travels to the cortical taste areas, which are Brodmann's area 43 (parietal lobe) and the adjacent parainsular cortex.

central tegmental tract

Chorda tympani ⟶ geniculate ganglion ⟶ nucleus tractus solitarius ⟶ VPM ⟶ cortical taste area

Taste involves 3 sets of "c.t."s: chorda tympani, central tegmental tract, and cortical taste area.

Parasympathetic Functions of CN VII

The parasympathetic fibers of CN VII innervate the lacrimal, parotid, sublingual, and submandibular glands.

The preganglionic parasympathetic neurons are located in the **superior salivatory nucleus**.

Reflexes Involving CN VII

Corneal Reflex

When the cornea is touched, the corneal reflex causes the eyelids to close. The afferent limb is the ophthalmic division of the trigeminal nerve **(V$_1$)**. The efferent limb is the facial nerve **(VII)**.

The Tearing (Lacrimal) Reflex

The afferent limb of the tearing reflex is V$_1$, and the efferent limb is the facial nerve **(VII)**.

Lesions of CN VII

Ramsay Hunt Syndrome (Herpes Zoster Oticus)

Ramsay Hunt syndrome is a Herpes zoster infection of the geniculate ganglion.

Patients have a unilateral facial palsy, pain in and behind the ear, and vesicles around the ear. They lose taste to the anterior 2/3 of the tongue. Spread of the infection may result in hearing loss.

Bell's Palsy

Bell's palsy is due to a lower motor neuron lesion of CN VII. It results in ipsilateral facial weakness, abnormal taste sensation, and hyperacusis.

CN VII

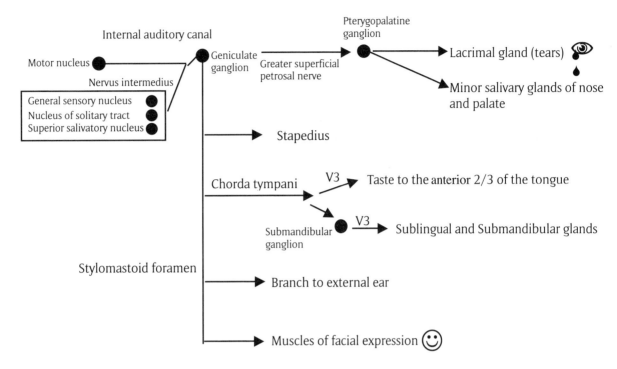

![HOT TIP] A lesion at the stylomastoid foramen causes paralysis of the muscles of facial expression, but taste is preserved.

CN VIII (Vestibulocochlear Nerve)

CN VIII has only sensory functions.

It has 2 components:

1. Vestibular nerve
2. Cochlear nerve.

Vestibular Nerve

The vestibular nerve is important for equilibrium.

Anatomy of the Vestibular System

The vestibular ganglion is in the internal auditory meatus.

 Bipolar cells in the vestibular ganglion innervate hair cells of the semicircular canals, saccule, and utricle.

Special receptors in the **utricle and saccule detect linear acceleration**. Cristae in the ampullae of the **semicircular canals respond to angular acceleration**.

Four subnuclei form the vestibular nuclear complex:
- Lateral vestibular nucleus
- Inferior vestibular nucleus
- Medial nucleus
- Superior nucleus

The lateral vestibular nucleus gives rise to the lateral vestibulospinal tract.

Fibers from the inferior and medial vestibular nuclei travel to the flocculonodular lobe of the cerebellum via the inferior cerebellar peduncle.

The medial nucleus is the main source of fibers for the medial vestibulospinal tract.

All four subnuclei contribute to the ascending medial longitudinal fasciculus, which helps with visual fixation when the head is moving.

Cochlear Nerve

The cochlear nerve is responsible for hearing. The cochlea is the organ of hearing.

Anatomy of Hearing

 Transmission of Sound
- Sound waves cause the tympanic membrane to vibrate.
- Sound is amplified by the middle ear ossicles (malleus, incus, and stapes).
- Sound waves then reach the oval window, which connects with the vestibule of the inner ear.
- Then sound travels in the scala vestibuli, which contains perilymph.
- Perilymph movements are transmitted to the cochlear duct. This results in movement of the basilar membrane relative to the tectorial membrane.

- This activates mechanoreceptor cilia on hair cells. (The base of the hair cells attach indirectly to the basilar membrane.)
- At the base of the hair cells, synapses activate the dendritic processes of bipolar cells of the cochlear division of CN VIII. Their cell bodies are located in the **spiral ganglion** in the temporal bone.

The hair cells of the cochlea and their supporting structures form the organ of Corti. **The hairs cells of the organ of Corti are the auditory receptor cells**.

The organ of Corti has a tonotopic organization. Hair cells at the base of the cochlea (near the oval window) are activated by higher frequency sounds, and hair cells at the apex of the cochlea are activated by low frequency sounds.

MNEMONIC

"NCSLIMA" is used to remember the peaks seen with Brainstem Auditory Evoked Potentials. It can also be used to remember the structures required for hearing.

I	**N**erve (Acoustic / 8th)

I   **N**erve (Acoustic / 8th)

II   **C**ochlear nuclei (medulla)

III   **S**uperior olivary complex (pons)

IV   **L**ateral lemniscus (pons)

V   **I**nferior colliculus (midbrain)

VI   **M**edial geniculate (thalamus)

VII   **A**uditory radiations (thalamocortical)

The primary auditory cortex (Brodmann's areas 41 and 42) is found in Heschl's gyrus in the temporal lobe.

HOT TIP

Above the level of the cochlear nuclei, unilateral lesions don't cause deafness due to bilateral connections.

The Weber Test

DEFINITION

The Weber test consists of placing a tuning fork on the vertex. It should be heard equally in both ears.

If there is conductive hearing loss, the vibration is better heard in the affected ear.

If there is sensorineural hearing loss, the vibration is better heard in the normal ear.

better in normal ear

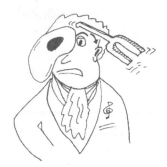

When a person with **sens**orineural hearing loss undergoes the Weber test, the results make **sense**; the vibration is better heard in the good ear. Andrew Lloyd **Weber** wrote the Phantom of the Opera, whose mask **sensibly** covers up his distorted face; think of the Weber test with a tuning fork on Phantom's face.

The Rinne Test

The Rinne test is performed by placing a vibrating tuning fork on the mastoid process. When it is no longer heard, it is placed near the ear. Normally, vibration can still be heard (air conduction persists after bone conduction).

If there is conductive hearing loss, the vibration is not heard in the diseased ear (bone conduction is better than air conduction).

If there is sensorineural hearing loss, the vibration can be heard (air conduction is better than bone conduction).

If a person with **conduct**ive hearing test undergoes the Rinne test, the **conduct**ion is messed up; bone conduction is better than air conduction, which isn't normally true.

CN IX (Glossopharyngeal Nerve)

The glossopharyngeal nerve has motor, sensory, and autonomic functions.

Motor Functions of CN IX

CN IX supplies one muscle: the stylopharyngeus.

To remember that the **gloss**opharyngeal nerve is associated with the **styl**opharyngeus muscle, think of In **Style** magazine, which has **gloss**y photos.

The **main motor nucleus of CN IX** is formed by part of the **nucleus ambiguus**.

Sensory Functions of CN IX

 CN IX provides sensation to middle and external ear, pharynx, and posterior 1/3 of the tongue. *(taste)*

The **sensory nucleus of CN IX** is part of the **nucleus of the tractus solitarius**.

Parasympathetic Functions of CN IX

 CN IX innervates the parotid gland.

The **parasympathetic nucleus of CN IX** is the **inferior salivatory nucleus**.

Reflexes Involving CN IX

 The carotid sinus reflex involves CN IX, which innervates the carotid body and sinus.

The glossopharyngeal nerve is responsible for the afferent limb of the gag reflex.

Lesions of CN IX

Glossopharyngeal neuralgia is characterized by episodes of brief sharp pain involving the tongue and radiating to the ear.

It is usually triggered by swallowing, but it may also result from talking.

It may be accompanied by bradycardia. Rarely, syncope may occur.

CN X (Vagus Nerve)

The vagus nerve has motor, sensory, and parasympathetic functions.

Motor Functions of CN X

ventral motor nucleus – ambiguus
dorsal motor nucleus – solitary

CN X innervates the muscles of the palate, pharyn**X**, and laryn**X** except the stylopharyngeus (which is innervated by CN IX) and the Tensor Veli Palatini (aka TVP, which is innervated by CN V).

CN X also innervates the **pal**atoglossus, which is the only muscle of the tongue that is not innervated by the hypoglossal nerve.

CN **X** supplies the **pal**ate, pharyn**X**, and laryn**X** including the **pal**atoglossus muscle of the tongue.

Your **X-pals**, pharyn**X** & laryn**X**, won't watch "Style TV." (X doesn't innervate the stylopharyngeus or the TVP).

Sensory Functions of CN X

CN **X** is responsible for taste sensation from the pharyn**X**.

Parasympathetic Functions of CN X

The parasympathetic nucleus of CN X is the dorsal motor nucleus of the vagus. Efferent fibers travel to the viscera (down to the distal 1/3 of the transverse colon).

Reflexes Involving CN X

CN X is the efferent limb of the oculocardiac and carotid sinus reflexes. (The oculocardiac reflex results in slowing of the heart rate when pressure is applied to the eye. The carotid sinus reflex results in heart rate slowing when pressure is applied to the carotid sinus. [I don't recommend testing these].)

CN X also is responsible for the efferent limb of the gag reflex. (You may not want to test this either.)

CN XI (Spinal Accessory Nerve)

The spinal accessory nerve is formed from cranial and spinal roots. Axons of nerve cells in the nucleus ambiguous form the cranial root. Recall that the right sternocleidomastoid turns the head to the left and vice versa.

The spinal accessory nerve innervates the trapezius and sternocleidomastoid muscles.

How do you recognize medial versus lateral winging of the scapula? By a *SALTy wings meal!* The Serratus Anterior muscle, innervated by the Long Thoracic nerve, causes **medial winging** (wings meal). Thus, you won't get caught in a *late, 11th hour, accessory trap!* (Yes, injury to the trapezius muscle, innervated by the accessory nerve – CN 11 – causes lateral scapular winging.)

The accessory portion of CN XI innervates the intrinsic muscles of the larynx except the cricothyroid muscle, which is supplied by a branch of the vagus nerve.

CN XII (Hypoglossal Nerve)

The hypoglossal nerve innervates the muscles of the tongue <u>except</u> the **pal**atoglossus muscle, which is innervated by CN **X**.

The tongue points toward the weak side when protruded.

Since corticobulbar fibers project to the contralateral hypoglossal nucleus, an upper motor neuron (UMN) lesion will cause deviation away from the lesion, and a lower motor neuron (LMN) lesion causes deviation toward the side of the lesion.

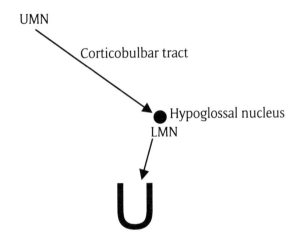

In the case of a **l**ower motor neuron lesion, the tongue could **l**ick the lesion because the tongue deviates toward the lesion.

Clinical Syndromes Involving Multiple Cranial Nerves

Site of lesion/Name of syndrome	Cranial nerves involved
Orbital apex lesion	2, 3, 4, 6, V_1
Superior orbital fissure lesion	3, 4, 6, V_1
Tolosa-Hunt and other causes of cavernous sinus syndrome	3, 4, 6, V_1, V_2

Orbital apex lesions, Tolosa-Hunt and other causes of cavernous sinus syndrome, and superior orbital fissure lesions can involve cranial nerves 3,4,6, V_1.

Orbital Apex Lesion

MNEMONIC   In an **Orbital apex lesion** you can have **CN II (O**ptic nerve**)** involvement and may have a **bulging eye.**

Cavernous Sinus Thrombosis

MNEMONIC   A cavernous sinus thrombosis presents with: **pap, prop, and pain-op! papilledema, proptosis, and painful ophthalmoplegia**

Recall that the cavernous sinus contains CN III, IV, V_1, V_2, VI, postganglionic sympathetic fibers, and the internal carotid artery.

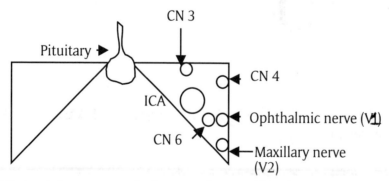

Cranial nerve VI, the abducens nerve, is closest to the carotid in the cavernous sinus. CN III, IV, and V_1 are further away, in the lateral wall.

The **ab**ducens nerve **ab**uts the artery (internal carotid artery) in the cavernous sinus.

Recall that the rhino-orbital-cerebral form of Mucormycosis, which can be found in diabetics, can cause cavernous sinus thrombosis and hemorrhagic brain infarction.

Tolosa-Hunt Syndrome

Tolosa-Hunt syndrome is granulomatous inflammation in the cavernous sinus that results in painful ophthalmoplegia. It is treated with prednisone.

In Tolosa-Hunt and other cavernous sinus syndromes you can have V2 (maxillary branch of the trigeminal nerve) involvement.

Hypothalamus

The hypothalamus is part of the diencephalon.

It is important for maintaining homeostasis.

Hypothalamic Nucleus	Function
Posterior	Heat conservation
Anterior	Detects elevated body temperature and triggers cooling mechanisms, stimulates the parasympathetic nervous system
Posterior lateral	Role in transition between wake and sleep
Lateral	Controls appetite
Ventromedial	Inhibits appetite
Paraventricular	Synthesizes antidiuretic hormone and oxytocin, responsible for neuroendocrine and autonomic responses to stress, provides excitatory input to preganglionic sympathetic neurons
Supraoptic	Synthesizes antidiuretic hormone (vasopressin) and oxytocin
Arcuate	Produces dopamine
Medial preoptic	Controls the release of gonadotropic hormones from the pituitary
Posterior tuberomammillary	Histaminergic innervation to cortex
Suprachiasmatic	Circadian rhythm

Mnemonics for remembering the functions of all the eleven (11) nuclei in the hypothalamus:

Anterior & Posterior = **A&P** (both regulate temp) - **A&P** convenience stores are either too hot (A) or too cold (P), respectively (not too convenient, eh?)

Posterior-**L**ateral (wakefulness and warmth) - **PLease** wake up warm!

VM and **Late**ral (both regulate appetite) - these nuclei are **Very Much Late** for dinner!

PV and **SON** (both make ADH and OT) - **Parents Versus SON** race to make ADequate Oxytocin for the baby, but the Parents STRESS out! (autonomic response to stress)

Arcuate (Dopamine) - think of all the **Dopes** that didn't listen to Noah and hop on his **Arc**!

Posterior **tub**eromammillary (histamine) - think of a **TUB** full of anti-Histamines like Benadryl!

Suprachias**matic** (circadian pacemaker) - auto**matic** timepiece of the brain

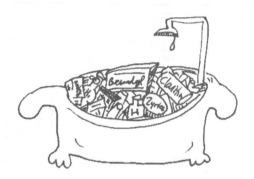

Hypothalamic Functions

Circadian Rhythms

The suprachiasmatic nucleus of the hypothalamus is responsible for circadian rhythms.

Suprachiasmatic - auto**matic** timepiece of the brain.

The retinosuprachiasmatic tract carries information from the retina to the suprachiasmatic nucleus.

Endocrine

The hypothalamus produces:

- Corticotropin-releasing hormone
- Growth hormone-inhibiting hormone

· Growth hormone-releasing hormone

· Luteinizing hormone-releasing hormone

· Prolactin-inhibiting hormone (dopamine)

· Prolactin-releasing hormone

· Thyrotropin-releasing hormone

Temperature Regulation

The anterior and posterior nuclei of the hypothalamus are involved in temperature control.

The anterior nucleus detects elevated body temperature and triggers cooling mechanisms. A lesion of the anterior nucleus of the hypothalamus causes increased temperature.

The posterior nucleus is responsible for heat conservation. A lesion of the posterior nucleus of the hypothalamus causes poikilothermia.

Anterior & Posterior = A&P (both regulate temp) - **A&P** convenience stores are either too hot (A) or too cold (P), respectively (not too convenient, eh?)

The **a**nterior nucleus **a**ctivates the **a**ir-conditioning. When it's broken, the "store" gets too hot.

The **p**osterior nucleus **p**reserves heat. When it's broken, the "store" gets cold.

Appetite

The medial, particularly ventromedial, and lateral hypothalamus affect appetite.

Stimulation of the lateral nuclei causes hunger/gluttony.

All of these nuclei are **Very Much Late** for dinner!

People **la**p up food when the **la**teral hypothalamus is stimulated.

Stimulation of the ventromedial nucleus (the satiety center) causes decreased appetite. Destruction of this nucleus results in obesity.

Stimulation of the **ve**ntromedial nucleus of the hypothalamus causes one to **ve**er away from food.

Water Balance

 The paraventricular (**PV**N) and supraoptic nuclei (**SON**) produce **A**nti**D**iuretic hormone (vasopressin) and Oxytocin. **Parents Versus SON** race to make **A**Dequate Oxytocin for the baby, but Parents STRESS out! The paraventricular nucleus also produces **co**rticotropin-releasing hormone. The Parents also try to **co**ax the **co**usin to release hormone.

Destruction of the paraventricular and supraoptic nuclei causes diabetes insipidus (**DI**). Destroying the Parents and the SON, and the entire family will DI.

Sleep

Please also see the sleep section in the Neurophysiology chapter for more information.

The anterior hypothalamus *promotes sleep*.

The posterior and lateral hypothalamus promote wakefulness. **PL**ease wake up warm!

Interestingly, the body is *colder when asleep*, and **warmer when awake**.

As previously mentioned, **Anterior & Posterior = A&P** (both regulate temp): **A&P** convenience stores are either too hot (A) or too cold (P), respectively.

And thus, the Anterior hypothalamus detects elevated body temperature, *triggers cooling mechanisms and promotes a nice cold sleep.*

The Posterior hypothalamus, triggers warming/wakefulness.

Neurons of the basal forebrain and anterior hypothalamus are important for sleep onset.

The ventrolateral preoptic (VLPO) area of the anterior hypothalamus and basal forebrain neurons produce GABA, which inhibits hypocretin neurons. This is important in the initiation of sleep.

Orexin/ hypocretin neurons, which are found in the posterior and lateral hypothalamus, promote wakefulness. They send projections to all the ascending arousal systems and to the cortex.

Deficient **O**rexin (also known as hypocretin) causes **Narco**lepsy.
No O? Become a Narco!

Sex

The medial preoptic area controls the release of gonadotropic hormones from the pituitary.

To remember that the medial **Pre-op**tic area controls the release of gonadotropic hormones:
Pre-op patients are stripped, and the gonads are exposed.

Also, the medial preoptic nucleus contains the sexually **di**morphic nucleus, which has twice as many neurons in males as females.

Limbic System

Limbic System Components

Components of the limbic system:
- Amygdala
- Basal forebrain
- Cingulate gyrus
- Habenula
- Hippocampal formation
    - Hippocampus, parahippocampal gyrus (including the entorhinal cortex), dentate gyrus, fornix, and subiculum
- Hypothalamus
- Mamillary bodies
- Olfactory cortex
- Septal nuclei
- Thalamus (anterior nucleus, mediodorsal nucleus)
- Ventral striatum

Limbic System Pathway

The Papez Circuit

 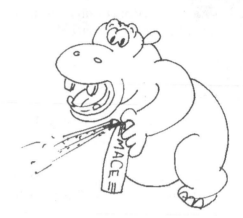

The Papez circuit includes:
- · Hippocampal formation
- · Fornix
- · Mammillary bodies
- · Anterior nucleus of the thalamus
- · Cingulate gyrus
- · Entorhinal cortex

The Papez circuit consists of hippocampal formation, fornix and MACE (**M**ammillary bodies, **A**nterior nucleus of the thalamus, **C**ingulate gyrus, and **E**ntorhinal area). Think of a hippopotamus named Pepe with a spraygun of MACE.

Remember that the A stands for anterior nucleus of the thalamus rather than amygdala.

The Papez Circuit

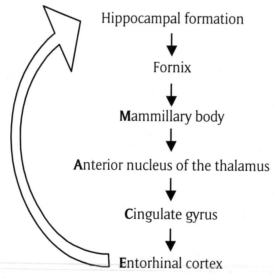

Hippocampal formation
↓
Fornix
↓
Mammillary body
↓
Anterior nucleus of the thalamus
↓
Cingulate gyrus
↓
Entorhinal cortex

Information exits the hippocampal formation through the fornix.

The **for**nix is the pathway by which information **for**ges out into limbic system from the hippocampal formation.

The mammillothalamic tract connects the mammillary body with the anterior nucleus of the thalamus.

The entorhinal cortex is how information enters the hippocampus.

 The **Entor**hinal cortex is how information **enter**s the hippocampus.

Stria Terminalis

 The stria terminalis travels from the amygdala to the septal nuclei and anterior hypothalamus.

Stria terminalis
Amygdala ⟶ septal nuclei and anterior hypothalamus

Stria Medullaris/ Stria Medullaris Thalami

 The stria medullaris travels from the septal nuclei and anterior hypothalamus to the habenula.

Stria medullaris
Septal nuclei and anterior hypothalamus ⟶ habenula

In summary,

Stria terminalis
Amygdala ⟶ septal nuclei and anterior hypothalamus ⟶ habenula.
Stria medullaris

Medial Forebrain Bundle

The median forebrain bundle connects the midbrain, orbitofrontal region, septal area, and hypothalamus.

 The medial forebrain bundle connects the Midbrain, Orbitofrontal region, Septal area, and Hypothalamus, which spell MOSH.

Clinical Conditions Affecting the Limbic System

Klüver-Bucy Syndrome

Klüver-Bucy Syndrome is due to **bilateral** anterior temporal lobe damage, which causes patients to be hyperoral, hypersexual, and placid: **the 2 dots over the ü represent bilateral anterior temporal lobe damage.**

Note that bilateral amygdala lesions can occur with **PHIL:** **P**ick's disease, **H**SV, **I**schemia, and **L**obectomies (gone awry).

Klüver-Bucy is a placid food-lover from PHILamygdala, Pennsylvania.

Korsakoff Psychosis

Korsakoff psychosis is an amnestic disorder in which patients have retrograde and anterograde amnesia and tend to confabulate. It is usually associated with malnutrition and alcoholism.

Think of Korsakoff as Of Course-akoff because Korsakoff patients will say "Of course I remember" even though they don't.

Wernicke Disease

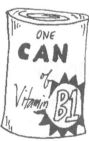

Wernicke Encephalopathy/Wernicke Disease is due to thiamine (vitamin B-1) deficiency.

Patients symptoms are: **C**onfusion, **A**taxia of gait, and extraocular movement abnormalities (**N**ystagmus). They need **one (1)** whole **CAN** of thiamine to improve.

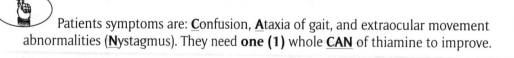

Peripheral Nerves

Spinal Nerves

 There are 31 pairs of spinal nerves: 8 cervical, 12 thoracic, 5 lumbar, 5 sacral, and 1 coccygeal.

Each spinal nerve is connected to the spinal cord by an anterior and posterior rootlet.

The dorsal rootlets are primarily sensory, and the ventral rootlets are primarily motor.

The spinal nerves divide into rami after leaving the intervertebral foramen.

The anterior rami are responsible for supplying the muscles and skin of the anterolateral body and appendicular muscles and skin.

The posterior rami are responsible for supplying the skin and muscles of the back.

In the **cervical region, the spinal nerves exit <u>above</u> the vertebrae.** (For example, the C3 nerve exits above the third cervical vertebra.) Since there are 7 cervical vertebra and 8 cervical nerves, **the nerve exits <u>below</u> the same numbered vertebrae in the thoracic, lumbar, and sacral regions**.

Cutaneous Receptors

Type of cutaneous receptor	Sensation	MNEMONIC
<u>**Free**</u> nerve **end**ings	<u>**P**</u>ain and <u>**T**</u>emperature	<u>**P**</u>arking and <u>**T**</u>ransportation is **free** at the **end** of the day
Paccinian	Touch, pressure, vibration	To play **Puccini**, you must apply perfect <u>touch, pressure, and vibration</u> on your instrument.
Merkel	**Light touch**	Angela **Merkel** is the first female Chancellor of Germany and so she has a **light touch**.
Meissner	<u>**Two-point discrimination**</u>	A **Meiser** is someone who is cheap and **discriminates** their **two cents** for everything!

Dermatomes

C5 shoulder
C6 thumb
C7 middle finger
C8 little finger
T2 axilla
T4 nipple
T10 umbilicus
L2 anterior thigh
L3 knee
L5 great toe
S1 small toe, sole
S2 posterior thigh
S3/4/5 perianal, genitals

 T2 innervates the axilla, and armpit odor can be deadly like T2 (Terminator 2).

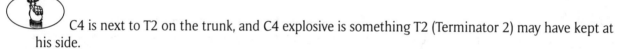 C4 is next to T2 on the trunk, and C4 explosive is something T2 (Terminator 2) may have kept at his side.

 L2 innervates the anterior thigh and S2 innervates the posterior thigh.

 S1 innervates the Sole, which one scrapes when checking for a Babinski.

Please see the Neuromuscular Diseases chapter.

Pituitary

 The anterior pituitary produces a **FLAT PiG**:
- **F**ollicle-stimulating hormone (**F**SH)
- **L**uteinizing hormone (**L**H)
- **A**drenocorticotropic hormone (**A**CTH)
- **T**hyroid-stimulating hormone (**T**SH)

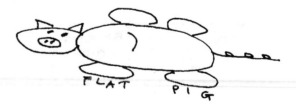

· **P**rolactin

· **i**=*ignore*

· **G**rowth hormone (**GH**)

The posterior pituitary releases oxytocin and vasopressin (ADH), which are produced in the hypothalamus by Parents Versus SON.

Spinal Cord

The anterior horn arises from the basal plate, and the posterior horn arises from the alar plate.

Cord segment	Importance
Mid-thoracic cord	Region of cord most vulnerable to ischemia
S2	Where lumbar cistern ends
L1	Where conus medullaris terminates in adults
L3	Where conus medullaris terminates in newborns

Area of cord	Cord segment	Importance
Clarke's column	C8-L3	Where the dorsal spinocerebellar tract arises
Ciliospinal center of Budge	C8-T2	Sympathetic innervation of the eye
Intermediolateral cell column	T1-L2	Sympathetic innervation of the body
Intermediolateral cell column	S2-S4	Gives rise to the sacral outflow of the parasympathetic nervous system.

Blood Supply to the Spinal Cord

The cord is supplied by an anterior spinal artery and two posterior spinal arteries.

The anterior spinal artery, which arises from the vertebral arteries, supplies the anterior 2/3 of the cord. This includes the lateral corticospinal tracts, lateral spinothalamic tracts, and anterior horns.

Therefore, infarction causes paralysis and loss of pain and temperature sensation. Patients have urinary and fecal incontinence. (The dorsal columns are supplied by branches of the posterior spinal arteries, so vibration and position sense are preserved.)

Radicular arteries arising from local arteries help to supply the cord.
They enter the vertebral canal from intervertebral foramina.

The **great radicular artery of <u>Adamkiewicz</u>** provides most of the blood supply to the lumbar and sacral cord.

<u>Adam</u>kiewicz is a **<u>rad</u>**icular artery arising from a **branch** of the **descending** aorta, usually between **<u>T</u>**9 -12 on the **<u>left</u>**.

<u>Adam left</u> between <u>9 and 12 red</u> apples on the <u>Tree's</u> branches before he <u>descended</u> from Eden. (By the way, Adam's last name could've been Kiewicz for all we know…)

Venous return from the cord enters epidural veins, called **Batson's plexus**.

These veins lack valves and allow the spread of infection or cancer into the epidural space.

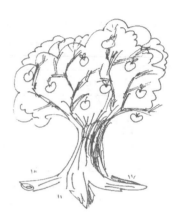

Lamina of the Spinal Cord

Lamina	Nuclei
I	Marginal zone
II	Substantia **gelatin**osa
III, IV	Nucleus proprius dorsalis
V	Neck of dorsal horn
VI	Base of dorsal horn
VII	Clarke's nucleus, intermediolateral nucleus
VIII	Commissural nucleus
IX	Motor nuclei
X	Grisea centralis

Lamina II, the substantia **gelatin**osa, is the area where spinothalamic fibers synapse when they enter the cord – it is **too (II) painful** (Lamina II = spinothalamic pain) to see how they make gelatin.

Lamina IX is the location of the anterior horn cells, where the corticospinal fibers synapse.

Lamina X is the grisea centralis, which is gray matter around the central canal.

Spinal Cord Tracts

Ascending Tracts of the Spinal Cord

 Major ascending tracts of the cord:

- Cuneocerebellar tract
- Dorsal columns
- Dorsal spinocerebellar tract
- Rostral spinocerebellar tract
- Spinothalamic tract
- Ventral spinocerebellar tract

Cuneocerebellar Tract

The cuneocerebellar tract carries afferent information about movement of the ipsilateral upper extremity and rostral body to the cerebellum.

Dorsal Columns

The **Dorsal Columns** carry **V**ibration, **P**roprioception, and **L**ight touch.

The nerves that carry this information are large, myelinated, fast-conducting nerve fibers.

Information travels in the ipsilateral **Dorsal Column** in the fasciculus gracilis or cuneatus. In the lower medulla, the nerves synapse in the nucleus gracilis or cuneatus. The arcuate fibers carry information to the contralateral medial lemniscus. The information then travels to the VPL nucleus of the thalamus, where there is another synapse. Then information travels through the posterior limb of the internal capsule to the postcentral gyrus of the cortex (Brodmann's areas 3,1,2).

Information regarding **V**ibration, **P**roprioception, and **L**ight touch travels through the **VPL** nucleus of the thalamus and the **V**ice **P**resident **L**ives in **D.C. (Dorsal Columns)**.

Dorsal Spinocerebellar Tract

 This tract carries unconscious proprioceptive information from the lower limbs and trunk.

It originates in the dorsal nucleus of Clarke (C8-L3). It transmits information from the muscle spindles, tendon organs, and joint receptors to the cerebellum via the ipsilateral inferior cerebellar peduncle.

 ## Rostral Spinocerebellar Tract

The rostral spinocerebellar tract carries unconscious proprioceptive information from the upper limbs and rostral body to the cerebellum, similar to the cuneocerebellar tract.

Spinothalamic Tract (ST)

 The spinothalamic tract carries pain and temperature.

 To remember that the ST tract carries pain sensation: when you hurt yourself, you may say S–T.

This information is carried in small, myelinated (Aδ) and unmyelinated (C) nerves.

To remember that C fibers carry pain sensation: pain may make you Cuss.

Spinothalamic fibers synapse in lamina II (the substantia gelatinosa) of the spinal cord and then cross in the anterior white commissure. The information travels in the contralateral spinothalamic tract to the VPL nucleus of the thalamus, where there is a synapse. Then the information travels in the posterior limb of the internal capsule to the postcentral gyrus of the cortex (Brodmann's areas 3,1,2).

Ventral Spinocerebellar Tract

 The ventral spinocerebellar tract carries the same type of information that the dorsal spinocerebellar tract carries. However, it enters the cerebellum via the superior cerebellar peduncle and some fibers cross.

Descending Tracts of the Spinal Cord

Descending tracts of the spinal cord include:
- Corticospinal tracts (lateral and ventral)
- Intermediolateral columns
- Reticulospinal tracts (lateral and medial)
- Rubrospinal tract
- Vestibulospinal tracts (lateral and medial)

Corticospinal Tracts

The **Lateral Cortical Spinal Tract** is responsible for **V**oluntary motor activity.

It arises from layer **V** of the cerebral cortex. Fibers from the primary motor cortex, lateral premotor cortex, and supplementary motor cortex are the main contributors to the **Cortical Spinal Tract**.

These fibers travel through the corona radiata, the internal capsule (posterior limb), and **V**entral brainstem. In the caudal medulla, 90% of the fibers cross, to descend in the **Lateral Cortical Spinal Tract**.

The remaining 10% fibers travel in the **Ventral Cortical Spinal Tract** (which is ipsilateral). These fibers in the ventral cortical spinal tract cross in the ventral white commissure and terminate in the cervical and upper thoracic regions.

Intermediolateral Columns

The intermediolateral columns extend from T1 to L2 segments of the spinal cord. Preganglionic sympathetic autonomic fibers for the body arise from this region.

Reticulospinal Tracts

The **medial reticulospinal tract** facilitates antigravity muscles.

The **lateral reticulospinal tract** does the opposite; it inhibits antigravity muscles and facilitates the antagonizing muscles.

Rubrospinal Tract

Similar to the corticospinal tract and lateral reticulospinal tract, the rubrospinal tract inhibits antigravity muscles and facilitates their antagonists.

Vestibulospinal Tracts

The **medial vestibulospinal tract** arises primarily from the medial vestibular nucleus. Some fibers cross as the tract descends to the anterior horn cells. This tract is responsible for changes in head and trunk position in response to information from the semicircular canals.

The **lateral vestibulospinal tract** arises from the ipsilateral lateral vestibular nucleus. Like the medial reticulospinal tract, it facilitates antigravity muscles.

Facilitate anti-gravity muscles	Antagonize anti-gravity muscles
Lateral vestibulospinal tract	Corticospinal tract
Medial reticulospinal tract	Lateral reticulospinal tract
	Rubrospinal tract

Diseases Affecting the Spinal Cord

Condition	Site of lesion/ Tracts involved
Brown-Sequard	Spinal cord hemisection. Affects the lateral corticospinal tract, lateral spinothalamic tract, anterior horn, and dorsal column.
B12 deficiency	Dorsal columns, lateral corticospinal tracts, spinocerebellar tracts
Friedreich's	Dorsal columns, lateral corticospinal tracts, spinocerebellar tracts
Polio	Anterior horns
Syphilis (Tabes dorsalis)	Dorsal columns
Syringomyelia	Cavitation of the cervical cord. Affects decussating lateral spinothalamic axons, anterior horns.
Ventral spinal artery occlusion	Anterior 2/3 of the cord. Affects lateral corticospinal tracts, lateral spinothalamic tracts, anterior horns.
Spinal muscular atrophy	Anterior horns
Amyotrophic lateral sclerosis (ALS)	Anterior horns and corticospinal tracts

Brown-Sequard is the worst, can you **C** how **SAD** it is?
Affects the lateral **C**orticospinal tract, lateral **S**pinothalamic tract, **A**nterior horn, and **D**orsal column.

If you are suspicious for subacute combined degeneration and the B12 level is normal, check serum homocysteine and methylmalonic acid levels.

Thalamus

The thalamus arises from the diencephalon.

The thalamus is like a truck stop. There is lots of traffic/information that comes from all over, stops, and moves on to other parts of the CNS.

Recall that one exception is the olfactory nerve, CN1, which has no relay through the thalamus.

The Thalamus

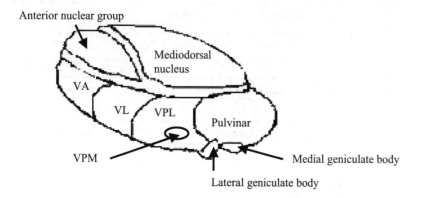

VA= ventral anterior nucleus, VL = ventral lateral nucleus, VPL = ventral posterior lateral nucleus, VPM= ventral posterior medial nucleus

Thalamic Nuclei

Anterior Nuclear Group

Anterior Nucleus

The anterior nucleus of the thalamus is important in limbic function. It is part of the **Papez circuit**.

The anterior nucleus receives input from the mamillary bodies of the hypothalamus (through the mamillothalamic tract).

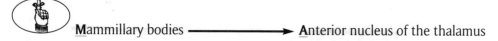

Mammillary bodies ⟶ **A**nterior nucleus of the thalamus

It sends information to the cingulate gyrus.

Anterior nucleus of the thalamus ⟶ **C**ingulate gyrus (part of the MACE mnemonic)

Intralaminar Nuclear Group

The intralaminar nuclear group, especially the centromedian and parafascicular nucleus, provide input to the striatum.

The internal segment of the globus pallidus (GPi) projects to the centromedian nucleus of the thalamus, which is the largest intralaminar nucleus.

Medial Nuclear Group

Mediodorsal Nucleus/Dorsomedial Nucleus

The mediodorsal nucleus has many important roles.

 It is the major thalamic nucleus involved in relaying information to the frontal association cortex. It has reciprocal connections with the prefrontal cortex.

It also receives information from the amygdala, temporal lobe, and substantia nigra.

It has a role in limbic function. Lesions of the mediodorsal thalamus, especially if bilateral, can affect motivation.

 The **me**diodorsal thalamus affects **m**otivation.

Destruction of the mediodorsal nucleus causes amnesia.

 The **me**diodorsal nucleus affects **me**mory.

Lateral Nuclear Group

Pulvinar

 The pulvinar is the largest thalamic nucleus. It is involved in visual attention.

To remember that the pulvinar is associated with visual attention, imagine that it became the largest thalamic nucleus to attract visual attention.

Ventral Posterior Lateral (VPL) Nucleus

Sensory information from the limbs meets in the ventral posterior lateral nucleus (VPL).

 Think of the VPL as VPLimbs.

The VPL projects to the postcentral gyrus (Brodmann's areas 3,2,1).

Ventral Posteromedial (VPM) Nucleus

The Trigeminal Nerve and the VPM

 Pain and temperature, fine touch, and position sense <u>for the face</u> first converge in the ventral posterior medial nucleus (VPM). The VPM projects to postcentral gyrus.

The various modalities of CN V meet in the VPM, which could be thought of as VPMeeting.

Recall from above:

Nucleus	Function
Chief sensory nucleus of V	Fine touch
Spinal nucleus of V	Pain and temperature sensation
Mesencephalic nucleus of V	Position sense

The VPM and Taste

The VPM also receives information about taste from nucleus tractus solitarius (NTS).

Since taste travels through it, the VPM could also be called the VPyum or VPmmm good nucleus.

Cranial nerves 7, 9, and 10 carry taste to the nucleus tractus solitarius (NTS). From there, taste travels to the VPM. Then it travels to the cortical taste areas, which are Brodmann's area 43 and the adjacent parainsular cortex.

Anterior 2/3 tongue----- CN7-------geniculate nucleus
Posterior 1/3 tongue---- CN9-------inferior nucleus 9   } ⇨ NTS ⇨ VPM ⇨ area 43 and parainsular cortex
Epiglottis, esophagus--- CN 10----inferior nucleus 10

Lateral Geniculate Nucleus (LGN)

The **LGN receives visual information** from the optic tract. It projects to the primary visual cortex (Brodmann's area 17). Please see the Neuro-ophthalmology chapter.

Medial Geniculate Nucleus (MGN)

The **MGN receives auditory information from the inferior colliculi**. (It is the M in NSCLIMA.)

It projects to the primary auditory cortex (Brodmann's areas 41).

Ventral Anterior Nucleus (VA)

The ventral anterior (VA) and ventral lateral (VL) nuclei have an important role in movement.

The VA and VL nuclei receive input from the internal segment of the globus pallidus (GPi) and the substantia nigra pars reticulata (SNr). Output from these regions is inhibitory; GABA is the neurotransmitter.

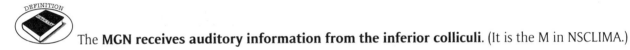

GPi/SNr ⸻⸻⸻⸻⸻⸻⟶ ventral thalamic nuclei (VA and VL)
              GABA

Then, there are excitatory connections from the ventral anterior and ventrolateral thalamic nuclei to the cortex. Thalamocortical fibers travel to the premotor cortex, supplementary motor area, and primary motor cortex for motor control.

Ventral Lateral Nucleus (VL)

Like the VA nucleus, the ventral lateral nucleus is important in movement.

The ventral lateral nucleus is part of the dentatorubrothalamic pathway, which is how the cerebellum influences synergy of movement.

The dentatorubrothalamic pathway:

Purkinje cells ⇨ dentate nucleus ⇨ contralateral red nucleus ⇨ VL thalamus ⇨ areas 4,6 motor cortex

Ventricular System

CSF Flow

Lateral ventricles ⟶ 3rd ventricle ⟶ 4th ventricle ⟶ subarachnoid space

Interventricular foramina of Monro   **Sylvian aqueduct**   Foramina of Luschka and Magendie

Then the CSF is absorbed from the arachnoid space into the dural venous sinuses by arachnoid granulations.

Adults have 150 cc of CSF.

CSF is produced by the choroid plexus at 20 cc/hour or 500 cc/day.

If you get a job in the **choir (choroid plexus)** making **$20/hr**, then you'll have $500 at the end of a 24-hour period!

The CSF pressure in the lateral recumbent position: 10-15 cm of water.

If you are **lying down** on the job (napping in the **lateral recumbent** position) you'll only make **$10-15**.

Circumventricular Organs

Circumventricular organs typically have an extensive vasculature and a **B**roken (interrupted) **B**lood-**B**rain **B**arrier (**BBB**) which allows for the linkage between the central nervous system and peripheral blood flow.

Circumventricular organs include:
- Area postrema
- Median eminence
- Neurohypophysis
- Organum vasculosum
- Pineal gland
- Subcommissural organ
- Subfornical organ

To remember the regions with a **B**roken **B**lood-**B**rain-**B**arrier (**BBB**) remember the phrase NO SPAM about fornication:

Neurohypophysis
Organum vasculosum

Subcommissural organ
Pineal gland
Area postrema
Median eminence

Sub**forn**ical organ

The **area postrema**, which is on the surface of the medulla adjacent to the 4th ventricle, detects toxins and causes vomiting. It connects to the nucleus tractus solitarius.

The area postrema (otherwise known as the chemotactic trigger zone) is the only paired circumventricular organ.

Unfortunately, there are 2 vomit-inducing regions since the area postrema is a paired circumventricular organ.

The **median eminence** is where the hypothalamus releases hormones that are carried to the anterior pituitary.

The **neurohypophysis** is the posterior pituitary, which secretes oxytocin and vasopressin that have been synthesized in the hypothalamus.

Eating 2 pastrami sandwiches in one area would make anyone want to vomit.

The Only

The area postrema is the only paired circumventricular organ.

The olfactory nerve (CN I) is the only sensory cranial nerve with no relay through the thalamus.

Neuroanatomy Quiz

(Answers on page 731)

1. Which cranial nerve has no relay through the thalamus?
    A. CN I
    B. CN II
    C. CN V
    D. CN VIII

2. Which lobe of the cerebellum is responsible for vestibular function?
    A. Anterior
    B. Flocculonodular
    C. Posterior

3. Which cells carry output from the cerebellum?
    A. Basket
    B. Granule
    C. Golgi
    D. Purkinje
    E. Stellate

4. Which structure is part of the Triangle of Mollaret?
    A. Dentate nucleus
    B. Emboliform nucleus
    C. Fastigial nucleus
    D. Globiform nucleus

5. In the circuit of Papez, what structure receives information from the mammillary bodies and sends information to the cingulate gyrus?
    A. Anterior nucleus of the thalamus
    B. Amygdala
    C. Entorhinal area
    D. Ventral lateral thalamus

6. The dentatorubrothalamic tract, which is important in synergy of movement, involves which area of the thalamus?

        A. Anterior nucleus of the thalamus

        B. Lateral geniculate nucleus

        C. Ventral lateral nucleus

        D. Ventral posterior lateral nucleus

        D. Ventral posterior medial nucleus

7. Match the cranial nerve with the structure it innervates.

        1. Muscles of mastication   A. Trigeminal nerve

        2. Muscles of facial expression   B. Facial nerve

        3. Stapedius

        4. Tensor tympani

        5. Stylohyoid

        6. Mylohyoid

8. What do macules in the utricle and saccule detect?

        A. Angular acceleration

        B. Linear acceleration

        C. Changes in barometric pressure

        D. Low frequency sounds

Chapter 2

Behavioral Neurology

Aphasia and Related Disorders

Aphemia

 Aphemia is a problem with speech production. In fact, some patients are mute. **The ability to write is preserved**.

Aphemia is due to a small lesion in Broca's area or its subcortical white matter.

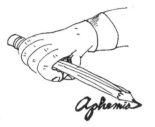

 A man with aphemia could write an affidavit but could not say clearly what it says.

The ability to write sets patients with aphemia apart from patients with the aphasias described below.

Broca's Aphasia

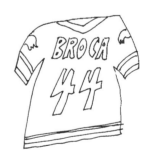

Broca's aphasia is an expressive aphasia. Patients have nonfluent speech and can't name or repeat. Written language is also affected. Comprehension is intact.

Broca's aphasia is due to a lesion in the posterior part of the dominant inferior frontal gyrus (Brodmann's areas 44 and 45). (This is anterior to the area of primary motor cortex that represents face.)

Broca's patients have *few words* like **broke** people have *few dollars*.

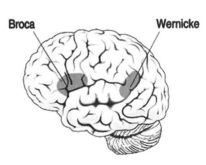

Wernicke's Aphasia

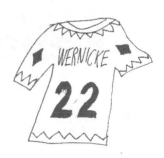

 Wernicke's aphasia is a receptive aphasia. Comprehension is severely impaired. Naming and repetition are also affected. Speech is fluent but nonsensical.

Wernicke's aphasia is due to a lesion in the posterior portion of the dominant superior temporal gyrus (Brodmann's area 22).

Conduction Aphasia

 Conduction aphasia is characterized by impaired **repetition**. Speech is fluent but not perfect, and patients can comprehend the spoken word. Naming and writing are affected.

Conduction aphasia is due to a lesion of the fibers connecting Broca's and Wernicke's areas e.g. the arcuate fasciculus.

 Don't **repeat** that **conduct**!

Global Aphasia

 Global aphasia is expressive and receptive aphasia due to a lesion of the dominant perisylvian area, involving Broca's and Wernicke's areas. Patients have nonfluent speech, poor comprehension, poor repetition, and poor naming.

Transcortical Aphasias

 Transcortical aphasia patients *can repeat* what is said to them.

 Transcortical aphasias can occur with watershed infarcts.

TransCortical Motor Aphasia (TCM)

 Like Broca's aphasia, TransCortical Motor aphasia is an expressive aphasia; however, patients with TCM can repeat.

TCM is due to a lesion in the dominant supplementary motor area (SMA), the connections between the SMA and Broca's area, or above or anterior to Broca's area.

It may be due to a stroke involving the watershed territory between the anterior cerebral artery (ACA) and middle cerebral artery (MCA).

On the **TCM** channel (Turner Classic Movies), you can watch **reruns** of **silent** films (TCM patients can repeat but not speak).

TransCortical Sensory Aphasia (TCS)

TransCortical Sensory aphasia is due to a lesion at the junction of the temporal, parietal, and occipital lobes.

TiCS at the TOP (Temporal, Occipital, and Parietal lobe junction).

Like Wernicke's aphasia, transcortical sensory aphasia is a receptive aphasia; however, patients with transcortical sensory aphasia can repeat.

TransCortical Mixed Aphasia

Patients with transcortical mixed aphasia have nonfluent speech like the transcortical motor aphasia patients and poor comprehension like the transcortical sensory aphasia patients. Repetition is preserved, as in all transcortical aphasia patients.

Transcortical mixed aphasia can occur with a stroke causing both ACA-MCA and MCA-PCA (posterior cerebral artery) watershed infarcts.

Disconnection Syndromes

Alexia <u>without</u> Agraphia (Pure Alexia)

Pure alexia can be due to a lesion of the *medial region of the dominant occipital lobe and splenium of the corpus callosum.* It can also occur with a lesion of the *periventricular white matter around the occipital horn* of the lateral ventricle in the dominant hemisphere.

The shorthand of the word "without" is **s** with a bar over it. Thus, alexia **s** agraphia is due to **s**plenium **s**trokes.

Pure alexia is often due to a posterior cerebral artery (PCA) infarct.

Alexia **A**nd **A**graphia is due to a lesion of the dominant **A**ngular gyrus. **(Brodmann's area 39).** **A**ll the **39 A**ngles are covered when a patient has **A**lexia **A**nd **A**graphia.

Bálint's Syndrome

Bálint's syndrome is a disconnection syndrome characterized by oculomotor-apraxia, optic-ataxia, simultagnosia, and problems with depth perception due to bilateral parietal-occipital damage.

Optic-ataxia is inability to move the hand to an object with vision, oculomotor-apraxia is inability to voluntarily control gaze, and simultanagnosia is inability to recognize 2 objects or more simultaneously in a visual field.

In Bálint's syndrome, the eyeball is off balance (off Bálint's) - patients have optic-ataxia. They also have oculomotor-apraxia and simultagnosia, which can be remembered with the following mnemonic:

When you see **BAL** in **Bál**int's syndrome, think of base**Bál**l and the Boston Red **S.O.X.** who have difficulty getting 3 outs sometimes because of 3 visual deficits:

- **S**imultagnosia (they cannot perceive simultaneous objects -- only focusing on their huge salary and not the baseball),
- **O**culomotor-apra**X**ia (they cannot change to a new location of visual fixation -- the fielder cannot look over to see the baserunner), and
- **O**ptic-ata**X**ia (they cannot guide their hand toward an object using visual information -- the fielder is unable to tag the runner out!)

Occipito*parietal* lesions cause problems determining *where* an object is, and occipito<u>temporal</u> lesions cause problems determining <u>what</u> an object is.

Pure Word Deafness/Auditory Verbal Agnosia

Patients with auditory verbal agnosia can hear sounds but can't understand words or repeat. They <u>can</u> read and write.

This can occur with a deep dominant superior temporal lesion or bilateral lesions of the midportion of the superior temporal gyrus.

Other Behavioral Syndromes

Alien Limb Syndrome

Patients with alien hand/limb syndrome may not recognize their own limb or may feel that they can't control it. There may appear to be involuntary movement of the limb.

Conditions that cause alien hand syndrome include: a lesion of the **C**orpus callosum, **A**CA infarct, and **B**asal ganglionic degeneration: think of an alien hailing a **CAB** with its Alien limb/hand.

> ### Alien Hand Syndrome
> When alien limb syndrome involves a hand, which is not atypical, it is called alien hand. In this case there can be intermanual conflict.
> *Talk about one hand not knowing what the other is doing!*

Anton's Syndrome

Patients with Anton's syndrome have cortical blindness but deny that they can't see. This is due to bilateral occipital lobe damage.

This can occur with bilateral PCA infarcts.

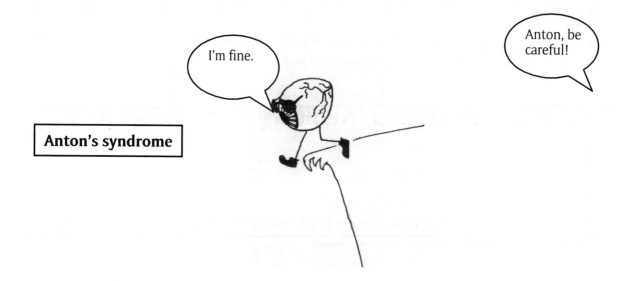

Anton's syndrome

HOT TIP Patients with cortical blindness do not blink to threat and have no optokinetic responses.

EITHER OR CHOICES To differentiate cortical blindness from pregeniculate lesions: patients with cortical blindness have pupillary responses to light.

Capgras' Syndrome

DEFINITION Patients with Capgras' syndrome have a delusion that people around them have been replaced by imposters.

MNEMONIC In **Ca**pgras' syndrome, patients believe people around them have been **cap**tured and replaced with imposters.

Alternatively, *crabgrass tries to replace real grass, and in Capgras' syndrome imposters replace people.*

Charles Bonnet's Syndrome

 In Charles Bonnet's syndrome patients with vision loss see things in the space where vision was lost. Complex visual hallucinations can be seen with profound interruption of visual input into the occipital cortex (ie, optic nerve/pathway damage or occipital stroke).

Patients are typically elderly, with normal cognition, who know they're having hallucinations.

The hallucinations usually are **colored patterns, images of people, animals, plants or inanimate objects.**

They often fit into the surroundings although are characterized as "lilliput" (smaller than normal).

Charles Bonnet's Syndrome is abbreviated **CBS**, which is a TV network that advertises an "Eye on America" – quite appropriate for this disorder! To remember the lilliput images associated with Charles Bonnet Syndrome, think of **CBS** airing the TV movie "Gulliver's Travels" which featured the miniature people known as Lilliputians from the island of **Lilliput**!

Ganser Syndrome

Ganser syndrome is also known as the syndrome of approximate but wrong answers *(e.g. "2 + 2 = 5").*

The DSM-IV-TR classifies Ganser syndrome as a **diss**ociative disorder, not associated with amnesia or fugue.

Patient's with *Ganser* syndrome *dance* around the answer. **Ganser, the "answer dancer," got dissed!**

Gerstmann's Syndrome

Patients with Gerstmann's syndrome have:
- Finger agnosia
- Agraphia
- Acalculia
- Right-left confusion

Gerstmann's syndrome is due to a lesion of the **Angular gyrus** Brodmann's area **39** (in the parietal lobe) of the dominant hemisphere.

Since they can't recognize their finger, patients with Gerstmann's syndrome have difficulty writing, can't use a calculator, and can't point right or left.

An **A** for every finger:

> **A**graphia
>
> **A**calculia
>
> **A**gnosia (finger)
>
> **AA**A (need to call American Automobile Association because can't tell left from right)
>
> **A**ngular gyrus

A lesion of the dominant **A**ngular gyrus is one of the causes of **A**nomic **A**phasia, which is characterized by difficulty with naming, but this is not part of Gerstmann syndrome. – **A**ll the 39 **A**ngles are covered when a patient has **A**lexia **A**nd **A**graphia (as mentioned earlier).

Kluver-Bucy Syndrome

Klüver-Bucy syndrome is due to **bilateral** anterior temporal lobe damage, *which causes patients to be hyperoral, hypersexual, and placid.*

Kl**ü**ver-**Buc**y contains **luver** and **buc**. These patients luv/love to put things in their buccal cavity/mouth. **The 2 dots over the ü represent bilateral anterior temporal lobe damage.**

Note that bilateral amygdala lesions can occur with **PHIL**: **P**ick's disease, **H**SV, **I**schemia, and **L**obectomies (gone awry).

PHIL took ü on a trip to lake Placid because he was thirsty (hyperoral). Alternatively, **Kluver-Bucy is a placid food-lover living in PHILamydala, Pennsylvania.**

Korsakoff Psychosis/Korsakoff Amnestic State

 Korsakoff psychosis is an amnestic disorder in which patients have retrograde and anterograde amnesia and tend to confabulate. It is usually associated with malnutrition and alcoholism.

Think of Korsakoff as **Of Course-akoff** because Korsakoff patients will say **"Of course I remember" even though they don't.**

Wernicke Encephalopathy/Wernicke Disease

Wernicke Encephalopathy/Wernicke Disease is due to thiamine (vitamin B-1) deficiency.

Patients symptoms are: **C**onfusion, **A**taxia of gait, and extraocular movement abnormalities (**N**ystagmus).

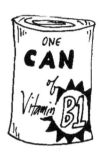

They need a whole **CAN** of thiamine to improve.

Lesions are seen in the **MMPP: M**ammillary bodies, **M**edial thalamic nuclei, **P**eriaqueductal gray, and **P**ontine tegmentum.

Patients with Wernicke disease have **extraocular movement abnormalities, ataxia of gait,** and **confusion.**

> ### Wernicke-Korsakoff syndrome
>
> When there's a lasting impairment in learning and memory, the patient has Wernicke-Korsakoff syndrome.

Wernicke encephalopathy may be seen in alcoholics with thiamine deficiency who receive glucose. *This is why thiamine is given before glucose in the ER...*

Terms

Abulia

 Patients with abulia lack initiative and have delayed, slowed responses.

 Think of this as **Able-LIA**. Patients are **Able but Lack Initiative to Act.**

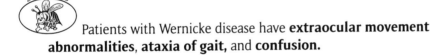

Akinetic Mutism

 Patients with akinetic mutism remain silent and still but are physically able to speak and move. (This is more severe than abulia.)

 Akinetic mutism may occur with bilateral medial frontal damage e.g. to the **cing**ulate gyrus. Patients with Akinetic mutism won't be able to **cing**, either!

Anosodiaphoria

 Anosodiaphoria is lack of concern about one's impairment.

 Lack of concern = **NO SWEAT!** Anosodiaphoria is similar to A-DIAPHORESIS (without sweating)!

Patients with anosodiaphoria **ain't so diaphoretic** about their condition. They don't sweat the small stuff, or the big stuff for that matter.

Anosognosia

Anosognosia is denial/lack of awareness of one's impairment.

It is often seen with right parietal lesions.

If you tell a man with anosognosia that he has a neurological problem, he will say, "**It ain't so**".

The Cats

Catalepsy

Patients with catalepsy remain in the position in which they are placed. This may be seen in catatonia.

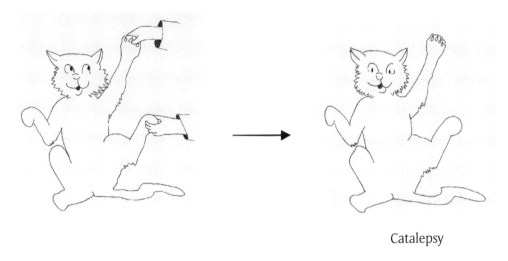

Catalepsy

Cataplexy

Cataplexy is seen in narcolepsy. It is sudden loss of tone following an emotion such as laughter or fear.

A patient with **catap**lexy is **catap**ulted to the floor when she experiences strong emotion.

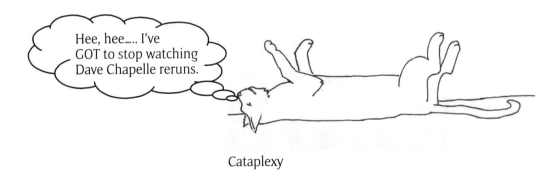

Hee, hee..... I've GOT to stop watching Dave Chapelle reruns.

Cataplexy

Catatonia

Two major types of catatonia are seen.

Stuporous Catatonia

Patients are mute, immobile, and may demonstrate echolalia, echopraxia, posturing, or catalepsy.

Excited Catatonia

Patients demonstrate purposeless frenetic activity.

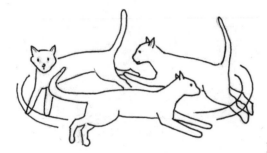

Excited catatonia

Cortical Deafness

Cortical deafness is characterized by deficits found in pure word deafness and deficits associated with auditory sound agnosia. In addition, these patients are unable to recognize vocal prosody, and the electrophysiological response of the primary auditory cortices to sound is absent.

It's due to bilateral lesions of the primary auditory cortex (like bilateral embolic strokes to Heschl's gyri).

Patients cannot interpret either verbal or nonverbal sounds, but are aware of the occurrence of sound.

Ideational Apraxia

In ideational apraxia, the patient can perform each individual component of a sequence but cannot perform the sequence (summ**ation**) of the components..

Ideomotor Apraxia

In ideomotor apraxia, the patient can physically perform a movement but can't if commanded.

Moto is a "No-go" to commands.

Ideational versus Ideomotor Apraxia

In idea**tion**al apraxia, the patient can perform each component of the idea but not the summa**tion.**

In ideo**motor** apraxia, patients can perform the **motor task**, but it's a **moto**-no-go if patients are commanded to do it.

Logorrhea

Logorrhea is pressured, abundant speech.

Logorrhea is **diarrhea of the mouth/words**.

Mental Retardation

The DSM-IV categorizes five different levels of mental retardation as listed below in this chart.

Diagnosis	I.Q. score
Borderline M.R	70-85
Mild M.R.	50 to 70
Moderate M.R.	35 to 50
Severe M.R.	20 to 35
Profound M.R.	Below 20

The DSM-V uses the terms "Intellectual Disability" and "Intellectual Developmental Disorder" rather than the term "Mental Retardation".

Prosopagnosia

 Prosopagnosia is the inability to recognize familiar faces. It is due to bilateral inferior occipitotemporal lesions.

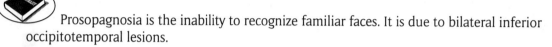 Patients with prosopagnosia **can't recognize some poor sap's face.**

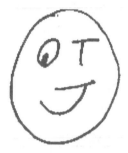

*To remember prosopagnosia is associated with **O**ccipito-**T**emporal lesions, draw a picture of a face with one eye as an **O** and the other as a **T**. It works!*

Wisconsin Card Sort Test

The Wisconsin card sort test is a neuropsychological test of executive function. It is good for assessing frontal lobe damage.

 The subject must match cards based on color, shape, or number. Feedback is given so that the subject can determine the pattern. After a certain number of trials, the rules are changed without notice. For instance, the subject may at first be required to match cards based on color. Then, without notification, the subject will be required to match cards by shape. Patients with frontal lobe damage continue to match cards based on color, even though they are told that they are wrong.

 You'd have to have frontal lobe damage to go to Wisconsin to play cards instead of Vegas.

Witzelsucht

 Witzelsucht is inappropriate jocularity, laughing/horsing around in inappropriate situations.

When you find something **witty/funny that sucks**, that's witzelsucht.

Patients with orbitofrontal lesions may demonstrate witzelsucht.

Echopraxia
_____

involuntary mimicking observed movements

lesion – lateral orbitofrontal

Behavioral Neurology Quiz

(Answers on page 733)

1. Match the condition with its description.

1) Aphemia	A) Not concerned about impairment
2) Abulia	B) Difficulty with producing speech
3) Anosodiaphoria	C) Delayed responses
4) Anosognosia	D) Not aware of impairment

2. Match the condition with the lesion.

1) Anton's syndrome	A) Bilateral parietal-occipital
2) Balint's syndrome	B) Arcuate fasciculus
3) Gerstmann syndrome	C) Bilateral occipital
4) Conduction aphasia	D) Dominant angular gyrus
5) Kluver-Bucy syndrome	E) Bilateral anterior temporal

3. Match the term with its definition.

1) Witzelsucht	A) Inability to recognize a familiar face
2) Logorrhea	B) Pressured, abundant speech
3) Prosopagnosia	C) Syndrome of approximate answers
4) Ganser syndrome	D) Inappropriate mirth

4. A patient with an IQ of 45 has:

    A. Mild mental retardation "Intellectual Disability"

    B. Moderate mental retardation "Intellectual Disability"

    C. Severe mental retardation "Intellectual Disability"

Chapter 3

Epilepsy

Seizure Types

In 2010, the International League Against Epilepsy (ILAE) recommended that the classification of seizures be changed.[1] There has been some resistance to these changes. Therefore, the 2010 and prior classifications are both discussed.

Classification of Seizures Prior to 2010 ILAE Statement	
Generalized	**Partial**
Absence	Simple partial
Atypical absence	Complex partial
Tonic	Secondarily generalized
Tonic-clonic	
Clonic	
Myoclonic	
Atonic	

Atypical Absence versus Absence Seizures

Atypical **A**bsence seizures are slower than absence seizures (1.5-2.5 Hz versus 3 Hz), **L**ast **L**onger, and tend to occur in children with **D**evelopmental **D**elay/neurologic deficits.

It's typical for a delinquent to skip school, but a **LAD** being **A**bsent is **A**typical.

Simple Partial versus Complex Partial Seizures

· With simple partial seizures the patient is aware.

· With complex partial seizures there is an alteration in awareness.

---

1 Berg AT, Berkovic SF, Brodie MJ, et al. Revised terminology and concepts for organization of seizures and epilepsies: report of the ILAE Commission on Classification and Terminology, 2005–2009. *Epilepsia* 2010;51:676–685.

Auras

Auras are simple partial seizures.

Auditory

Auditory auras tend to arise from the *temporal lobe*.

 If your aura has a *tempo*, it is likely from the *temporal* lobe.

Olfactory

 Patients describe a smell like burning rubber or other unpleasant odors.

Olfactory auras tend to arise from the *medial temporal lobe*.

Visual

 Formed visual auras arise from the *temporal-occipital region*.

Simple, unformed visual auras, such as spots, arise from the occipital lobe.

Epilepsy Classification

Definitions*

Symptomatic

There is a structural lesion, delayed development/less than normal intelligence, or a history of a neurologic problem (meningitis, head trauma, etc).

---

* = Prior to 2010 ILAE Statement

Idiopathic

 Presumed to be genetic. Patients are normal apart from having seizures and have a normal MRI.

Cryptogenic

 Thought to be symptomatic, but the underlying cause is unknown.

Classification of Seizures by the ILAE in 2010

The 2010 ILAE statement classified seizures as **generalized seizures, focal seizures,** or **unknown.**

Focal seizures are those arising within one hemisphere. They can evolve into a bilateral convulsive seizure. The terms simple and complex partial seizures were discarded.

Generalized seizures are those thought to begin and spread rapidly within bilateral networks.

GENERALIZED SEIZURE TYPES PER ILAE 2010 STATEMENT
Absence · Typical · Atypical · Absence with special features
Tonic
Tonic-clonic
Clonic
Myoclonic · Myoclonic · Myoclonic-atonic · Myoclonic-tonic
Atonic

Epilepsy Syndromes

Infantile Spasms

Clinical Features/Infantile Spasms

This is a generalized epilepsy that presents between 3 and 7 months with flexor and/or extensor spasms (myoclonic-tonic seizures), often called "Salaam" or "Jackknife" attacks.

There is rapid bending of the head and torso forward and simultaneous raising and bending of the arms while drawing the hands together in front of the chest – similar to the ceremonial greeting "Salaam."

Diagnosis/Infantile Spasms

West syndrome is defined by a triad:

1) **H**ypsarrhythmia
2) **I**nfantile spasms
3) **D**evelopmental delay

In the old **West**, when an infant seized, people yelled, "**ACTH!**" and they **HID**.

EEG/Infantile Spasms

The characteristic EEG pattern in infantile spasms is **hypsarrhythmia**.

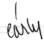

Hypsarrhythmia is asynchronous, chaotic high amplitude slow activity with multifocal spikes.

early

later, more synchrony

Notice that the EEG looks the same if you flip it upside down.

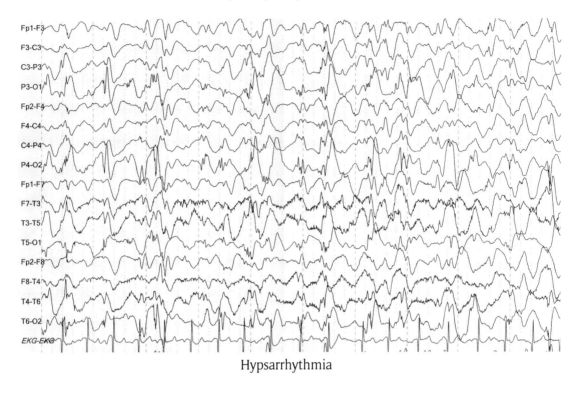

Hypsarrhythmia

Infantile spasms are the seizures found in West syndrome.

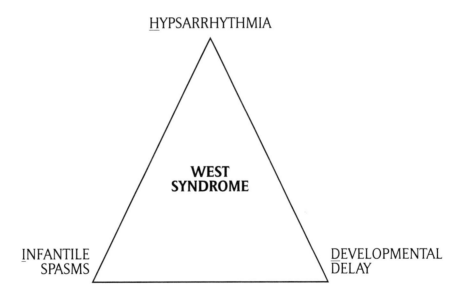

Treatment/Infantile Spasms

Remember to rule out metabolic causes, which require specific treatment e.g. phenylketonuria, maple syrup urine disease, biotinidase deficiency, Menkes' disease, glucose transporter deficiency.

Infantile spasms are often treated with ACTH. Vigabatrin is used to treat infantile spasms in tuberous sclerosis. Topamax and Keppra are second-line agents. The ketogenic diet is also effective – giving up to 70% of children a 50% or more reduction in seizures.

Lennox-Gastaut Syndrome

Lennox-Gastaut syndrome is a generalized epilepsy characterized by a triad:

1) At least **2 seizure types** including tonic, atonic, and atypical absence (remember the **LAD** above).
2) Specific EEG: generalized 1.5-2.5 Hz spike and wave discharges.
3) Developmental delay

Clinical features of Lennox-Gastaut syndrome:

· Onset is 1 to 8 years.
· May be preceded by infantile spasms.
· Difficult to treat. — VPA, clonazepam

To remember the details of Lennox-Gastaut syndrome: **Lenox** (the company that makes expensive dishes) had the **Greatest** sale: **buy one seizure type, get one free!**

Draret syndrome

o/w ne infant
sz c̄ fever – 1st yr – clonic/ T-C
dev. delay
usv. fever-related sz   SCN1A mutation
resistant to tx

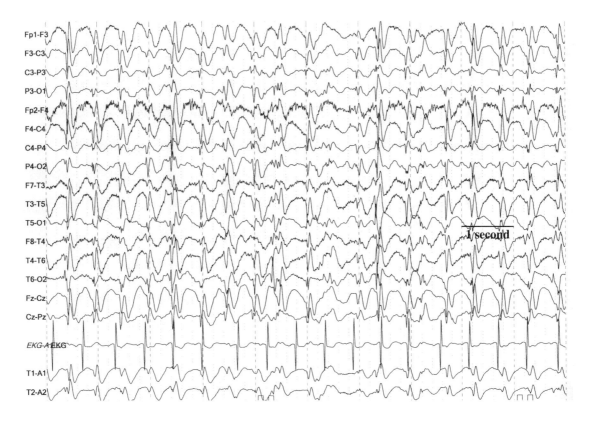

Slow spike-and-wave discharges seen in Lennox-Gastaut syndrome.

Landau-Kleffner Syndrome (Acquired Epileptic Aphasia)

Landau-Kleffner syndrome is a condition associated with language disturbances, which appear at 3 to 7 years of age. Patients develop word deafness. Receptive language is affected more than expressive, but speech output may decrease significantly as well.

Patients may have partial or generalized seizures.

The EEG may show epileptiform discharges over the temporal or parietal regions. During sleep, **electrical status epilepticus of sleep (ESES)** may be seen.

Landau sounds like **Lambeau**, the stadium where the Green Bay Packers football team plays; The fans at **Lambeau** field scream **disturbing language** during football games **deaf**eningly loud!

Thus, it's easy to remember **Landau** syndrome is associated with **word deafness** and **language disturbances**.

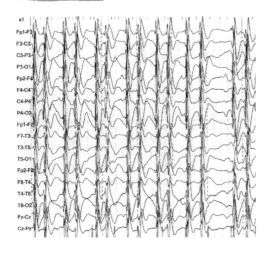

ESES

This pattern is seen in at least 85% of slow wave sleep.

Childhood Absence Epilepsy (CAE)

Clinical Features/CAE

CAE is a generalized epilepsy that presents at 4 to 8 years of age with brief staring episodes.

EEG/CAE

In CAE, the EEG shows generalized 3 Hz spike and slow wave discharges.

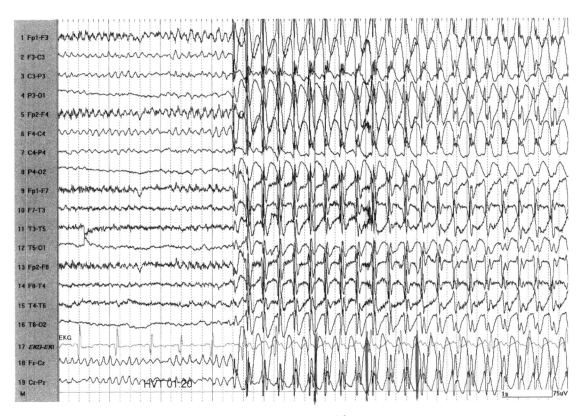

Seizure in a patient with CAE.

Treatment/CAE

Ethosuximide can treat absence seizures, but it is not effective at treating generalized tonic-clonic seizures.

Classically, **valproic acid** would be used in patients with absence seizures **and** generalized tonic-clonic seizures. Lamotrigine is also an option.

Juvenile Myoclonic Epilepsy (JME)

Clinical Features/JME

JME often presents with generalized tonic-clonic seizures at 13 to 20 years of age. *The seizure may follow sleep deprivation and/or drinking alcohol.* Patients often have myoclonic jerks (particularly in the morning) before the generalized tonic-clonic seizure but have ignored them. The usual onset of myoclonic jerks is 12 to 18 years. Patients may also have absence seizures. These tend to present at 7 to 13 years.

— no cognitive decline

JME patients **J**erk **M**ore with the 3 **E**'s:

Ethanol

Elimination of sleep, and[2]

Electric Light (photic stimulation or disco).[3]

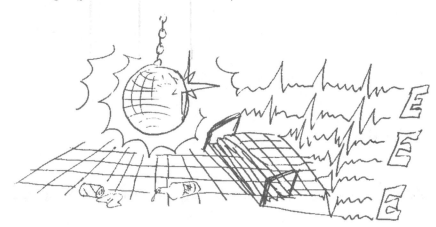

---

[2] Mnemonic courtesy of Dr. James Wheless with permission

[3] Mnemonic courtesy of Dr. James Wheless with permission.

EEG /JME

In JME, the EEG shows generalized 3.5-4.5 spike/polyspike and wave discharges. There may be a photoparoxysmal response.

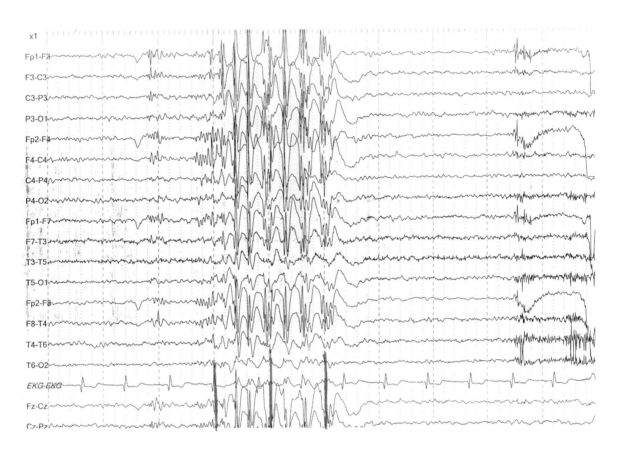

EEG of a patient with JME.

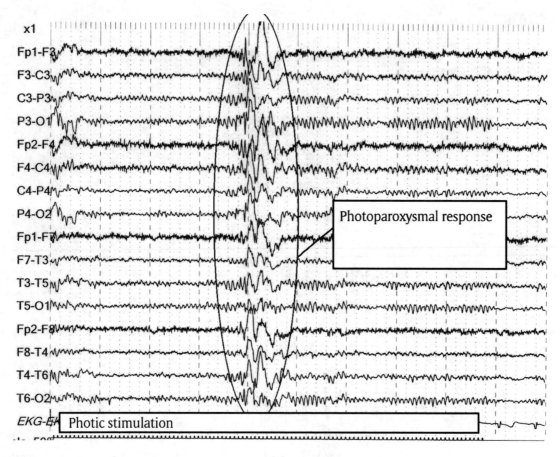

Photoparoxysmal response in JME patient undergoing photic stimulation.

Benign Rolandic Epilepsy of Childhood (BREC)

Clinical Features/BREC

BREC is the most common form of ~~benign partial epilepsy~~ of childhood.

BREC presents at 4 to 12 years of age. Patients present with **nocturnal generalized tonic-clonic seizures**. They also have ~~simple partial seizures with motor symptoms involving the face~~, which tend to ~~occur during sleep or upon awakening.~~ These may be associated with prominent **drooling and speech arrest**.

EEG/BREC

In BREC, the EEG shows **centro-temporal spikes**, which can be seen bilaterally and **increase in sleep**.

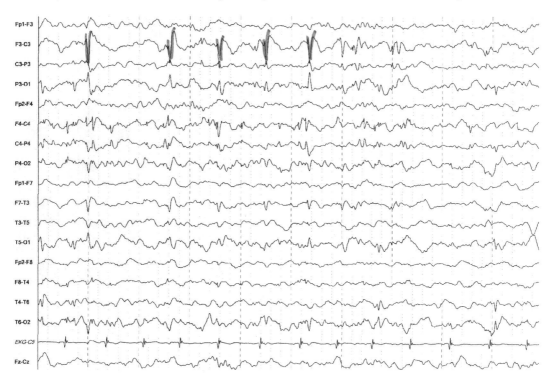

EEG from a patient with BREC showing a run of left centro-temporal spikes.

Neurophysiology fellows should know that a **horizontal dipole** is seen in this condition. **Frontal positivity** is seen.

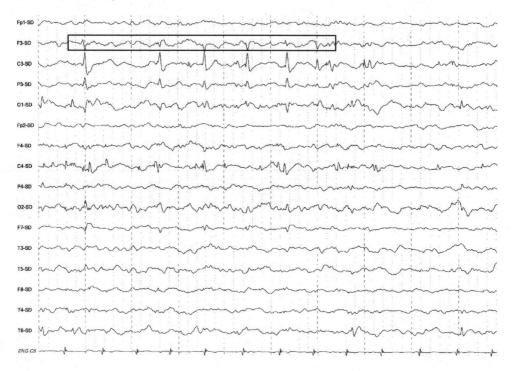

EEG from a patient with BREC in a referential (Laplacian montage) showing frontal positivity.

Frontal Lobe Epilepsy

In frontal lobe epilepsy, the seizure semiology depends upon where the seizures start.

In general, seizures occur most often at night, and patients may have **multiple seizures per night**.

Seizures tend to be brief, with rapid recovery.

Bizarre movements such as pelvic thrusting and frenetic activity can be seen.

aura - HA, dizzyness, odd feeling
may not show up on EEG (large area)

Temporal Lobe Epilepsy

lateral temporal - formed hallucinations
more motor automatisms

The most common pathologic findings in a temporal lobe removed for intractable seizures is **mesial temporal sclerosis**/ **Ammon's horn sclerosis**.

Recall that the anterior choroidal artery supplies the hippocampus.

Classically, patients have an aura of a **rising epigastric sensation**. Then they have automatisms.

(An epigastric aura can be seen with seizures arising from other lobes.)

Occipital Lobe Epilepsy

Early Onset Benign Epilepsy of Childhood with Occipital Paroxysms

This is also known as **Panayiotopoulus Syndrome**.

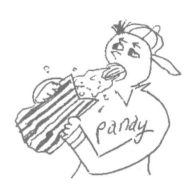

The age of onset of this condition is 2 to 8 years.

Seizures usually occur at night and can be prolonged. **Vomiting** and **tonic eye deviation** are seen. This may be followed by hemiclonic activity or secondary generalization.

Late Onset Benign Epilepsy of Childhood with Occipital Paroxysms

This is also known as **Gastaut type**.

The age of onset of Gastaut type may occur in adolescence.

Seizures consist of **visual symptoms** e.g. hemianopsia, blindness, hallucinations, or illusions. The seizures may secondarily generalize.

Seizures may be triggered by changes in light intensity and may be followed by migraine-type headaches.

Progressive Myoclonic Epilepsy (PME)

As a group, PME is characterized by: **Progressively SLUMiN' it!**

1) Seizures e.g. generalized tonic-clonic and myoclonic
2) Myoclonic jerks
3) Neurological decline, especially cerebellar and cognitive

Progressive Myoclonic Epilepsy	Chromosome	Gene Defect	Unique feature
Sialidoses	6p	Neuraminidase	Cherry-red spot
Lafora disease	6q (EPM2A) 6p (EPM2B)	Laforin (Protein encoded is a tyrosine phosphatase) Malin	Intracellular polyglucosan-containing inclusions in skin, muscle, liver, and brain
Unverricht-Lundborg disease (EPM1)	21q	Cystatin B	Membrane bound vacuoles on eccrine gland biopsy
Myoclonic Epilepsy with Ragged-Red Fibers	Maternally-inherited mutation at position 8344 in the mitochondrial genome in over 80% of cases	tRNA lysine	Ragged red fibers Elevated lactate and pyruvate
Neuronal Ceroid Lipofuscinoses (NCL)	Multiple	Multiple	Unique patterns on electron microscopy

Modified from Chyung ASC, Ptácek LJ. Genetics of epilepsy. Continuum Lifelong Learning Neurol 2005;11(2);79-94 (with permission). Conroy JA. Progressive Myoclonic Epilepsies. J Child Neurol 2002;17:S80-84. Leppik IE. Classification of the myoclonic epilepsies. Epilepsia 2003;44(Suppl 11):2-6.

Unverricht-Lundborg Disease

Unverricht-**L**undborg is the most common type of PME. It is due to a mutation in the **Cys**tatin **B** gene on chromosome **21**.

It presents between 6 and 18 years of age with stimulus-sensitive myoclonic jerks, which usually occur in the morning.

Intellect remains relatively intact and cerebellar deterioration is late.

To remember **U**nverricht-**L**undborg disease, think of your smart but messy 21-year-old, younger sister: **U, Little Cys, Be intelligent at age 21, and try to stop Progressively SLUMiN' it!**

Somatosensory evoked potentials (SSEPs) may be high in amplitude.

It is diagnosed with skin biopsy from the axillary region, which shows **membrane-bound vacuoles in eccrine sweat glands**.

Lafora's Disease

These patients do tend to have dementia. *(early)*
ataxia, spasticity (later)

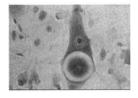

Patients may have occipital seizures with **visual hallucinations**. **Lafora bodies** are found in various tissues, especially eccrine **sweat** glands. **Lafora bodies** are polyglucosan bodies → see photo, which looks like a "Mercedes Benz sign" →

PAS⊕

Compared to **U**nverricht-**L**undborg, **Lafora's disease progresses faster**.

The new "**Lafora**" – made by **Mercedes Benz** – is much **faster** than U**r Little Cys**'s car. It's so fast, you'll **hallucinate** the images going by and **sweat** profusely!

Neuronal Ceroid Lipofuscinoses (NCL)

NCL are autosomal recessive lysosomal storage disorders characterized by **accumulation of abnormal amounts of lipopigment**.

Vision loss occurs. Electron microscopy on skin, rectal, or conjunctival tissue may show granular **osmiophilic deposits, curvilinear bodies, fingerprint profiles, or rectilinear complexes**.

Photo: Jeffrey A. Golden & Brian N. Harding. (2004). Developmental Neuropathology. *The International Society of Neuropathology.*

NCL also stands for **N**orwegian **C**ruise **L**ines (they paint **NCL** on all their boats). On a cruise, you'll see:

- as you board, **fingerprint profiles** for security purposes;
- guests in the ship's casino, placing cash **osmiophilic deposits** into **rectilinear complexes** (slot machines);
- on deck, **curvilinear bodies** bathing in the sun;
- **vision loss** if they don't wear their sunglasses; and
- everyone **accumulating lots of lipo-pigment** -- pigment from the sun, and fat (= lipo) at the all-you-can-eat buffet!

Infantile NCL

Infantile NCL is due to a defect in CLN1 gene at 1p, which codes for palmitoyl protein thioesterase (PPT1). It presents between 6 months and 2 years. Microcephaly, epilepsy, and regression are seen.

The adult form is called Kuf's disease.

Myoclonic Epilepsy and Ragged Red Fibers (MERRF)

MERRF is a mitochondrial disease characterized by myoclonic epilepsy clinically and by ragged red fibers on muscle biopsy. Patients may also have deafness, optic atrophy, lipomas, short stature, myopathy, or neuropathy.

As with other **m**itochondrial diseases, the condition is **m**aternally inherited and lactate and pyruvate are elevated.

A mutation in the tRNA^{Lys} gene is responsible for most of the cases.

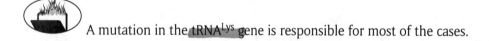

To remember that MERRF is associated with Lys, remember the phrase **Merve has lice.** Poor Merve also has lipomas, deafness, optic atrophy, short stature, myopathy, and neuropathy. At least his mother, who passed on her mitochondrial DNA, still loves him.

Sialidosis Type I

 Sialidosis Type I is due to a defect in **NeurA**minidase, which cleaves **S**ialic **A**cid from **gal**actose.

 Patients have cherry-red spots and little cognitive deterioration.

Elevated sialyloligosaccharides in urine can help to confirm the diagnosis.

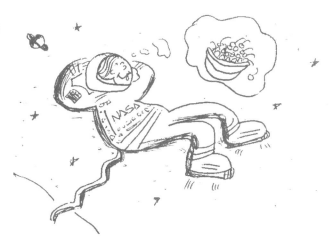

To remember that sialidosis type I is associated with a cherry-red spot, think of a **gal** astronaut (working for **NASA**) who is **sal**ivating for **cherries**.

Genetics

Epilepsy	Gene product	Gene	Locus
Benign Familial Neonatal Convulsions (EBN1)	Voltage-gated potassium channel	KCNQ2	20q13.3
Benign Familial Neonatal Convulsions (EBN2)	Voltage-gated potassium channel	KCNQ3	8q24
Benign Familial Neonatal-Infantile Seizures	Voltage-gated sodium channel	SCN2A	2q24
Generalized Epilepsy with Febrile Seizures Plus (Type 1)	Voltage-gated sodium channel	SCN1B	19q13
Generalized Epilepsy with Febrile Seizures Plus (Type 2)	Voltage-gated sodium channel	SCN1A	2q24
Generalized Epilepsy with Febrile Seizures Plus	Voltage-gated sodium channel	SCN2A	2q24
Generalized Epilepsy with Febrile Seizures Plus (Type 3)	GABA A receptor	GABRG2	5q31
Childhood Absence Epilepsy and Febrile Seizures	GABA A receptor	GABRG2	5q31
Autosomal Dominant Nocturnal Frontal Lobe Epilepsy	Nicotinic acetylcholine receptor	CHRNA4	20q13
Autosomal Dominant Nocturnal Frontal Lobe Epilepsy	Nicotinic acetylcholine receptor	CHRNB2	1q21
Autosomal Dominant Lateral Temporal Lobe Epilepsy or Autosomal Dominant Partial Epilepsy with Auditory Features	LGI1 (leucine-rich, glioma inactivated 1 gene)	LGI1	10q24
Autosomal Dominant Juvenile Myoclonic Epilepsy	GABA A receptor	GABRA1	5q34
Juvenile Myoclonic Epilepsy		EFHC1	6p12
Severe Myoclonic Epilepsy of Infancy	Voltage-gated sodium channel	SCN1A	2q24

Modified from Chyung ASC, Ptácek LJ. Genetics of epilepsy. Continuum Lifelong Learning Neurol 2005;11(2);79-94 (with permission). Ottman R. Analysis of Genetically Complex Epilepsies. Epilepsia 2005;46(Suppl 10):7-14.

MNEMONIC

To remember that benign neonatal convulsions are associated with potassium (K$^+$) channel mutations, recall that neonates receive vitamin K at birth.

HOT TIP

Mutations in the SCN1A gene on chromosome 2q24 are responsible for severe myoclonic epilepsy of infancy and generalized epilepsy with febrile seizures plus type 2.

V-G Na$^+$ ©

Anti-Epileptic Drugs

Side Effects/Complications

Antiepileptic drug	Characteristic Side Effects
ACTH (Acthar gel)	Can cause hyperglycemia, hypertension, and immune suppression.
Carbamazepine (Tegretol, Carbatrol)	Hyponatremia, agranulocytosis, liver inducer, autoinduction. *Skin rash*
Ethosuximide (Zarontin)	Gastrointestinal side effects.
Felbamate (Felbatol)	Liver failure, aplastic anemia, insomnia.
Gabapentin (Neurontin)	Peripheral edema may worsen myoclonus. *HA, fatigue, ataxia*
Lamotrigine (Lamictal)	Stevens-Johnson syndrome. *tremor @ ↑ doses*
Levetiracetam (Keppra)	May cause irritability. Rare cases of psychosis.
Oxcarbazepine (Trileptal)	Hyponatremia.
Phenobarbital	Hyperactivity and cognitive disturbances in children, Dupuytren's contractures.
Phenytoin (Dilantin)	Gum hyperplasia, hypertrichosis, nonlinear kinetics, lupus-like syndrome, cerebellar atrophy, coarsening of facial features. IV form can cause arrhythmias if given too fast and purple-glove syndrome.
Tiagabine (Gabitril)	Absence status.
Topiramate (Topamax)	Kidney stones, oligohydrosis, weight loss, glaucoma, metabolic acidosis, word finding difficulties at high doses.
Valproate (Depakote, Depacon, Depakene)	Hepatotoxicity, weight gain, polycystic ovary syndrome, alopecia, pancreatitis, tremor, hyperammonemia. There's an increased risk for liver failure if less than 2 years, developmentally delayed, and on multiple drugs.
Vigabatrin (Sabril)	Visual field defects.
Zonisamide (Zonegran)	Kidney stones, oligohydrosis, weight loss.

Oxcarbazepine versus Carbamazepine

 Oxcarbazepine (Trileptal) is rapidly metabolized to 10-monohydroxy derivative (MHD), an active metabolite.

During the metabolism of carbamazepine (Carbatrol, Tegretol), an epoxide is created, which is thought to be responsible for some of carbamazepine's side effects.

 Metabolism of oxcarbazepine does not create an epoxide.

Vigabatrin

Look at the name itself: **V-I-GABA-TR-IN.**

It's a **Vi**gorous, **I**rreversible **GABA TR**ansaminase **IN**hibitor.

It is the drug of choice for infants with **tuberous sclerosis** and **infantile spasms**.

It is not currently FDA approved due to a risk of causing visual field defects. It causes bilateral concentric visual field defects with relative temporal sparing.

Vigabatrin causes **Vi**sual field defects and is a **Vi**gorous, **I**rreversible **GABA TR**ansaminase **IN**hibitor.

> ### Topiramate and Zonisamide
>
> These antiepileptic medications have similar side effect profiles: kidney stones, oligohydrosis, hyperthermia, decreased appetite.
>
> Both inhibit carbonic anhydrase. (Recall that Diamox [acetazolamide] is a carbonic anhydrase inhibitor and was used in the past as an AED.)
>
> One difference is that zonisamide contains sulfa, so it should be avoided in patients with a sulfa allergy.

Antiepileptic Medications and Worsening of Seizures

Worsen Generalized Seizures

Carbamazepine can worsen generalized seizures e.g. absence, atonic, myoclonic.

 CBZ
Tiagabine can cause absence status.

Vigabatrin
baclofen
amitriptyline

Worsen Myoclonic Seizures

Antiepileptic medications that can worsen myoclonic seizures:

Carbamazepine

Phenytoin

Gabapentin

*Lamotrigine**

Tiagabine

Vigabatrin

Lamotrigine has been reported to worsen myoclonus but also has been used successfully in Juvenile Myoclonic Epilepsy.

Bonus Features

 Many antiepileptic medications have side effects that can be useful.

Mood Stabilizer

~~Carbamazepine~~

~~Lamotrigine~~

~~Oxcarbazepine~~

~~Valproate~~

To remember that **C**arbamazepine, **L**amotrigine, **O**xcarbazepine, and **V**alproate have a calming effect: some smokers smoke **CLOV**e cigarettes to calm down.

Weight Loss

Felbamate

Topiramate

Zonisamide

Like the **Zone diet**, Zonegran (zonisamide) can cause weight loss, as can topiramate and felbamate.

Weight Gain

> ~~Gabapentin~~
> ~~Pregabalin~~
> ~~Valproate~~

Migraine Prophylaxis

> Gabapentin
> Topiramate
> Valproate

Tremor

> ~~Primidone~~
> ~~Topiramate~~

 ~~Tremor~~ **prevention** with ~~topiramate~~ and **pr**imidone.

Drug Elimination

Gabapentin (Neurontin), vigabatrin, and levetiracetam (Keppra) are eliminated almost entirely by the kidneys.

 When you see **Neurontin**, think of **Nephron-tin** because Neurontin is eliminated by the kidney.

 ~~Keppra~~ is eliminated by the ~~kidneys.~~

 ~~Vigabatrin~~ is eliminated by ~~voiding.~~

In addition, note that a significant amount of topiramate is eliminated by the kidneys.

CBZ, VPA, PHY : not removed by dialysis

Drug Interactions

Drug interactions	AEDs
Inducers and inducible	Carbamazepine, phenobarbital, phenytoin
Inducible but usually don't induce	Oxcarbazepine, topiramate, lamotrigine, zonisamide
Usually inhibit other antiepileptic medications	Valproate, felbamate
Free of interactions	Gabapentin, levetiracetam, pregabalin, vigabatrin

Faught E. Pharmacokinetic considerations in prescribing antiepileptic drugs. Epilepsia 2001; 42 (Suppl 4):19-23.

Recall that carbamazepine also induces its own metabolism.

Lamotrigine's metabolism is inhibited by valproate, so lamotrigine should be increased even slower than usual in patients who are also taking valproate.

Remember that lamotrigine can cause **Stevens-Johnson Syndrome**, which is a **life threatening** rash, if increased rapidly.

— add valproate to phenytoin regimen → transient phenytoin tox 2/2 ↑ free phenytoin Uc displaced

salicylates
chloramphenicol
EtOH   Sulfa
amio   INH   ↑ phenytoin
trazodone   level

rifampin
antacids   ↓ phenytoin (free)
             level

phenytoin ↓   OCP
               quinidine
               chloramphenicol
               (levels)

Mechanism of Action

Most drugs have multiple mechanisms of action. This section is simplified for the sake of clarity and recognition on the exam.

Antiepileptic drug	Primary Mechanism(s)
Carbamazepine (Tegretol)	Sodium channel blockade
Diastat (rectal Valium)	Increases frequency of opening of GABA A chloride channel.
Ethosuximide (Zarontin)	Calcium channel blockade (voltage-dependent T-type calcium channel alpha-1G subunit).
Felbamate (Felbatol)	Sodium channel blockade, acts on NMDA receptor, acts at GABA A receptor.
Gabapentin (Neurontin)	Inhibits L-type calcium channels.
Lamotrigine (Lamictal)	Sodium channel blockade.
Levetiracetam (Keppra)	Binds to synaptic vesicle protein (SV2A). May block N-type calcium channels and inhibit delayed rectifier K+ current.
Oxcarbazepine (Trileptal)	Sodium channel blockade.
Phenobarbital	Increases frequency of opening of GABA A chloride channel.
Phenytoin (Dilantin)	Sodium channel blockade.
Pregabalin (Lyrica)	Modulates P/Q-type voltage-gated calcium channels.
Tiagabine (Gabitril)	Blocks GABA reuptake
Topiramate (Topamax)	Sodium channel blockade, acts on non-NMDA receptors, enhances chloride currents through GABA A receptor
Valproate (Depakote, Depacon, Depakene)	Sodium channel blockade, calcium channel blockade
Vigabatrin (Sabril)	Inhibits GABA-transaminase, which breaks down GABA
Zonisamide (Zonegran)	Sodium channel blockade, calcium channel blockade

Rho JM, Sankar R. The pharmacologic basis of antiepileptic drug action. Epilepsia 1999; 40:1471-1483.

Antiepileptic medications that act at voltage-dependent sodium channels:

> Carbamazepine
> Lamotrigine
> Phenytoin
> Topiramate
> (2) Valproate
> (2) Zonisamide

Antiepileptic medications that block T-type voltage-gated calcium channels:

> Ethosuximide
> (2) Valproate
> (2) Zonisamide

Barbiturates versus Benzodiazepines

Barbiturates and benzodiazepines both act at GABA A receptors.

Benzodiazepines increase the frequency of opening of the GABA channel.

Barbiturates increase the duration of time that the channel is open; they make it stay open longer.

To remember that **ben**zodiazepines increase the frequency and barbiturates increase the time that the GABA A receptor is open, remember that **Ben** Affleck is photographed frequently and bars stay open long into the night.

Protein Binding

Low Protein Binding (< 10%)	High Protein Binding (> 75%)
Ethosuximide	Carbamazepine
Gabapentin	Phenytoin
Levetiracetam	Tiagabine
Vigabatrin	Valproate

Low protein binding antiepileptic medications can be remembered by GLoVE:

Gabapentin
Levetiracetam
o = omit
Vigabatrin
Ethosuximide

Imagine that a slippery glove makes it hard to hold onto the protein.

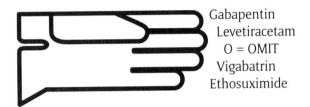

Gabapentin
Levetiracetam
O = OMIT
Vigabatrin
Ethosuximide

 High protein binding antiepileptic medications can be remembered with the phrase **Very Tight Protein Connection:**

Valproate
Tiagabine
Phenytoin
Carbamazepine

Other Epilepsy Treatments

Surgery

Resection

Surgical resection may be preceded by placement of grids, strips, or depth electrodes to localize the onset of the seizures. Grids and strips may also be used to map eloquent cortex.

Vagus Nerve Stimulation

Vagus nerve stimulation is used to treat intractable epilepsy in patients who are not candidates for, have failed, or refuse surgical resection. It is also being used to treat intractable depression.

Corpus Callosotomy

Corpus callosotomy is a palliative procedure used for generalized seizures, particularly those causing falls (e.g. atonic seizures).

Post-operatively patients can have a temporary left limb apraxia.

Hemispherectomy

Hemispherectomy is used to treat treat **S**turge-Weber Syndrome, **H**emimegalencephaly, **A**ntinatal MCA/ICA **S**trokes, intractable epilepsy due to **R**asmussen's encephalitis, and **D**iffuse cortical dysplasias.

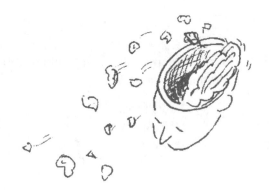

Removing one's hemisphere leaves **SHARDS** of brain tissue everywhere!

Rasmussen's Encephalitis

Rasmussen's encephalitis presents with epilepsia partialis continua (EPC), which is focal motor status epilepticus. This results in progressive hemiparesis. Progressive atrophy is seen on MRI.

Antibodies to the Glu-R3 receptor have been found in some patients.

Sturge-Weber

Please see the Neurocutaneous Disorders chapter.

Pyridoxine (B6)

Consider pyridoxine for treatment of neonatal seizures that do not respond to conventional therapy; the patient may have B6 dependency.

Some patients with infantile spasms also respond to B6.

Ketogenic Diet

The ketogenic diet is successfully used in some patients.

It is ideal for patients with a glucose transporter-1 defect (which is diagnosed with low CSF glucose).

It may also be useful in pyruvate dehydrogenase complex deficiency, and infantile spasms in tuberous sclerosis.

However, the ketogenic diet is contraindicated and may be lethal in other metabolic conditions, such as pyruvate carboxylase deficiency. Some additional diseases for which the ketogenic diet is contraindicated include: acute intermittent porphyria (AIP); some mitochondrial diseases such as myoclonic epilepsy with ragged red fibers (MERRF), mitochondrial encephalopathy with lactic acidosis and stroke-like episodes (MELAS), and cytochrome oxidase deficiency; carnitine deficiency; and defects in oxidation of free fatty acids.

To remember the diseases that contraindicate a ketogenic diet, think of it causing a **Peruvian COMA!**

Pyruvate carboxylase deficiency, **C**ytochrome oxidase deficiency; **C**arnitine deficiency; **O**xidation of FFAs; **M**ELAS/**M**ERRF, and **A**IP.

Complications of the diet include hypoglycemia during initiation of the diet, weight loss, constipation, kidney stones, and elevated cholesterol.

Recall that topiramate and zonisamide also increase the risk of kidney stones.

Women and Epilepsy

Special Considerations in Women with Epilepsy

Birth Control

CBZ, pheno-barb, phenytoin

Anti-epileptic drugs that are inducers can reduce the levels of oral contraceptives, which can result in pregnancy.

Folate

Consider giving folate to all girls/women of childbearing age to prevent neural tube defects.

Pregnancy and AEDs

This is a huge topic.

Key points:

During pregnancy the goal is to maintain seizure freedom with the lowest possible dose of AEDs. If possible, monotherapy is preferred.

AED levels change during pregnancy and in the post-natal period.

Certain antiepileptic medications are more likely to result in birth defects. There are ongoing studies/birth registries.

Infants of Women with Epilepsy

Infants born to women taking enzyme-inducing antiepileptic medications are at **higher risk for hemorrhagic disease of the newborn**. In the last month of pregnancy these mothers should take vitamin K daily. Infants should receive vitamin K intramuscularly at birth.

The Bare Bones of Bone Health

Bone health is a hot topic in epilepsy. Antiepileptic medications can adversely affect bone metabolism. Therefore, neurologists have started recommended calcium for patients on antiepileptic medications long-term.

The List of "Mosts"

- Unverricht-Lundborg is the most common progressive myoclonic epilepsy.

- Temporal lobe epilepsy is the most common epilepsy in adults.

- Mesial temporal sclerosis is the most common finding when temporal lobectomy is performed in adults.

Epilepsy Quiz

(Answers on page 735)

1. Match the mechanism with an anticonvulsant.

    1) Blocks reuptake of GABA into presynaptic neurons

    2) Blocks breakdown of GABA by GABA transaminase

    3) Sodium channel blocker

    4) Calcium channel blocker

    A. Ethosuximide

    B. Lamotrigine

    C. Vigabatrin

    D. Tiagabine

2. Match the antiepileptic medication with its mechanism.

    1) Phenytoin

    2) Carbamazepine

    3) Valproic acid

    4) Zonegran

    A. Sodium channel blocker

    B. Calcium channel blocker

    C. Both

3. Match the EEG to the condition.

    1) High-voltage, chaotic slow waves with multifocal admixed spikes

    2) 1.5-2.5 Hz generalized spike and wave discharges

    3) 4-6 Hz generalized spike/polyspike and wave discharges

    4) Centro-temporal spikes, often bilateral, sometimes associated with frontal positivity

    A. Infantile spasms

    B. Benign Rolandic Epilepsy

    C. Juvenile Myoclonic Epilepsy

    D. Lennox-Gastaut syndrome

4. Which of these antiepileptic medications is an inducer?

        A. Valproate

        B. Felbamate

        C. Carbamazepine

        D. Gabapentin

5. Which of these antiepileptic medications has the fewest drug interactions?

        A. Levetiracetam

        B. Topiramate

        C. Lamotrigine

        D. Zonisamide

        E. Oxcarbazepine

Chapter 4

Infectious Diseases

Bacterial Infections

Brain Abscess

A brain abscess is usually due to spread of infection from a contiguous infected site.

Often an abscess is a mixed infection, which may include anaerobes. Streptococci are most commonly isolated.

Bacterial Meningitis

Group B Streptococcus (GBS) is the most common cause of neonatal meningitis.

Escherichia coli (E. coli) is the **second** most common cause of neonatal meningitis.

Listeria is the **third** most common cause of neonatal meningitis.

To remember the top 3 causes of neonatal bacterial meningitis, remember **BELLA** (beautiful) Baby!
Group **B** Strep, **E.**coli, and **L**isteria (in order!)

Remember to add Ampicillin when treating neonatal meningitis to cover *Listeria.*

Neisseria meningitidis is the most common cause of bacterial meningitis **in children**.

It can cause meningitis outbreaks in college dorms and military barracks due to crowding.

Waterhouse-Friedreichsen syndrome is adrenal failure due to adrenal hemorrhage associated with meningococcemia.

Pneumococcus *(Streptococcus pneumoniae)* is the most **common cause** of bacterial meningitis in **adults**;

· the most common cause of meningitis in **patients with a CSF leak**;

· the most common cause of meningitis in **patients who have suffered from blunt head trauma**; and

· a common cause of meningitis in **patients who had a splenectomy** or **sickle cell disease** because **S. pneumoniae** is an encapsulated organism that asplenics/sicklers cannot handle well.

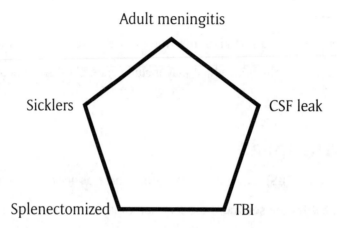

Adult meningitis

Sicklers   CSF leak

Splenectomized   TBI

Subdural Empyema

A subdural empyema is purulent exudate between the dura and arachnoid. It usually is secondary to ear or sinus infection.

Specific Bacterial Infections

Bartonella Henselae

Bartonella henselae causes Cat-scratch disease, which can result in encephalitis.

Patients have a papule or pustule at the site of injury and regional lymphadenitis.

Campylobacter Jejuni

Campylobacter jejuni is associated with the axonal form of Guillain-Barré Syndrome (GBS), the Miller-Fisher variant of GBS, and anti-GM1 antibodies.

To remember that *Campylobacter jejuni* is associated with the axonal form of GBS, the Miller-Fisher variant, and anti-GM1 antibodies remember this:

Take your GM™ truck to go camping where you sit on you're a** , drink Miller™ and Fish.

Take your GM (anti-GM1 antibodies) truck to go camping (*Campylobacter*), where you sit on you're a** (axonal), drink Miller and Fish (Miller-Fisher).

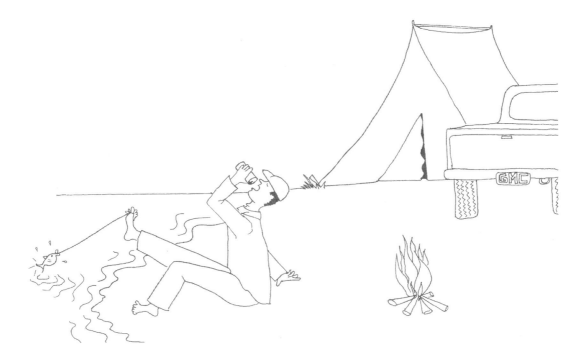

Clostridium Botulinum

Botulism in Adults

In adults, botulism is due to toxin produced by germinated Clostridium botulinum spores. Spores can be found in improperly prepared canned foods, undercooked food, or anaerobic wounds.

The toxin **blocks release of acetylcholine.**

Adults with botulism poisoning have a dry mouth, vomiting, ophthalmoplegia, loss of pupillary reflexes, and symmetric **descending** weakness, which can lead to respiratory failure.

If patients present at that point, they can look like Guillain-Barré patients. However, Guillain-Barré usually causes **ascending** weakness without loss of pupillary reflexes. EMG/NCS also differentiate the two diseases.

In botulism, EMG/NCS show low-amplitude muscle action potentials (CMAPs). With repetitive stimulation at 20-50 Hz, there is potentiation of the response. Posttetanic facilitation and absence of posttetanic exhaustion are seen in adult and infantile botulism.

Lambert-Eaton also interferes with acetylcholine release, can cause **dry mouth**, and has **similar EMG/NCS findings**. Please see the Neuromuscular Diseases chapter for more details.

Botulism in Infants

In infants, botulism is due to a toxin produced by **ingested** *Clostridium botulinum.*

Infants living near construction sites are at risk; however, on the exam, infantile botulism is usually associated with ingestion of honey. An infant is given honey and then develops **constipation**. Then they develop **generalized weakness** including **bulbar and skeletal muscles**, **hypotonia**, **decreased reflexes**, **ptosis**, and **dilated pupils**. They can have **respiratory failure**.

Stool cultures and EMG/NCS findings help with the diagnosis.

Posttetanic facilitation and absence of posttetanic exhaustion are seen in **both adult and infantile botulism.**

Clostridium Tetani (Tetanus)

Clostridium tetani causes **opisthotonus** and muscle spasms when spores enter a wound.

The **tetanus toxin (tetanospasmin)** **inhibits the release** of **Glycine** and **GABA**, which are the major inhibitory neurotransmitters in the CNS.

Inhibiting your friends **G**uy and **G**abby from playing **tennis** will cause them to **spaz, man**, and get **opissed off!**

Corynebacterium **D**iphtheriae (**D**iphtheria)   gram ⊕ bacillus

The exotoxin from *Corynebacterium diphtheriae* causes Diphtheria.

Diphtheria produces a **D**emyelinating neuropathy that may resemble Guillain-Barré Syndrome. (motor)

oculomotor/ciliary paralysis

10d → 3mo post infxn

Initially patients have **D**isgusting **pharyngitis** with a **D**eep **gray membrane** in the throat.

Mycobacterial Disease

Mycobacterium Tuberculosis

Mycobacterium tuberculosis is the acid-fast bacillus that causes tuberculosis (TB).

TB has many neurological complications such as meningitis, tuberculomas, stroke, cranial nerve palsies, and Pott's disease.

TB Meningitis

TB meningitis tends to localize to the base of the brain.

Complications include **cranial nerve palsies** and **hydrocephalus**.
Vasculitis and **ischemia/ infarction** also occur.

CSF shows a *lymphocytic pleocytosis*, *high protein*, and *low glucose (hypoglycorrhacia)*.

HIV is a major risk factor.

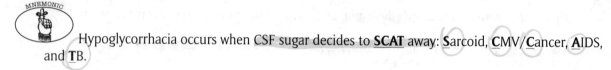 Hypoglycorrhacia occurs when CSF sugar decides to **SCAT** away: **S**arcoid, **C**MV/**C**ancer, **A**IDS, and **T**B.

Tuberculoma

 A tuberculoma is a mass of granulation tissue in the parenchyma containing TB. It can resemble a tumor.

Pott's Disease

 Pott's disease is a TB **infection of the spine** associated with **myelopathy**.

 To remember that <u>Pott</u>'s disease is due to *Tuber*culosis, recall that **Pot**atoes are *Tuber*s.

Neurological Side Effects of TB Medications

Ethambutol can cause optic neuropathy.

INH can cause *pyridoxine deficiency*, which can lead to **peripheral neuropathy** and **seizures**.

Mycobacterium Leprae (Leprosy)

Mycobacterium leprae (M. leprae) is the acid-fast bacterium that causes leprosy.

Findings suggestive of leprosy are **anesthetic skin lesions**, **neuropathy** and/or **nerve enlargement**, and the presence of **acid-fast bacilli in a skin biopsy**.

M. Leprae likes the peripheral nerves because it prefers cooler temperatures.

In the past, leprosy was most common cause of peripheral neuropathy worldwide. Today, diabetes mellitus, which is the number one cause in the US, is trying to take over the world as well.

Leprosy goes to the **periphery** just as lepers were ostracized to the periphery of society.

Patients can have **palpable peripheral nerves**.

Other causes of hypertrophic nerves are:
- **Amy**loidosis
- **C**hronic Inflammatory Demyelinating Polyneuropathy (CIDP)
- **C**harcot-Marie-Tooth Neuropathy Type 1/ **Here**ditary Motor and Sensory Neuropathy 1
- **Re**fsum's disease
- **S**arcoid

Because of her **big, palpable nerves, Amy Lloyd Resembles a Scary, Hairy Clown!** (**Amy**loid-**Re**fsum-**Sar**coid-HMSN1/**C**MT1-**C**IDP!)

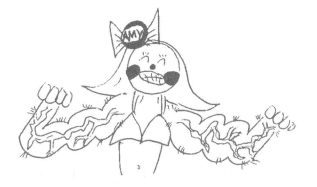

In leprosy, you have nerves you can see.

Lepromatous Leprosy

Lepromatous leprosy is the **systemic form of leprosy**. It occurs in patients with *reduced cell-mediated immunity.*

Patients have widely distributed, **nonanesthetic symmetric skin lesions**. The **skin may be shiny**.

It can cause **leonine facies** and **involves multiple organs**.

Patients develop a **distal symmetric sensory peripheral neuropathy.**

Lord love patients with lepromatous leprosy who have low immunity, lots of lesions, leonine facies, and loss of limb sensation.

If It's Not Too Hot In the Kitchen

Clinical Vignette: A patient presented to my clinic with a chief complaint of "I can't feel my own arms." The patient was an immigrant cook at a restaurant who discovered the patient's deficit when the patient leaned on a hot stove that the patient thought was off! The patient's co-workers screamed in horror as the patient inadvertently self-inflicted second-degree burns! The patient's skin biopsy by dermatology revealed "red snappers" consistent with Mycobacterium leprae. The patient was treated with dapsone and improved.

Tuberculoid Leprosy

Tuberculoid leprosy occurs in individuals with **normal** cell-mediated immunity.

Patients have a few asymmetric, **well-defined, dry, hypopigmented anesthetic plaques** or **macules**.

TL tends to cause **mononeuritis** or **mononeuritis multiplex**.

Dapsone is used to treat leprosy and can **cause a motor neuropathy**.

Second-line agents include Clofazimine and Rifampin.

Spirochetes

Treponema Pallidum

Treponema pallidum causes syphilis.

It looks like this (only smaller):

Clinical Features

Tabes dorsalis is the most common form of neurosyphilis. Patients have **lancinating pains (usually in the legs)** and **urinary incontinence**. Signs are **Argyll Robertson pupils**, **areflexia at the knees and ankles**, **decreased vibration and proprioception** in the feet and legs causing **ataxia** and a positive **Romberg**, and **Charcot joints**.

Argyll-Robertson pupils are small "LAP DANCER" pupils that accommodate but react poorly to light. Any LAP DANCER will **accommodate but not react** for you. Just watch out for syphilis!

To remember the clinical features of neurosyphilis: remember LAP DANCER.

Lancinating pains in **L**egs

Ataxia **A**nd **A**reflexia in **A**nkles **A**nd knees

Proprioception reduced in legs

Dorsalis, tabes

Argyll-Robertson pupils **A**ccommodate but don't react

Need **D**epends undergarments

Charcot joints

Eventual bone distruction and deformity (Charcot joint)

Romberg positive

Congenital Syphilis

Patients with congenital syphilis can have **interstitial keratitis**, **chorioretinitis**, a **saddle nose**, **saber shins**, **pseudoparalysis**, **peg-shaped incisors**, **osteochondritis**, **periostitis**, **rhinorrhea/snuffles**, **hepatosplenomegaly**.

RPR can help you remember some of the findings in congenital syphilis:

Rash (interstitial keratitis, condyloma lata, maculopapular rash)

Periostitis/osteochondritis

Rhinorrhea

There is a classic triad associated with congenital syphilis called **Hutchinson triad**:

1) Interstitial keratitis

2) Notching of central incisors

3) Nerve deafness

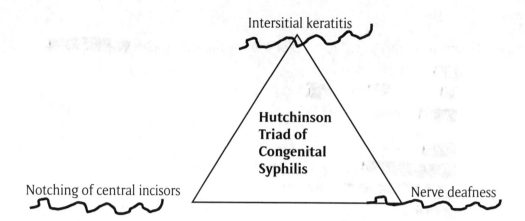

 Hutchinson triad also can be remembered as:

Dry dermis (interstitial keratitis)

Dentition problems (peg-shaped incisors)

Deafness

Sensitivities of VDRL vs. FTA-ABS:

	SENS	SPEC
VDRL	LO	HI
FTA-ABS	HI	LO

Borrelia Burgdorferi (Lyme Disease)

Borrelia burgdorferi, which is transmitted by deer ticks (Ixodes species), causes Lyme disease. **Lyme rhymes with nine and IX in Ixodes is = 9.**

Lyme Disease Stage I

Erythema chronicum migrans (ECM) is the characteristic rash. This is an erythematous area with a central clearing.

Headache, stiff neck, myalgias, fatigue can be seen.

Rule of 3's: Stage I may occur between 3 AND 33 days after tickbite

Lyme Disease Stage II

Systemic involvement occurs during Stage II.

Rule of 3's: Stage II may occur 3 weeks after tickbite

Lyme Disease Stage III

Chronic arthritis is part of Stage III.

Rule of 3's: Stage III may occur 3 months after tickbite

In addition, multiple neurological complications are seen. The most common neurologic finding in Lyme disease is **unilateral or bilateral facial nerve palsy**. It usually occurs within one month of the rash.

Tropheryma Whippelii (Whipple Disease)

Tropheryma whippelii is a gram-positive PAS-positive bacillus that causes Whipple disease.

Diagnosis is made by biopsy of duodenum via endoscopy, revealing presence of the organism as PAS-positive, non-acid-fast macrophage inclusions.

To remember the triad of Whipples disease, think of **My** **S**uper **D**uodenum.

Diagnostic **triad for Whipple disease**:
    1) Myoclonus
    2) Supranuclear gaze palsy
    3) Dementia

Oculomasticatory and skeletal myorhythmias are pathognomonic for Whipple disease.

Convergence-divergence nystagmus can also be seen.

Systemic symptoms of Whipple disease include **lymphadenopathy, steatorrhea**, and **weight loss**.

 Symptoms of Whipple's Disease *(triad first: My Super Duodenum)*
My Super Duodenum Smells Like We Can't Digest Nothing!

<u>Myoclonus-Supranuclear palsy-Dementia</u>, Steatorrhea, Lymphadeno, Weight loss, C/D-Nystagmus!

To remember that there's lots of **rhythm in this disease**, remember the song **"Whip it" by Devo**.

It may look like you are dancing and singing "Whip it" if you have Whipple's disease due to the oculomasticatory and skeletal myorhythmias.

Whipple Whipple Good

To remember the clinical findings in Whipple's disease I've reworded Devo's song "Whip it".

When you're running to the john	(diarrhea)
You have Whipple's	
When your poop comes out wrong	(steatorrhea)
You have Whipple's	
When your weight is all gone	(weight loss)
You have Whipple's	
(sing chorus here)	
When your eyes are moving wrong	(supranuclear gaze palsy and oculomasticatory myorhythmia)
You have Whipple's	
While your jaw goes up and down	
You have Whipple's	
Your memory goes away	(dementia)
Then you have Whipple's	

Fungus

The Fungus Among Us

Fungi are divided into the following categories:

1. **Yeasts**: *Blastomyces, Candida, Coccidioides, Cryptococcus, Histoplasma.*

 After eating yeasty bread, you'll say, "BLCCCH!"

2. **Branching hyphae**: *Aspergillus* (septate) and *Mucor* (non-septate).

 MA branches out to hyphae(have) friends;
*Also, there's an **S** in A**S**pergillus and **S**eptate and thus Mucor is non-septate.*

3. **Pseudohyphae**: *Candida.*

The book **Candide** by Voltaire is a satire about the **pseudo**-rationalist idea that optimism can overcome extremes of cruelty and evil..

Aspergillus

Aspergillus has branching, septate hyphae. *MA branches out to hyphae(have) friends.*

 Aspergillus may spread to the **CNS from the sinuses.**

Organ transplant patients are at risk for brain abscesses with this organism.

It is angioinvasive and can cause **hemorrhagic infarction**.

 Aspergillosis is **A**ngioinvasive. There's an S in a**S**pergillus and **S**eptate.

 Fungi **with hyphae**, such as *Aspergillus* and *Mucor*, **can obstruct arteries** and cause infarction.

Coccidioides

Coccidioides is ***a yeast ("BLCCCH!")*** found in the US in the Southwest, especially the San Joaquin Valley.

It forms large round spherules, which have a thick capsule.

Coccidioides forms capsulated circles.

Cryptococcus Neoformans

Cryptococcus neoformans is the **most common cause of fungal meningitis.**

It is **a yeast ("BLCCCH!")** that is found in immunocompetent and immunocompromised individuals.

It usually enters through the respiratory tract and is due to exposure to bird, especially pigeon, droppings.

Meningitis can be associated with hydrocephalus and increased intracranial pressure.

India ink stain and cryptococcal antigen testing can help with diagnosis.

Cryptococcus can cause cysts/ **"soap bubbles"** in the parenchyma.

Think of *Cryptococcus* as Cystococcus because it can cause cysts/ "soap bubbles" in your brain.

Histoplasma Capsulatum

Histoplasma capsulatum is **a yeast ("BLCCCH!")** found in the Ohio and Mississippi River valleys.

It causes **chronic meningitis** or **mass lesions**.

In meningitis, the basilar meninges are the most affected.

The yeast form is found in the cytoplasm of macrophages.

Histoplasma **h**ides in macrophages.

Histo is found in Ohio...and Mississippi River valleys.

Zygomycetes

Mucoraceae are in the *Zygomycetes* class and cause mucormycosis.
MA branches out to hyphae(have) friends.

Diabetic patients are at increased risk for infection with this fungus.

Spores are inhaled. Infection spreads from the nose and sinuses along blood vessels.

The rhino-orbital-cerebral form can cause **orbital cellulitis**, **cavernous sinus thrombosis**, **brain abscess**, and **hemorrhagic brain infarction**.

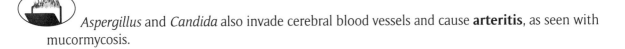

Aspergillus and *Candida* also invade cerebral blood vessels and cause **arteritis**, as seen with mucormycosis.

Black nasal discharge can be seen with mucormycosis. Histopathology shows non-septate, branching hyphae.

To remember that **sinusitis** is associated with Mucormycosis, think of Mucormycosis as **Mucusmycosis**.

Parasites

Naegleria Fowleri

Naegleria fowleri is an amoeba that causes hemorrhagic meningoencephalitis after swimming in a warm fresh water lake. CNS invasion occurs via nasal inoculation e.g. doing a cannonball.

Naegleria enters via the **Nares and lives in a Fresh Water Lake** *(FoWLeri).*

Taenia Solium

Taenia solium, which is a tapeworm found in pigs, causes cysticercosis, **the most common parasitic CNS infection**.

Think of this in someone with new onset seizures who was in Mexico.

Calcified cysts are seen on CT.

Cysticercosis is treated with albendazole or praziquantel.

To remember that cysticercosis is treated with praziquantel, I think of this as Sistercercosis. Sisters in the Catholic Church <u>bend</u> and *pray*, so sistercercosis is treated with al<u>bend</u>azole or *pray*ziquantel.

Plasmodium Falciparum

Cerebral malaria is due to *Plasmodium falciparum*.

To remember that cerebral malaria is due to *P. falciparum*, remember that there is a **falx in the head**.

Symptoms of <u>**Cerebral MALARIA**</u> include:

- **M**ental status changes and Seizures, progressing to Coma.
- **A**bnormal liver and spleen (Hepatosplenomegaly) due to destruction of RBCs ➔ iron and heme overloads organs
- **L**actic acid level elevated in the serum.
- **A**bnormal Extraocular movements,
- **R**etinal hemorrhages,
- **I**maging/CSF: Often MRI and lumbar puncture will be normal.
- **A**wful outcome: There is a 50% mortality with Cerebral malaria!

Toxoplasma

Toxoplasmosis is one of the TORCH infections, which include: **T**oxoplasmosis, **R**ubella, **C**ytomegalovirus, and **H**erpes simplex virus. Toxoplasma is an obligate intracellular protozoa, existing in either the bradyzooite stage (slow cyst) or the tachyzooite stage (free & fast).

Toxoplasmosis causes scattered calcifications in newborns (versus CMV, which causes periventricular calcifications). In adults, symptoms include headache, fever, and mental status change (like a subacute encephalitis picture).

Toxoplasmosis is in the differential diagnosis of a ring-enhancing mass in the brain, especially in AIDS patients. About 2/3 of toxo-infected patients will have multiple ring-enhancing lesions. The other major diagnosis on the differential is Primary CNS Lymphoma. While the workup is underway, remember to **"Treat for Toxo"** first, until biopsy, SPECT, or PET can determine otherwise. **Lumbar puncture may reveal elevated Lymphocytes and protein, IgG (not IgM). CSF PCR is 95% specific but only 50% sensitive for CNS toxoplasmosis.**

Toxoplasmosis is treated with 6 WEEKS OF <u>S&P</u>: <u>S</u>ulfadiazine and <u>P</u>yrimethamine (PLUS folate because pyriMethamine can Mess up the bone Marrow). In HIV patients, treatment persists until CD4>200.

Trichinella

Trichinella is the intestinal nematode that is found in undercooked pork and causes Trichinosis.

To remember that Trichinosis is due to undercooked pork, recall that Babe the pig knew tricks.

This is one situation where the saying **the way to a man's heart is through his stomach is true.**

A man eats undercooked pork and ends up with myocarditis and myositis.

To remember that Trichinosis comes from pigs and affects the heart: **Protecting one's heart is tricky** due to all the pigs out there.

Alternatively, recall that Hearts is a trick-taking card game.

The infection also spreads to other muscles causing **weakness** of extraocular, paraspinal, respiratory, and limb muscles.

It can spread to the brain and produce **eosinophilic meningitis, meningoencephalitis, stroke,** and **venous thrombosis.**

Patients have **elevated muscle enzymes** and **eosinophilia.**

To remember that trichinosis causes eosinophilia and eosinophilic meningitis, remember that it is associated with the heart, which is represented with a red ♥.

Viral

Cytomegalovirus (CMV)

CMV is another example of a TORCH infection.

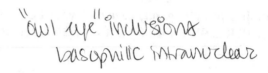

"owl eye" inclusions
basophilic intranuclear

Remember that the calcifications usually surround the ventricles in CMV, whereas Toxoplasmosis calcifications are widespread.

I remember CMV surrounds the ventricle by picturing a C around the lateral ventricles.

Alternatively, CM**V** is peri**v**entricular.

CMV can cause **Guillain-Barré Syndrome** or **aseptic meningitis** in **immunocompetent** **individuals**.

In **immunocompromised** hosts, CMV can also cause *retinitis, encephalitis, mononeuritis multiplex, lumbosacral polyradiculopathy,* or *myelitis.*

CMV retinitis is the most common cause of vision loss in AIDS patients.

CMV may cause you to not see if you have HIV.

CMV is often responsible for *subacute lumbosacral polyradiculomyelitis in HIV patients.*

Epstein-Barr Virus (EBV)

EBV causes **infectious mononucleosis,** which rarely can have neurological complications including *meningitis, encephalitis, transverse myelitis, Guillain-Barré Syndrome, cranial nerve palsies, optic neuritis,* and *cerebellitis.*

EBV is associated with *CNS lymphoma in immunocompromised individuals* such as *organ transplant patients* and patients with AIDS.

Herpes Simplex Virus (HSV)

HSV Encephalitis

HSV encephalitis has a predilection for the **L**imbic structures, **O**rbitofrontal cortex, and **T**emporal lobes. That's a **LOT** of areas.

The classic EEG finding in Herpes encephalitis is **periodic lateralized epileptiform discharges (PLEDs).** Sharp or sharp-and-slow wave complexes are seen every 1 to 3 seconds in the temporal regions. They may be seen bilaterally. If they are bilateral they may be independent or synchronous.

CSF findings in Herpes encephalitis: *elevated protein, increased RBCs (usually less than 500),* and *lymphocytic pleocytosis (although PMNs may predominate if CSF checked very early, like less than 48 hours).*

HSV 1 versus HSV 2

HSV 1 is the most common focal encephalitis in the US.
HSV 2 is the most common neonatal encephalitis.

HSV 2 is usually sexually transmitted or due to vertical transmission from a mother to a child.

To remember that HSV 2 is sexually transmitted, remember that <u>usually</u> 2 people are involved in sex.

Human Immunodeficiency Virus (HIV)

Central Nervous System Complications of HIV

Dementia

HIV-associated dementia is a subcortical dementia. Patients are forgetful and have psychomotor slowing, **slowed thinking, gait disturbances such as stumbling**, and **deterioration in fine motor skills.**

MRI shows *cortical atrophy* and *symmetric white matter signal abnormalities.*

Meningitis

The most common organisms that cause meningitis in HIV patients are:

· *Cryptococcus neoformans*
· *Treponema pallidum* syphilis
· TB.

Toxoplasma Encephalitis

Toxoplasma encephalitis causes brain abscess(es).

The most common cause of focal brain lesions with edema and enhancement in an HIV patient is *Toxoplasma*, which is treated with **S&P**: **S**ulfadiazine and **P**yrimethamine PLUS folate -- because pyri**M**ethamine can **M**ess up the bone **M**arrow.

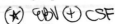

CNS Lymphoma

Toxoplasmosis causes **multiple lesions** -- 2/3 of the time!
CNS lymphoma tends to cause a **single lesion**.

(*) EBV (+) CSF

Progressive Multifocal Leukoencephalopathy (PML)

 The most common cause of brain lesions without mass effect is **progressive multifocal leukoencephalopathy (PML),** which is caused by JC virus. PML tends to cause multiple areas of subcortical demyelination that are asymmetrical.

Recall that HIV-associated dementia causes <u>symmetric</u> white matter abnormalities.

Vacuolar Myelopathy

 HIV can cause **vacuolar myelopathy**, which is the **most common cause of spinal cord dysfunction in AIDS patients**.

Peripheral Nervous System Complications of HIV

Distal Sensory Polyneuropathy

The most common neuropathy in AIDS is a **distal sensory polyneuropathy**, which is axonal.

Patients frequently complain about **pain involving the soles of the feet**.

AIDP/CIDP

Both Guillain-Barré Syndrome/ AIDP (Acute Inflammatory Demyelinating Polyradiculoneuropathy) and CIDP (Chronic Inflammatory Demyelinating Polyneuropathy) due to HIV are associated with CSF pleocytosis.

Cauda Equina Syndrome (Ascending Polyradiculopathy)

CMV can cause a cauda equina syndrome in patients with AIDS.

Mononeuritis Multiplex

CMV can also cause mononeuritis multiplex (frequently with **hoarseness due to laryngeal nerve involvement**) in AIDS patients.

Neurological Complications of AIDS Treatments

HAART (highly active antiretroviral therapy) reduces opportunistic CNS infections in HIV patients. However, some antiretrovirals have neurologic side effects.

Myopathy

AZT can cause a myopathy with ragged-red fibers due to mitochondrial toxicity.

Neuropathy

Nucleosides used to treat AIDS can cause a **peripheral neuropathy**: ddC (zalcitabine), ddI (dideoxyinosine), d4T (stavudine), and 3TC (lamivudine). Like HIV itself, they can cause a distal sensory neuropathy.

An elevated lactate and abrupt onset help to differentiate neuropathy due to nucleosides from HIV distal sensory polyneuropathy.

Human T-Cell Lymphotropic Virus Type 1

Human T-Cell Lymphotropic Virus Type 1 causes **T-cell leukemia or lymphoma** in adults and a **myelopathy (HTLV-1 associated myelopathy-tropical spastic paraparesis)**.

JC Virus

JC virus, which is a human polyomavirus, causes **progressive multifocal leukoencephalopathy (PML)**.

The **pathology of PML**:
- Oligodendrocytes have Intranuclear Inclusions.
- Astrocytes are bizarre.
- Asymmetric multifocal demyelination that begins in the Occipital lobes.

PML is seen in the late stages of AIDS and in other immunocompromised patients.

Hopefully one day, when **AIDS** **IS** **OVER**, then PML will be less prevalent too!

     A: **A**strocytes are bizarre & **A**symmetric multifocal demyelination starts as...

     I: **I**ntranuclear **I**nclusions initiate in...

     O: **O**ligodendrocytes with **O**ccipital lobes' demyelination.

Measles (Rubeola)

Measles is a paramyxovirus that can cause encephalitis or later result in subacute sclerosing panencephalitis. Most children get immunized against measles by age 18 months with the MMR vaccine (measles, mumps, and rubella), making it very rare in developed countries these days.

Subacute Sclerosing Panencephalitis (SSPE)

SSPE is a neurodegenerative condition secondary to chronic measles infection.

The age of onset is 5 to 15 years.

Children who contract measles at an early age are at higher risk.

\multicolumn{2}{Stages of SSPE}	
Stage	**Signs and symptoms**
I	Personality changes and grades fall
II	Myoclonic jerks and further intellectual deterioration
III	Stupor, extrapyramidal signs, autonomic instability, rigidity, hyperactive reflexes
IV	Chronic vegetative state

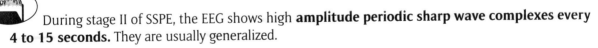 During stage II of SSPE, the EEG shows high **amplitude periodic sharp wave complexes every 4 to 15 seconds.** They are usually generalized.

 There are **elevated antibodies to rubeola** in the serum and CSF.

MRI shows subcortical white matter lesions, followed by periventricular lesions, and then cortical atrophy.

For SSPE, remember the **5-15 Rule: periodic sharp wave complexes are every ~5-15 sec, in kids age 5-15 yrs.**

Polio

Polio is a type of enterovirus that **infects anterior horn cells**.

Acute polio is associated with **Cowdry B inclusions**, whereas other viruses are usually associated with Cowdry type A inclusions.

Besides **P**olio, other viral infections which spread to the CNS from the peripheral nerves via retrograde axonal transport are: **Rabies, HSV,** and **VZV.** You can remember the 4 viruses that have retrograde transport by this mnemonic: **P**lease **R**everse **H**is **V**irus!

Rhabdovirus

Rabies is caused by a rhabdovirus that travels to the CNS by axonal transport along nerves. (**P**lease **R**everse **H**is **V**irus)

It is due to bite from an infected animal. Symptoms begin 3-8 weeks after the bite.

The clinical findings of rabies include **tingling at the site of the bite.** Patients foam at the mouth, are unable to swallow fluids due to **laryngeal spasm**, have **seizures**, and **exhibit unusual behavior – such as extreme hydrophobia (fear of water)**. Patients progress to coma and death.

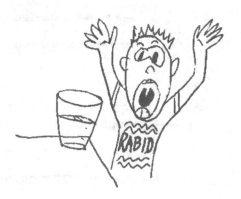

Pathologic findings of rabies: **Negri bodies** are seen in the cytoplasm of neurons, especially Purkinje cells, pyramidal cells (hippocampus), and brainstem nuclei.

Dumb rabies is a less common form of rabies. It causes a Guillain-Barré Syndrome picture.

Varicella-Zoster Virus (VZV)

VZV causes chickenpox, which may be followed by acute cerebellar ataxia.

 Other neurologic complications are meningitis, brainstem encephalitis, myelitis, and a granulomatous arteritis that can cause infarcts.

 Reye's syndrome has been associated with patients with VZV or influenza B who received aspirin.

Herpes Zoster (Shingles)

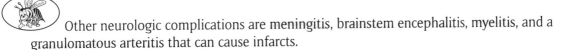 **Post-herpetic neuralgia** is the most common neurologic complication of Herpes zoster.

It is due to reactivation of virus that has been latent in the dorsal root ganglion.

Most often T5-T12 dermatomes are involved.

Ramsay Hunt Syndrome (Herpes Zoster Oticus)

Ramsay Hunt Syndrome (Herpes Zoster Oticus) is due to Herpes zoster infection of the **geniculate ganglion.**

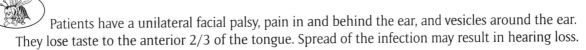 Patients have a unilateral facial palsy, pain in and behind the ear, and vesicles around the ear. They lose taste to the anterior 2/3 of the tongue. Spread of the infection may result in hearing loss.

 There is a second Ramsay Hunt syndrome, which is a type of **progressive myoclonic ataxia**.

West Nile Virus

West Nile Virus is an arbovirus that causes an influenza-like illness.

 This may be associated with a **maculopapular rash**, which starts on the trunk and may spread to the limbs and face.

West Nile Virus can cause multiple neurologic conditions including **meningitis, encephalitis, a Guillain-Barré** type picture, and a **polio-like syndrome** due to involvement of anterior horn cells. There is asymmetric muscle weakness, absent deep tendon reflexes, and often a tremor or myoclonus.

 West Nile Virus (**WNV**) causes encephalitis plus <u>**W**</u>**eakness,** <u>**N**</u>**o reflexes, and** <u>**V**</u>**ery bad tremors**.

Japanese encephalitis is the most common cause of arboviral encephalitis worldwide.

Prion Diseases

 A gene on chromosome 20 encodes human prion protein (PrP). PrP^c is normal.
In prion diseases, the metabolism of the prion protein PrP is abnormal.
PrP^{sc} is an abnormal form. Sc stands for scrapie.
In prion diseases, abnormal prion protein (PrP^{sc}) accumulates in neurons.
PrP^{sc} (β-pleated sheet) converts PrP^c (α helix) to PrP^{sc}.

 PrP^c is normal. (Think of c as standing for correct). Think of sc as standing for screwed up.
The beta-pleated sheet is a bad influence, which converts the correct form (PrP^c) to the screwed up form (PrP^{sc}).

Creutzfeldt-Jakob Disease

Pathologic Features of CJD:

· **Spongiform change**/ vacuolation of neuropil

· Loss of neurons

· Proliferation of astrocytes

· Loss of synapses on electron microscopy

· Deposition of prion protein

To remember that Creutzfeldt-Jakob disease is associated with spongiform change:

Creutzfeldt sounds like Seinfeld, which had an episode about sponges.

For CJD, there are **Four Forms -- all lead to the end (el Fin) -- so the mnemonic is FINS:**
- · **F**amilial
- · **I**atrogenic
- · **N**ew variant
- · **S**poradic

Sporadic CJD

Sporadic is the most common of all the FINS (85% of all cases of CJD).

Homozygosity for valine (**V**al) or methionine (**M**et) at codon 129 confers increased risk for sporadic CJD.

Sporadic CJD is Very Much common.

Clinical Findings in Sporadic CJD:

Dementia, myoclonic jerks, ataxia, and pyramidal and extrapyramidal signs.

EEG Findings in Sporadic CJD:

Generalized periodic sharp wave complexes that occur every 0.5- 1.6 seconds.[1]
These EEG findings are not seen with New variant CJD.

CSF Findings in Sporadic CJD: 14-3-3 protein.

This is a nonspecific finding, but in the right clinical scenario it helps with the diagnosis.
This protein is not seen with New variant CJD.

Iatrogenic CJD

Sources of infection have included human cadavaric growth hormone, human gonadotrophin, dura matter grafts, depth electrodes, neurosurgical instruments, and corneal transplants.

---

1 Markand ON, Brenner RP. Organic Brain Syndromes and Dementias. In: Ebersole JS, Pedley TA eds. Current Practice of Clinical Electroencephalography, 3rd edition. Philadelphia: Lippincott Williams & Wilkins, 2003;396.

Remember that if you think someone has CJD and he/she is undergoing surgery, special precautions must be taken.

Familial CJD

Familial CJD is autosomal dominant. It is due to a mutation in the prion protein gene. The clinical course is longer than in patients with sporadic CJD.

Familial CJD lasts **F**ar longer than the other FINS.
And because it's autosomal dominant, it dominates (and devastates) the family.

New Variant CJD

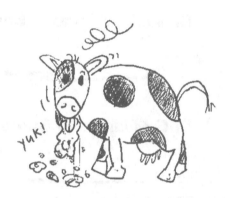

New Variant CJD is thought to be due to consumption of beef infected with the agent that causes bovine spongiform encephalopathy (mad cow disease). Patients usually are homozygous for methionine **(Met-Met)** at codon 129.

People with **New Variant Never Vary** from their meal: it's always **Meat, Meat (Met-Met)** until they eat a **bad cow**!

New Variant CJD versus Sporadic CJD:

The age of onset is younger and the clinical course is longer for patients with variant CJD.

Patients with variant CJD tend to present with psychiatric symptoms. Sensory symptoms such as pain and paresthesias are also seen early in the course of vCJD.

As mentioned above, 14-3-3 protein and generalized periodic sharp wave complexes are seen in sporadic CJD but not in variant CJD.

New variant CJD can be diagnosed with tonsil biopsy, which may show PrP^{sc}.

Florid plaques are seen in vCJD. A florid plaque consists of an amyloid plaque surrounded by vacuolation.

MRI shows **bilateral pulvinar hyperintensity in variant CJD**, whereas **basal ganglia hyperintensity is seen with sporadic CJD**.

To remember that variant CJD is associated with increased signal in the pulvinar thalamic nuclei: people who vary from the norm (variants) are often pulverized (pulvinar).

Other Prion Diseases

Kuru

Discovered in New Guinea. Due to cannibalism.

progressive cerebellar ataxia usu. absent dementia

Symptoms include a profound sense of euphoria and severe pains in the legs.

Gerstmann-Sträussler-Scheinker

Autosomal dominant.

PrP → leucine

The typical patient for the boards with GSS is 50 years old, with memory loss, euphoria, supranuclear gaze palsy, and cerebellar atrophy on MRI.

prion - amyloid plaques

Can you GueSS what happened to your super cerebellum?

Fatal Familial Insomnia

Autosomal dominant.

PrP → methionine

Patients also may present around age 50 years and symptoms last about 15 months before death occurs. Symptoms include **ataxia, dementia, dysautonomia**, and of course, severe **insomnia** refractory to treatment. MRI may reveal degeneration of **thalamic subnuclei** (specifically the **VA and MD**).

Families in **VA** and **MD can't sleep** with all the **demented** congressmen arguing nearby at the capitol!

anterior & dorsomedial

Recurrent Meningitis

Behçet Disease

 Behçet disease is a type of vasculitis that can be associated with recurrent meningoencephalitis.

It is characterized by **triad** of:

· Oral ulcers

· Genital ulcers

· Uveitis

Mollaret Meningitis

 Mollaret meningitis is recurrent aseptic meningitis associated with headache, neck stiffness, and low-grade fever. Patients are asymptomatic between attacks.

Mollaret's cells (large endothelial cells thought to be a type of monocyte) are found in the CSF.

Some cases are associated with HSV.

Neurosarcoidosis

Neurosarcoidosis is found in 5% of patients with systemic sarcoidosis.

Neurosarcoidosis can cause recurrent meningitis, but it is rare.

The most common neurological findings in neurosarcoidosis are cranial nerve palsies due to basal meningitis. Most often the facial nerve is involved, at times bilaterally.

> Recall that besides Sarcoid, TB and Histoplasma can all cause a basal meningitis and cranial nerve palsies.

CSF shows increased protein and a mild lymphocytic pleocytosis. There may be an elevation in **angiotensin-converting enzyme**.

Most patients with neurosarcoidosis have abnormal chest x-rays.

It can be diagnosed by lymph node, lung, or conjunctival biopsy.

Basal leptomeningitis or **granulomas** may be seen on MRI in patients with neurosarcoidosis.

 The MRI can resemble multiple sclerosis.

Vogt-Koyanagi-Harada (VHK) syndrome

Patients with Vogt-Koyanagi-Harada **(VHK)** syndrome have **recurrent meningitis, uveitis, depigmentation of the skin and hair, and hearing loss**.

VKH patients have **Very Krazy Hair, Very Krappy Hearing,** and **Very Kopied Headaches** (recurrent meningitis)!

The Most

Group B streptococcus is the most common cause of neonatal meningitis.

Neisseria meningitidis is the most common cause of bacterial meningitis in children.

Streptococcus meningitis is the most common cause of bacterial meningitis in adults.

The most common cause of meningitis in a patient with a CSF leak is *Streptococcus pneumoniae*.

Enteroviruses are the number one cause of aseptic meningitis.

HSV1 is the most common focal encephalitis in the US.

HSV2 is the most common neonatal encephalitis.

CMV is the most common nonheritable cause of hearing loss.

CMV retinitis is the most common cause of vision loss in AIDS patients.

Cysticercosis is the most common parasitic CNS infection.

Mycotic aneurysms are most commonly found in the distal branches of the middle cerebral artery.

The most common organism responsible found in a spinal epidural abscess is *Staphylococcus aureus*.

Japanese encephalitis is the most common cause of arboviral encephalitis worldwide.

Infectious Diseases Quiz

(Answers on page 737)

1. Which statement is false?

    A. Variant CJD is not associated with periodic sharp wave complexes.

    B. Variant CJD is not associated with 14-3-3 protein.

    C. Variant CJD is associated with signal change in the pulvinar.

    D. Florid plaques are seen in variant CJD.

    E. Initial symptoms in patients with variant CJD are psychiatric and sensory.

    F. Variant CJD has a younger age of onset than sporadic CJD.

    G. Variant CJD has a shorter clinical course than sporadic CJD.

2. Match the region to the fungus.

    1) Southwest US   A. Histoplasma

    2) Ohio and Mississippi River valleys   B. Coccidioides

3. Match the animal to the infection.

    1) Cow   A. Cryptococcosis

    2) Pig   B. New variant CJD

    3) Pigeon   C. Trichinosis

    4) Cat   D. *Bartonella henselae*

4. Which diseases are usually associated with meningitis at the base of the brain?

    A. Neurosarcoidosis

    B. Tuberculosis

    C. Mollaret meningitis

    D. A and B

    E. B and C

5. Diabetic patients are at increased risk for infection with which fungus?

    A. *Aspergillus*

    B. *Blastomyces*

    C. *Cryptococcus*

    D. *Histoplasma*

    E. *Mucoraceae*

6. Which has not been associated with a Guillain-Barré Syndrome-like picture?

    A. Botulism

    B. Diphtheria

    C. Rabies

    D. Tetanus

    E. West Nile Virus

7. Match the organism to its description.

    1) Causes hemorrhagic meningoencephalitis after swimming in a fresh water lake.

    2) Can cause supranuclear palsy, myoclonus, and dementia.

    3) Causes soap bubbles in the parenchyma.

    4) Prefers the peripheral nerves due to cooler temperatures there.

    5) Most common cause of neonatal bacterial meningitis.

    6) Most common cause of meningitis in children.

    7) Most common cause of meningitis in adults.

    A. *Cryptococus*

    B. Group B streptococcus

    C. *Mycobacterium leprae*

    D. *Naegleria fowleri*

    E. *Neisseria meningitidis*

    F. *Streptococcus pneumoniae*

    G. *Tropheryma whippelii*

Chapter 5

Metabolic Diseases

Categories of Metabolic Disease

Aminoacidopathies

Aminoacidopathies tend to present in infancy or times of illness with altered mental status, vomiting, and poor feeding. **The ammonia level is usually normal** except in urea cycle disorders (see separate section).

The aminoacidopathies include the disorders listed in the table below.

Aminoacidopathies
Hartnup disease
Homocystinuria
Maple syrup urine disease
Nonketotic hyperglycinemia
Phenylketonuria
Sulfite oxidase deficiency

Glycogen Storage Diseases (GSD)

The glycogen storage diseases are listed in the table below.

GSD Type	Enzyme Defect	Eponym
I	Glucose-6-phosphatase	Von Gierke
II	Acid maltase (1,4 glucosidase)	Pompe
III	Debranching	Cori-Forbes
IV	Transglucosidase	Andersen
V	Muscle phosphorylase	McArdle
VI	Liver phosphorylase	Hers

GSD Type	Enzyme Defect	Eponym
VII	Muscle phosphofructokinase	Tarui
VIII	Phosphorylase kinase	
IX	Phosphoglycerate kinase	
X	Phosphoglycerate mutase	
XI	Lactic dehydrogenase	

All of the glycogenoses are **autosomal recessive** except phosphoglycerate kinase deficiency (Type IX), which is X-linked recessive.

Most of the glycogen storage diseases, except Types I and VI, involve muscle.

Acid maltase deficiency is also a lysosomal storage disease.

Lysosomal Storage Diseases

LSD = MPS + NCL + SLD = **M**uco**P**oly**S**acchrid**oses** + **N**euronal **C**eroid **L**ipofuscin**oses** + **S**phingolipid**oses**

To remember the 3 groups of LSDs, think that **My Niece Sells LSD** – which we don't encourage!

Also, all 3 groups end in the suffix **'oses'** which makes it even easier to remember!

Mucopolysaccharidoses

See below.

Neuronal Ceroid Lipofuscinoses

See below.

Sphingolipidoses

Disease	Enzyme Defect
Fabry's disease	Alpha-galactosidase
Farber's disease	Ceramidase
Gaucher's disease	Beta-glucosidase (glucocerebrosidase)
Krabbe disease *(globoid cell)*	Galactosyl ceramide beta galactosidase *(galacto cerebrosidase)*
Metachromatic leukodystrophy	Arylsulfatase A
Niemann-Pick disease Types A and B	Sphingomyelinase
Sandhoff disease *(GM2)*	Hexosaminidase A and B deficiency
Tay-Sachs disease *(GM2)*	Hexosaminidase A deficiency

all As
cherry

cherry
cherry, HSM
cherry, ↓HSM

These are discussed individually below.   *Beta - galactosidase*   *cherry*
GM1 gangliosidosis

Mitochondrial Diseases

Mitochondrial diseases may be due to mutations in the mitochondrial genome or due to abnormalities of the mitochondria, such as respiratory chain enzyme abnormalities. The inheritance pattern depends on the genome and gene product affected. Lactate and pyruvate may be elevated.

Mitochondrial Diseases	Abbreviation
Chronic Progressive External Ophthalmoplegia	CPEO
Kearns-Sayre Syndrome	KSS
Leber's Hereditary Optic Neuropathy	LHON
Leigh's Syndrome	
Mitochondrial Encephalopathy, Lactic Acidosis, and Stroke	MELAS
Myoclonic Epilepsy and Ragged Red Fiber Disease	MERRF
Neuropathy, Ataxia, Retinitis Pigmentosa	NARP

These are described below.

Neurotransmitter-related Disorders

Neurotransmitter-related Disorders
Aromatic L-amino acid decarboxylase deficiency
Dopamine β-hydroxylase deficiency
GTP cyclohydrolase deficiency
Succinic semialdehyde dehydrogenase deficiency (Gamma-hydroxybutyric aciduria)
Tyrosine hydroxylase deficiency

Organic Acidemias

Patients with organic acidemias tend to present in infancy or times of stress with refusal to feed, emesis, hypoglycemia, acidosis, and hyperammonemia.

Some patients have neutropenia and/or thrombocytopenia.

Ketosis is found in some organic acidemias such as isovaleric acidemia, methylmalonic acidemia, multiple carboxylase deficiency, and propionic acidemia.

Organic Acid Disorders
Glutaric acidemia type I
Isovaleric acidemia
Methylmalonic acidemia
Multiple carboxylase deficiency (Biotinidase deficiency, Holocarboxylase synthase deficiency)
Propionic acidemia
Pyruvate dehydrogenase deficiency

(handwritten note bracketing Isovaleric through Propionic: "ketosis")

These diseases are discussed below. Pyruvate dehydrogenase deficiency is one of the causes of Leigh syndrome.

Peroxisomal Disorders

Peroxisomal disorders are divided into categories.

Peroxisomal Biogenesis Disorders

The first category is characterized by defective peroxisome assembly or biogenesis. This category includes **Zellweger syndrome, neonatal adrenoleukodystrophy,** and **infantile Refsum disease.** These are autosomal recessive.

Defects that Affect a Single Peroxisomal Enzyme

The second category is characterized by defects that affect a single peroxisomal enzyme. This includes **classic Refsum disease** and **X-linked adrenoleukodystrophy**.

Urea Cycle Disorders

The urea cycle converts ammonia to urea. Multiple enzymes are involved in this process.

 Patients with complete absence of any of these enzymes present in the **neonatal period** with **coma** and **hyperammonemia**. They may have a **respiratory alkalosis due to tachypnea.**

They have a **normal glucose** and are **not acidotic.**

Patients with **partial deficiency** of these enzymes, including **female heterozygotes** with OTC deficiency, present at times of illness/stress with **hyperammonemia**. Urea cycle defects can present for the first time in adulthood with stressor events.

Urea Cycle Defects
Carbamyl phosphate synthetase I (CPS I) deficiency
Ornithine transcarbamylase (OTC) deficiency
Citrullinemia (Arginosuccinic acid synthetase [ASS] deficiency)
Arginosuccinicaciduria (Arginosuccinate lyase [ASL] deficiency)
Arginemia (Arginase deficiency)

OTC deficiency is the most common urea cycle defect.

Inheritance of OTC deficiency is X-linked; the other urea cycle disorders are inherited in an autosomal recessive manner.

The Urea Cycle

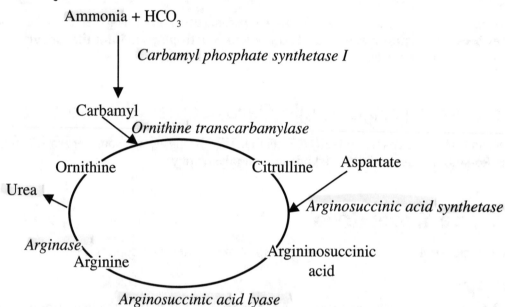

Ammonia + HCO_3

Carbamyl phosphate synthetase I

Carbamyl

Ornithine transcarbamylase

Ornithine   Citrulline   Aspartate

Urea

Arginosuccinic acid synthetase

Arginase

Arginine   Argininosuccinic acid

Arginosuccinic acid lyase

To remember the **enzyme order** in the **Urea Cycle: Ammonia Came (CPS-I) Over The Counter (OTC) synthesized (Arginosuccinic acid Synthetase), And SLid** (Argino-Succinic-Lyase) **Away as** (Arginase) **Urea** (Urea).

Specific Metabolic Diseases

(In alphabetical order)

Abetalipoproteinemia/Bassen-Kornzweig Syndrome

Abetalipoproteinemia is an autosomal recessive disorder due to mutations in the gene that encodes for **microsomal triglyceride transfer protein (MTP)** on chromosome 4. Deficiency of MTP results in near absence of apo-B-containing lipoproteins in the plasma.

Abetalipoproteinemia primarily affects the posterior columns and spinocerebellar tracts.

Patients with abetalipoproteinemia have **ataxia, neuropathy, steatorrhea, retinitis pigmentosa,** and **acanthocytosis**.

Loss of fat-soluble vitamins (A,D,E,K) in the stool causes deficiencies of these vitamins.

Vitamin E deficiency results in neurologic symptoms such as areflexia, a sensory neuropathy affecting large fiber modalities (vibration and proprioception), and sensory ataxia.

Acanthocytosis is seen on peripheral smear.

Total cholesterol and triglyceride levels are very low, and chylomicrons, VLDL, LDL, and apoB are absent in the plasma.

Abetalipoproteinemia is associated with lots of **A**s: **A**canthocytosis, **A**taxia, **A**reflexia, and loss of vitamin **A** (and vitamins D, E, and K).

To remember some of the characteristics of abetalipoproteinemia/ Bassen-Kornzweig disease use BASSEN-K:

> **B** apolipoprotein (apolipoprotein B) is deficient
>
> **A**canthocytosis, **A**taxia, **A**reflexia, vitamin **A** deficiency
>
> **S**teatorrhea
>
> **S**ensory loss (vibratory and proprioception), **S**pinocerebellar degeneration
>
> **E**ye findings: pigmentary retinopathy, vitamin **E** deficiency
>
> **N**europathy
>
> K vitamin **K** deficiency

Abeta sounds like **"I better"** . When you see abeta, think *I better* **head to the bathroom due to diarrhea/steatorrhea.** If you can't get to a bathroom, **you'd better look for a basin (Bassen)** or hope there's a **field of corn (Kornzweig).**

As mentioned above, abetalipoproteinemia is due to a deficiency in microsomal triglyceride transfer protein.

MTP transfers lipids to nascent apolipoprotein-B-containing lipoproteins. Deficiency of MTP interferes with assembly of apo-B-containing lipoproteins such as low-density lipoproteins and chylomicrons.

MTP could stand for **More TP (More Toilet Paper),** which patients with abetalipoproteinemia/ Bassen-Kornzweig need due to steatorrhea.

Acid Maltase Deficiency

Acid maltase deficiency is also known as Pompe's disease and Glycogen Storage Disease Type II. It is autosomal recessive.

Infantile-Type Acid Maltase Deficiency

Infantile-onset acid maltase deficiency/ **Pompe's disease** presents with **neonatal hypotonia.** The patients also have **macroglossia, cardiomegaly**, and **hepatomegaly**.

They tend to die by age 2 years from **cardiorespiratory failure** or **aspiration pneumonia** without treatment.

Membrane-bound vacuoles, which are **PAS (periodic acid-Schiff)-positive**, are found in muscle, liver, and Schwann cells.

Patients with infantile-onset glycogen storage **disease type II (2),** usually **die by age 2 years** without treatment.

Think of this as **Pump's disease** because they have a **defective heart, which is a pump.**

Or think of this as **Plump's disease**. They have a **plump heart, liver, and tongue.**

Enzyme replacement therapy is now available.

Adult-Type Acid Maltase Deficiency

Adults with acid maltase deficiency usually present in their 20s or 30s.

In **younger adults**, acid maltase deficiency may present with **fatigue**.

In **older adults**, it may present with leg and trunk weakness.

Some patients present with **respiratory failure** or develop it later.

Adults with acid maltase deficiency have an **increased CK** and **myotonia** on EMG particularly in the **paraspinal** muscles.

They may have **intracranial aneurysms** due to glycogen deposition.

A **vacuolar myopathy** is seen on muscle biopsy. Due to glycogen storage, **lysosomes stain with PAS**.

Acid **M**altase deficiency in adults is associated with **A**neurysms and **M**yopathy (vacuolar), and **A**symptomatic **M**yotonia (in the paraspinal muscles on EMG). Folks with **AM** say, "I **AM** what I **AM**."

Acute Intermittent Porphyria (AIP)

Acute intermittent porphyria is due to a defect in heme biosynthesis. Specifically, **porphobilinogen deaminase** is deficient. This results in increased production of porphobilinogen and δ-aminolevulinic acid.

Heme Synthesis:

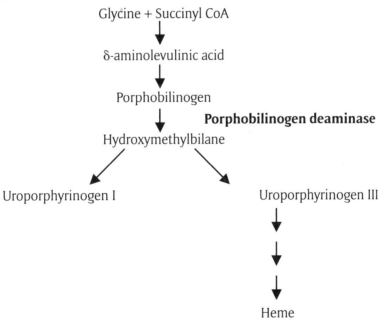

Glycine + Succinyl CoA

↓

δ-aminolevulinic acid

↓

Porphobilinogen

↓ **Porphobilinogen deaminase**

Hydroxymethylbilane

↙   ↘

Uroporphyrinogen I   Uroporphyrinogen III

↓

↓

↓

Heme

AIP is autosomal dominant, and the gene is on 11q.

The onset of AIP is usually in adolescence and early adulthood.

Attacks are periodic and may be triggered by certain medications, fasting, infection, or hormonal changes such as pregnancy.

Patients with AIP have **severe abdominal pain** during attacks. They may have **fever, tachycardia**, and **hypertension**.

Weakness occurs due to a **motor neuropathy**. It may progress to **quadriparesis** and **respiratory failure, resembling Guillain-Barré syndrome. Reflexes are decreased**.

In addition to peripheral nervous system abnormalities, central nervous system abnormalities are seen such as **confusion, delirium, psychosis**, or **seizures**.

Laboratory findings include *elevated δ-aminolevulinic acid, porphobilinogen*, and *several porphyrins in urine*.

Barbiturates, carbamazepine, clonazepam, phenytoin, and valproate should be avoided in patients with acute intermittent porphyria.

Attacks are treated with intravenous dextrose and propranolol (for tachycardia and hypertension). Hematin has also been used to treat attacks.

Variegate Porphyria is clinically similar except these patients can have a rash.

Aromatic L-Amino Acid Decarboxylase Deficiency (AADC Deficiency)

AADC deficiency is a autosomal recessive disorder of neurotransmitter metabolism.

Recall that AADC is important in the synthesis of dopamine and serotonin:

$$Dopa \xrightarrow{AADC} dopamine$$

$$\text{5-HTP (5-hydroxytryptophan)} \xrightarrow{AADC} \text{5-HT (serotonin)}$$

AADC deficiency presents in the **first few months of life**.

Patients have **dystonia, athetosis, tongue thrusting, torticollis, oculogyric crises, ptosis**, and *autonomic dysfunction* such as **apnea, hypothermia**, and **sweating**.

Gross motor milestones and expressive speech are delayed.

Later, ataxia is seen.

Autonomic symptoms

Athetosis, **A**taxia

Dystonia

C (see): ptosis, oculogyric crisis

Aromatic L-Amino Acid Decarboxylase Deficiency is diagnosed by sending CSF for neurotransmitters.

Adrenoleukodystrophy (ALD)

Neonatal Adrenoleukodystrophy

Like Zellweger syndrome, infantile Refsum disease, and rhizomelic chondrodysplasia punctata, neonatal adrenoleukodystrophy is due a disorder of peroxisomal biogenesis, and multiple peroxisomal enzymes are deficient. There is clinical overlap with Zellweger syndrome; however, neonatal adrenoleukodystrophy is less severe.

Neonatal adrenoleukodystrophy is an **autosomal recessive condition** that presents in the first few months of life.

Patients are **dysmorphic, weak,** and **hypotonic**. They **feed poorly**. They have **seizures, hepatomegaly, retinal degeneration,** and a **hearing deficit**.

Laboratory findings are similar to Zellweger syndrome: *phytanic acid, pipecolic acid,* and *very long chain fatty acids (VLCFA)* are elevated. Urinary pipecolic acid is also elevated.

To remember which diseases elevate VLCFA's, think of **RAZ** (**R**efsum disease, **R**hizomelic chondrodysplasia punctata, A**L**D, and **Z**ellweger syndrome), the weak, sickly dog on a **Very Long Chain Far Away**.

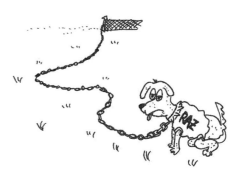

Adrenoleukodystrophy (Sudanophilic Cerebral Sclerosis)

Adrenoleukodystrophy is a neurodegenerative, demyelinating disease.

 Unlike the neonatal form, this is **X-linked recessive**.

It is due to mutations in the *ABCD1* gene on Xq28. This gene encodes an **ATP-binding cassette protein**.

There are multiple phenotypes:

- Cerebral form (child, adolescent, and adult onset)
- Adrenomyeloneuropathy
- Addison's disease
- Asymptomatic.

Childhood Cerebral Form

The childhood cerebral form of adrenoleukodystrophy is the most common form of X-linked adrenoleukodystrophy.

 This presents at **4-8 years of age** with **behavior problems and difficulties in school**. At first, the patient may appear to have ADHD. However, **speech and handwriting deteriorate**. **Problems with spatial orientation and auditory discrimination** develop. **Seizures** may be seen.

Then patients develop **spastic quadriparesis**, **difficulty swallowing**, and **vision loss**.

The **skin may appear bronze** due to adrenal involvement.

MRI first shows **demyelination in the occipital region**. As the disease progresses, demyelination spreads frontally.

CSF protein may be increased. Patients may have some white cells in the CSF.

Very long chain fatty acids are increased in the blood.

Brain and adrenal macrophages show **lamellar cytoplasmic inclusions**, which consist of very long chain fatty acid esters.

This has been treated with **bone marrow transplant** (before neurologic involvement).

Adolescent Cerebral Form

 The adolescent cerebral form is similar; however, it presents between ages 10 and 21 years.

Adult Cerebral Form

The adult form presents after age 21 years.

Patients may appear to have schizophrenia. Dementia and spasticity are seen.

Adrenomyeloneuropathy (AMN)

 Adrenomyeloneuropathy presents in the **third decade**.

Patients have progressive **spastic paraparesis, decreased vibration in the lower extremities, bowel or bladder problems, sexual dysfunction**, and sometimes **abnormal adrenocortical function**.

Alexander Disease

Alexander disease is an **autosomal dominant** hypomyelinating leukoencephalopathy due to a mutation in the gene that encodes **glial fibrillary acid protein (GFAP)**.

 The infantile form can present in the **first weeks of life**.

Patients have **megalencephaly, seizures,** and **progressive spastic quadriparesis**. Death is in childhood.

To remember that patients with **Alexander disease** have **megalencephaly** and **seizures**, recall that Alexander the Great had a **big head/ large ego** and **seized lots of land**.

MRI in Alexander disease shows **demyelination**, particularly over the **frontal regions**.

Jason Alexander from Seinfeld has **frontal balding**, and patients with Alexander disease have **frontal demyelination**.

Alex, Can-U remember the 2 diseases that pathologically involve U-fibers? (**Alex**ander's and **Can**avan's).

Rosenthal fibers are found in astrocytes in patients with Alexander disease.

 Rosenthal fibers are also characteristic of juvenile pilocytic astrocytoma.

Ataxia with Isolated Vitamin E Deficiency (AVED)

Ataxia with isolated vitamin E deficiency, which is autosomal recessive, is also known as **Friedreich-like ataxia** because the phenotype is similar to Friedreich's ataxia. It is due to a mutation in the gene that encodes **alpha-tocopherol transfer protein (ATTP)** on chromosome 8q.

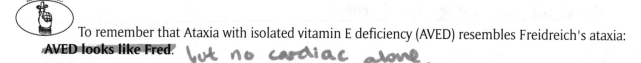 To remember that Ataxia with isolated vitamin E deficiency (AVED) resembles Freidreich's ataxia: **AVED looks like Fred**. *but no cardiac alone.*

 Symptoms usually begin in puberty. Patients have a **progressive ataxia, loss of proprioception, areflexia**, and **upgoing toes**.

Some patients have **titubation, deafness, tendon xanthomas**, or **retinitis pigmentosa**.

 AVED can be used to remember the characteristics of this disease:

>   Ataxia, Areflexia
>   Vitamin E deficiency
>   Eye findings (retinitis pigmentosa)
>   Deafness

Vitamin E prevents progression and **may reverse some deficits**.

Bassen-Kornzweig Syndrome

See Abetalipoproteinemia above.

Biotinidase Deficiency

See multiple carboxylase deficiencies below.

Canavan Disease

Canavan disease is an autosomal recessive disorder characterized by **spongy degeneration of the cerebral white matter.** It is due to deficiency of **aspartoacylase,** which hydrolyzes N-acetyl-L-aspartic acid (NAA) to aspartic acid and acetic acid.

 Symptoms start around 2 months including **hypotonia and regression. Seizures, optic atrophy**, and **macrocephaly** are then seen. **Tone gradually increases**, and late in the course, **spasticity, opisthotonus**, and **posturing** can be seen.

N-acetylaspartic acid is increased in the plasma and urine.

MR spectroscopy shows an **elevated NAA** to creatine and choline ratio.

MRI shows **diffuse degeneration of the white matter**. On T2-weighted images, there is **increased signal in the white matter.**

To remember that <u>Canavan</u> disease is due to *aspart*oacylase deficiency: **Living in a <u>caravan</u> can be *a Spart*an lifestyle.**

Alex, Can-U remember the 2 diseases that pathologically involve U-fibers? (**Alex**ander's and **Can**avan's).

Think of Canavan disease as Ca<u>NAA</u>van disease because NAA is increased.

Patients with Canavan disease have **macrocephaly, but MRI shows loss of white matter** and **pathology shows cystic/spongy degeneration**.

Carbohydrate-Deficient Glycoprotein Syndromes

These are also known as congenital disorders of glycosylation (CDG).

They are characterized by abnormal glycosylation of N-linked oligosaccharides and are diagnosed by **isoelectric focusing** of serum transferrin isoforms.

Consider this diagnosis in patients with seizures or developmental delay who have coagulopathy or GI symptoms.

CDG-la

CDG-Ia is the most common CDG.

It is due to a defect in the gene *PMM2*, which encodes phosphomannomutase (PMM).

Characteristic features **are inverted nipples** and **an abnormal fat distribution** (over the buttocks and suprapubic region). These are found in infancy.

Infants with CDG-Ia may have pure neurologic symptoms or neurologic and systemic systems.

As far as *neurologic symptoms*, **strabismus, developmental delay**, and **cerebellar hypoplasia** may be seen.

Systemic manifestations include **coagulopathy, liver failure, pericardial effusion, nephrotic syndrome**, and **renal cysts**.

Children may have **seizures or stroke-like episodes**, particularly associated with infection. *Later*, **cerebellar ataxia** and **progressive vision loss** occurs.

Adults have **mental retardation** and **hypogonadism**. **Skeletal deformities** may be present.

If you see fat above the bum, think of CDG #1. Phosphomannomutase! That's a weird place to get fat!

ATKINS can be used to remember some of the findings in CDG-Ia:

    Ataxia, **A**bnormal fat distribution

    Transferrin is deficient of carbohydrate, **T**one is low (hypotonia)

    Koagulopathy

    Inverted

    Nipples

    Seizures, **S**troke-like episodes

Cerebral Folate Deficiency

 Cerebral folate deficiency presents around **4 months of age** with **irritability** and **sleep disturbances**.[1]

Then **psychomotor retardation** is seen with **cerebellar ataxia, dyskinesia, spastic paraplegia,** and sometimes **seizures. Head growth slows**.

Around **age 3 years, vision disturbances** occur.

Hearing loss develops around **age 6 years**.

CSF shows a **low concentration of 5-methyltetrahydrofolate**.

 Cerebral folate deficiency is **treated** with **folinic acid (leucovorin).**

Many of the patients have **autoantibodies to the folate receptors found on the choroid plexus**[2].

Cerebral folate deficiency may also result from mutations in the folate receptor 1 (FOLR1) gene.[3]

Cerebrotendinous Xanthomatosis

Cerebrotendinous xanthomatosis is an autosomal recessive disease of lipid metabolism. It is due to a mutation in the **sterol 27-hydroxylase gene**, on chromosome 2, which results in absence of the bile acid chenodeoxycholic acid. This leads to **increased cholestanol in the plasma and tissues**, including the central nervous system.

Patients with **cerebrotendinous xanthomatosis** have **cataracts, xanthomas, ataxia,** and **dementia**.

Cerebrotendinous xanthomatosis presents with **diffuse white matter abnormalities**, including the white matter of the cerebellum. In fact, *CT* demonstrates **hyperdense nodules in the cerebellum**.

Cerebrotendinous xanthomatosis is treated with chenodeoxycholic acid.

1 Ramaekers VT, Blau N. Cerebral folate deficiency. Dev Med Child Neurol 2004; 46:843-851.

2 Ramaekers VT, Rothenberg SP, Sequeira JN, et al. Autoantibodies to folate receptors in the cerebral folate deficiency syndrome. N Engl J Med 2005; 352:1985-1991.

3 Hyland K, Shoffner J, Heales SJ. Cerebral folate deficiency. J Inherit Metab Dis 2010;33:563-570.

To remember that cerebrotendinous xanthomatosis is associated with **white** matter abnormalities, due to a mutation on chromosome **2** and is treated with **chenodeoxycholic acid**, picture **2** big globs of **white** lipid on former Vice-President Dick **Cheney**'s face.

Chronic Progressive External Ophthalmoplegia (CPEO)

CPEO is a mitochondrial disease that begins after age 20. It is characterized by progressive bilateral ptosis and loss of eye movements.

Patients with CPEO have ragged red fibers.

Creatine Deficiency

Creatine deficiency may be due to arginine-glycine aminotransferase (AGAT) deficiency, guanidinoacetate methyl transferase (GAMT) deficiency, or a mutation in the creatine transporter gene.

- Arginine-glycine aminotransferase (AGAT) deficiency
- Guanidinoacetate methyl transferase (GAMT) deficiency } Automosal recessive
- Mutation in the creatine transporter gene--------------------------------- X linked recessive

Creatine deficiency causes **mental retardation**, **epilepsy**, **movement disorders**, and **autistic behavior**.[4]

Patients have an increased urine creatine/creatinine ratio. Also, *MR spectroscopy* shows low creatine levels. The two *autosomal recessive forms* can be treated with creatine supplementation.

To remember the two enzymes associated with treatable **Creat def**iciency, remember that **A'GAT GAM**e **T**ickets to watch the **Creat**ures **def**eated.

---

[4] Lion-François L, Cheillan D, Pitelet G, et al. High frequency of creatine deficiency syndromes in patients with unexplained mental retardation. Neurology 2006;67:1713-1714.

Dopamine β-Hydroxylase Deficiency

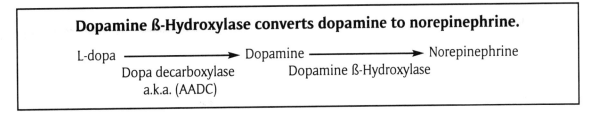

Dopamine ß-Hydroxylase converts dopamine to norepinephrine.

L-dopa ————————→ Dopamine ————————→ Norepinephrine
      Dopa decarboxylase   Dopamine ß-Hydroxylase
      a.k.a. (AADC)

The gene for dopamine ß-Hydroxylase deficiency has been mapped to chromosome 9q. It is an autosomal recessive condition.

In **neonates**, dopamine ß-Hydroxylase deficiency causes episodes of **hypothermia, hypoglycemia**, and **hypotension**, which may be lethal.

Neonates with dopamine ß-**Hy**droxylase deficiency have **hy**pothermia, **hy**poglycemia, and **hy**potensive episodes.

Dopamine ß-Hydroxylase deficiency is **treated with L-Dops (DL-threo-dihydroxyphenylserine)**, which is decarboxylated by dopa decarboxylase (also known as AADC) to norepinephrine

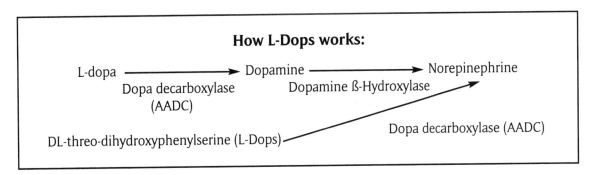

How L-Dops works:

L-dopa ————————→ Dopamine ————————→ Norepinephrine
     Dopa decarboxylase   Dopamine ß-Hydroxylase
     (AADC)

DL-threo-dihydroxyphenylserine (L-Dops)   Dopa decarboxylase (AADC)

Fabry's Disease
(Angiokeratoma Corporis Diffusum)

Fabry's disease is an **X-linked recessive** sphingolipidosis due to **alpha-galactosidase A deficiency**. This results in accumulation of glycosphingolipids such as globotriaosylceramide.

"Rash" is often the first manifestation. **Angiokeratomas**, which are dark red/purple papules, appear in the groin area and around the umbilicus.

Corneal deposits also are seen.

Patients with Fabry's disease have **autonomic dysfunction**. They have hypohidrosis, decreased tear and saliva production, impotence, and gastrointestinal dysmotility. Other GI complications include abdominal pain and episodes of diarrhea.

Patients also have a small fiber neuropathy that results in lancinating pains in the distal extremities called **acroparesthesias**. *Fever, hot weather, and exercise worsen this pain.* **Hand and foot edema** can be seen.

Cardiac complications include **arrhythmia, hypertrophic cardiomyopathy**, and **heart failure**.

Cerebrovascular complications include hemorrhage and thrombosis.

Renal failure is the most common cause of morbidity.

Enzyme replacement is available.

Fabry's disease is associated with **All A's: A**lpha-galactosidase A, **A**croparesthesias, **A**utonomic dysfunction, **A**ngiokeratomas, **A**nhidrosis, **A**rrhythmia, **A**cute renal failure, and **A**bdominal pain.

Farber's Disease

Farber's disease, which is also known as **lipogranulomatosis**, is an autosomal recessive degenerative disease that affects gray matter and is accompanied by visceral storage of the lipid ceramide.

It is due to **ceramidase deficiency**, which causes accumulation of ceramide in tissue, particularly the joints.

Farber's disease presents in the first few weeks to months of life. The characteristic features are worsening **hoarseness, subcutaneous nodules, macular cherry-red spots,** and **progressive arthropathy**.

Neurological findings include **hypotonia, weakness**, and **developmental delay**.

To remember a few details of Farber's disease think of this mnemonic: **Farber and Arthur both like grey ceramic horses!** (arthropathy, grey matter, ceramide, and hoarseness = Farber's disease)

Patients with Farber's disease develop difficulty swallowing and aspirate. They also develop respiratory insufficiency. They tend to die in the first 2 years of life.

Cerise means **cherry in French**, and **ce**ramidase deficiency causes a **cherry-red spot**.

The diseases with a cherry-red spot: Farber Salivates Getting **cherry-picked**, half-off Sales at Sacks Fifth Ave & Nieman Marcus! **(Farber's disease, Sialidosis, GM1-Gangliosidosis, Sandhoff's, Tay-Sachs, and Niemann-Pick type A)**.

Galactosemia

Galactosemia is a disorder of carbohydrate metabolism.

Multiple enzyme deficiencies in galactose metabolism can cause galactosemia in newborns. All are autosomal recessively inherited.

The most severe cause of galactosemia is complete deficiency of galactose-1-phosphate uridyltransferase, which can be associated with mental retardation if untreated. This is also called classical galactosemia.

Symptoms of classical galactosemia **present in the newborn period after feeding**. Patients have **vomiting, diarrhea, jaundice, and hepatomegaly**.

Patients with this type of galactosemia are **hypotonic** and **lethargic** and may have **cerebral edema**.

Cataracts develop by 1-2 months of age.

Escherichia coli **sepsis is common in classical galactosemia**.

Gamma-Hydroxybutyric Aciduria

See Succinic semialdehyde dehydrogenase deficiency below.

Gaucher's Disease

Gaucher's disease is a lipid storage disorder due to a defect in **glucocerebrosidase**.

To remember that Gaucher's disease is due to a defect in glucocerebrosidase: It may be gauche (Gaucher) but I always have sugar (glucose) on my mind (cerebrum).

All forms are associated with **Gaucher cells**, which are histiocytes containing lipid. (They are PAS+). They can be found in spleen, liver, lymph nodes, and bone marrow.

Type 1

Type 1 is **nonneuropathic**. It is **the most common form**.

Type 2

Type 2 is the acute neuropathic form.

It presents before one year of life with visceral organomegaly and developmental delay.

It is associated with **trismus, strabismus, opisthotonus, and spasticity**.

Laryngeal stridor and **aspiration pneumonia** are seen.

Death usually occurs by age 2 years.

Type 3

Type 3 is the **chronic neuropathic form**.

It presents in the first decade and is characterized by **cognitive deterioration**, **seizures**, **rigidity**, and **ataxia**. **Horizontal supranuclear gaze palsy** is a manifestation of the disease.

Patients have **hepatosplenomegaly**. **Interstitial lung disease** may be present.

 Enzyme replacement is used for types 1 and 3.

Glucose Transporter Defect

Glucose Transporter Type 1 (GLUT1) Deficiency (De Vivo disease)

Glucose transporter type 1 deficiency is due to a mutation in the *SLC2A1* gene, which encodes the protein GLUT1, a glucose transporter. It is also called De Vivo disease.

Patients with glucose transporter type 1 deficiency develop **seizures between one and 4 months of age** that are difficult to control.

They may have **apnea and eye movements resembling opsoclonus**.

Also, they have **delayed milestones** and develop **microcephaly**, **spasticity**, and **ataxia**.

Glucose transporter type 1 deficiency is diagnosed by lumbar puncture. Patients have a **low CSF glucose (< 40), a low ratio of CSF glucose to blood glucose (about 1/3), and a normal CSF lactate.**

low CSF glucose

Sarcoid Cancu/CMV AIDS TB

 Glucose transporter type 1 deficiency is treated with the **ketogenic diet**.

To remember GLUT1 deficiency: De Vivo, low-low gluco, opso, micro, treat with keto!

GLUT1 deficiency due to mutations in SLC2A1 is also associated with early-onset absence epilepsy.[5]

---

[5] Suls A, Mullen SA, Weber YG, et al. Early-onset absence epilepsy caused by mutations in the glucose transporter GLUT1. Ann Neurol 2009;66:415-419.

Glutaric Acidemia

Glutaric Acidemia Type I

Glutaric acidemia type 1 is an autosomal recessive organic acidemia due to deficiency of glutaryl-coenzyme A dehydrogenase.

Glutaric acidemia type 1 causes an extrapyramidal syndrome in infancy. Patients with glutaric acidemia type 1 have **dystonia, dyskinesias,** and **developmental delay**. They may also have **hypotonia** or **opisthotonus**.

Macrocephaly may be present at birth or develop in early infancy.

At the time of infection, the patient may decompensate and develop encephalopathy, seizures, vomiting, acidosis, hyperammonemia, and ketotic hypoglycemia.

Retinal hemorrhages and **subdural effusions** can be seen in glutaric acidemia type 1, resulting in **confusion with child abuse.** Menkes' kinky hair disease is another metabolic condition confused with abuse.

MRI shows **frontotemporal atrophy** with prominent Sylvian fissures. This results in a **bat wing** appearance.

Infants with **glu**taric acidemia type 1 may wish that they could be **glu**ed to the crib due to dystonia, dyskinesias, and opisthotonus, which must make them batty.

Glutaric Acidemia Type II

Glutaric acidemia type II is also known as **multiple acyl-CoA dehydrogenase deficiency**.

Glutaric acidemia type II is a disorder of fatty acid oxidation. It is due to deficiency of **electron transport flavoprotein (ETF)** or **ETF-ubiquinone oxidoreductase**.

Neonatal Forms

There are 2 neonatal forms. Only one will be discussed.

One neonatal form of glutaric acidemia type II presents with hypotonia and metabolic abnormalities. They have **hypoglycemia and metabolic acidosis.** They do not have ketosis. They have a **sweaty**

socks/sweaty feet odor (similar to patients with isovaleric acidemia due to deficiency of isovaleryl dehydrogenase).

This form is fatal in the first month of life.

 To remember that glutaric acidemia type **II** (rather than type I) is associated with a sweaty odor, think of **2** sweaty feet.

Ethylmalonic-adipicaciduria

There is also a form of glutaric acidemia type II (ethylmalonic-adipicaciduria) that presents later in life similar to **Reye syndrome**. The infant or child presents with intermittent encephalopathy, hepatomegaly, hypoglycemia, and metabolic acidosis.

Ethylmalonic-adipicaciduria may respond to **riboflavin (Vitamin B2)**.

To remember Ethylmalonic-adipicaciduria, think of the chocolate maker Ethyl-M's (yummy!) **Buying 2 (vitamin B2) much chocolate at Ethyl-M's (Ethyl**malonic-adipicaciduria), **will burst your liver (hepatomegaly)!**

GTP Cyclohydrolase Deficiency

GTP cyclohydrolase deficiency is the most common cause of Dopa-Responsive Dystonia (DRD). The gene for GTP cyclohydrolase is located on chromosome 14q. **It is Autosomal Dominant.**

Recall that **GTP cyclohydrolase catalyzes the rate-limiting step in tetrahydrobiopterin (BH$_4$) synthesis.**

HARP Syndrome

HARP syndrome has its own mnemonic! **HARP** stands for: **Hypobetalipoproteinemia, Acanthocytosis, Retinitis pigmentosa,** and **Pallidal degeneration.**

Some patients with HARP syndrome have a mutation in the *PANK2* gene, which is responsible for pantothenate kinase-associated neurodegeneration with brain iron accumulation, or NBIA.

When you see HARP, think of TWO pink harps being played in a palace. This may remind you that it is associated with the *PANK2* gene and pallidal degeneration..

Hartnup Disease

Hartnup disease is an aminoaciduria due to a **defect in transport of neutral amino acids** in the kidney and small intestine.

Hartnup disease causes **intermittent ataxia,** which may be associated with nystagmus. Altered mental status may be seen. The patient may be hypotonic.

Patients with Hartnup disease may have a **photosensitive rash** that resembles pellagra. This is because poor tryptophan absorption leads to niacin deficiency.

Elevated levels of neutral amino acids are found in urine and stool.

Hartnup disease is **treated with a high-protein diet.** Other treatments include tryptophan or nicotinic acid.

The word HARTNUP can be used to remember the clinical characteristics of the disease:

    Hat needed because photosensitive

    Aminoaciduria, **A**taxia, **A**MS (altered mental status)

    Rash after sun exposed

    Tryptophan is deficient

    Nicotinamide needed

    Urine and

    Poop have elevated neutral amino acids

Other metabolic defects that can cause intermittent ataxia: maple syrup urine disease, pyruvate dehydrogenase deficiency, some urea cycle defects.

Holocarboxylase Synthase Deficiency

See multiple carboxylase deficiencies below.

Homocystinuria

Multiple enzyme deficiencies in methionine metabolism can cause homocystinuria including deficiency of cystathionine beta-synthase, methylenetetrahydrofolate reductase (MTHFR), methionine synthase reductase (MTRR), or methionine synthase (also known as 5-methyltetrahydrofolate-homocysteine methyltransferase [MTR]). Defective methylcobalamin synthesis is also associated with homocystinuria. All are autosomal recessively inherited.

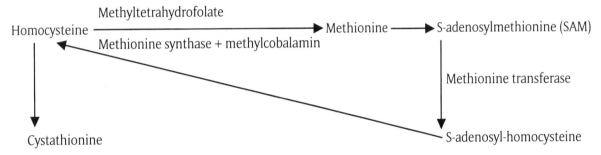

Nitrous oxide (laughing gas from the dentist) inhibits methionine synthase, and thus increases plasma total homocysteine. Prolonged exposure to nitrous oxide (N_2O) can lead to neuropathy and spinal cord degeneration.

Homocystinuria due to Cystathionine Beta-Synthase Deficiency

This is the most common genetic form of homocystinuria.

It is due to a defect in the gene CBS on 21q, which encodes cystathionine beta synthase.

cystathionine β-synthase
Homocysteine ————————→ cystathionine ————————→ cysteine
Pyridoxine (B6)   Pyridoxine (B6)

If untreated, it is characterized by **Marfanoid features, ectopia lentis and/or myopia, mental retardation, seizures, livedo reticularis, codfish vertebra, a malar flush, and a risk for thromboembolism**.

Laboratory findings include an increased methionine and homocystine in the blood, increased urinary homocystine, and a positive urinary cyanide-nitroprusside reaction.

· In homocystinuria, the lens of the eye deviates downward.

· In Marfan syndrome it deviates upward.

To remember that Marfan syndrome is associated with upward lens deviation and homocystinuria with downward deviation:

· Remember Marfan syndrome patients are really, really **tall**, so their lens dislocation is **upwards**.

· Vitamin treatment for the Homocysteinemic patient should bring **down their homocysteine level**, so their lens dislocation is **downwards**!

· **Alternatively, you look up to see Mars and down to see urine.**

Homocysteine causes injury to endothelium and premature atherosclerosis.

Some patients respond to pyridoxine (B6). Sometimes a cocktail of B6, folic acid, and B12 may be prescribed to lower homocysteine.

Betaine has also been used to convert homocysteine to methionine.

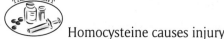

Isovaleric Acidemia

Isovaleric acidemia is an autosomal recessive organic acidemia that is due to a deficiency in isovaleryl-CoA dehydrogenase. This enzyme is a mitochondrial enzyme and is involved in leucine catabolism.

Isovaleric acidemia presents in 2 forms:

· **Acute neonatal form**

· **Chronic form**.

The **neonatal form** of isovaleric acidemia may present with **acidosis and coma in the first week of life**. The patent may have **seizures**.

The tip-off that this is isovaleric acidemia is that the **urine smells like sweaty feet**. **Pancytopenia** may occur in patients with isovaleric acidemia.

Think of isovaleric acidemia as it's so vile acidemia, which would characterize the patient's urine odor. **If I smelled like sweaty socks, I'd probably seize too**. Maybe the **bone marrow is knocked out by the odor**.

The **chronic form** of isovaleric acidemia is associated with **recurrent episodes of vomiting**, **ketoacidosis**, and **lethargy**. *These patients also have the sweaty feet odor.*

Kearns-Sayre Syndrome

Kearns-Sayre syndrome is a mitochondrial disorder characterized by progressive external ophthalmoplegia and pigmentary retinopathy.

Symptoms start before age 20 years. **Symptoms** may include **heart block**, **mitochondrial myopathy**, a **cerebellar syndrome**, **elevated CSF protein**, and **endocrine abnormalities**.

To remember that KSS is associated with eye findings, think of KSS as **KiSS** and recall the saying that love is blind.

How to associate KSS with **Pig**mentary retinopathy, **end**ocrine problems, and **heart block**?

Because love is blind, you'll need to KiSS the Pig in the end or else you'll break his heart.

Krabbe Disease (Globoid Cell Leukodystrophy)

Krabbe disease is an autosomal recessive neurodegenerative lysosomal storage disease of glycosphingolipid metabolism that causes central and peripheral demyelination.

It is due to mutations in the **GALC gene** on chromosome on 14q which result in deficiency of **galactocerebrosidase**, otherwise known as galactosylceramide β-galactosidase.

Gauchers = glucocerebrosidase

The infantile form presents between 3 and 6 months of life.

Initially, **irritability** and rigidity are seen – **that is one krabby baby!**

Patients with Krabbe disease may **feed poorly** and have **unexplained episodes of fever**.

Later **optic atrophy, blindness,** and **deafness** develop. **Psychomotor regression** occurs.

Patients with Krabbe disease have a **progressive demyelinating peripheral neuropathy**.

Deep tendon reflexes are lost, but bilateral Babinski signs are present. This is also seen in adrenoleukodystrophy and metachromatic leukodystrophy.

Nerve conduction velocities are decreased.

CSF protein is elevated.

Early in the course, CT shows **increased density of the basal ganglia, thalami, corona radiata, brainstem,** and **cerebellum.**

Globoid cells, which are PAS-positive multinucleated macrophages, are found in the white matter.

Krabbe disease has been treated with hematopoietic stem cell transplant and bone marrow transplant.

>
> **The ups and downs in Krabbe disease** (which would explain why these babies are so krabby):
>
> - **Krabbe up:** temperature, Babinskis, CSF protein, and CT density of the basal ganglia, thalamus, corona radiata, brainstem and cerebellum.
>
> - **Krabbe down:** Nerve conduction velocities, deep tendon reflexes, and hearing/sight.
>
> Death occurs around 13 months of age and is often due to a respiratory infection.

Leber's Hereditary Optic Neuropathy

This bilateral optic neuropathy is due to a mitochondrial DNA point mutation.

It causes painless loss of **central vision usually beginning in adolescence or early adulthood**.

Leigh Syndrome   *subacute necrotizing encephalomyelopathy*

Leigh syndrome is a neurodegenerative disorder that has multiple etiologies including (but not limited to) mutations in the ATPase 6 gene of mtDNA, cytochrome-c oxidase deficiency, and pyruvate dehydrogenase deficiency.

Leigh syndrome typically presents in the **first year of life with hypotonia and developmental delay**.

Abnormal extraocular movements and **ataxia** are seen.

Vomiting, respiratory disturbances (**hyperventilation or apnea**), **seizures**, **movement disorders**, **peripheral neuropathy**, or **retinitis pigmentosa** may be seen.

Lactate is elevated.

MRI shows symmetric **abnormalities in the putamen on T2-weighted imaging**. Lesions may also be seen in the thalamus and brainstem. *midbrain tectum, spares mammillary bodies and red nuclei*

 LEIGH can be used to remember the features of Leigh syndrome:

> **L**actic acidosis
> **E**pilepsy, **E**xtraocular movements abnormal
> **I**ncreased T2 signal in the putamen
> **G**ag/vomit
> **H**yperventilation or apnea, **H**ypotonia

tx - Thiamine (B1)

Lesch-Nyhan Syndrome

Lesch-Nyhan syndrome an **X-linked recessive** neurodegenerative condition due to a defect in purine metabolism. Specifically, patients with Lesch-Nyhan syndrome have a **deficiency of HGPRT (hypoxanthine guanine phosphoribosyl transferase)**.

Lesch-Nyhan syndrome presents in the **first year of life with developmental delay**.

Patients develop movement disorders such as **dystonia** and **choreoathetosis**. Also, compulsive and **self-mutilating behaviors** are seen. For instance, **patients bite their lips and fingers**.

Seizures and **vocal tics** can also be seen.

Patients have **hematuria** and **renal calculi**. Renal failure and gouty arthritis can be seen late in the course.

Labs show **hyperuricemia** and an elevated urine uric acid to creatinine ratio.

The letters of HGPRT, the enzyme deficient in Lesch-Nyhan syndrome, can be used to remember the clinical features of the disease:

Hematuria

Gouty arthritis, **G**naw fingers

Psychomotor retardation in first year

Renal calculi, **R**enal failure (later)

Tics

Patients with Lesch-Nyhan disease can have vocal tics. Maybe they say, "Bite me".

Lowe Syndrome (Oculocerebrorenal Syndrome)

Lowe syndrome is an **X-linked recessive** condition due to a mutation in the *OCRL1* gene on Xq26.1. (The *OCRL* gene encodes a phosphatidylinositol 4,5-bisphosphate-5-phosphatase.)

Lowe syndrome is also known as **oculocerebrorenal syndrome** due to abnormalities of the eyes, brain, and kidneys found in this disease.

Eye findings include **bilateral congenital cataracts**, **glaucoma** *with or without* **buphthalmos** (big bulging eyes), **corneal cheloids**, and **blindness**.

When you go to **Lowe's**® Home Improvement stores, your **eyes will bulge out** at the **O**utstanding **C**ollection of **R**emodeling **S**tuff (**O**culo**C**erebro**R**enal Syndrome).

Neurologic abnormalities include **neonatal hypotonia, delayed motor milestones**, possible **mental retardation, seizures, peripheral neuropathy**, and **decreased reflexes**. Behavior problems and **obsessive-compulsive behaviors** may be seen.

MRI may show **periventricular cysts or increased signal in the periventricular region** on T2-weighted images.

Renal findings include: **proximal renal tubular acidosis** and a **renal Fanconi syndrome**.

Patients with Lowe syndrome may develop **rickets**.

Maple Syrup Urine Disease (MSUD)

MSUD is an autosomal recessive aminoacidopathy. It is due to decreased activity of **branched-chain keto-acid dehydrogenase** (BCKAD), which metabolizes the keto-acid forms of leucine, isoleucine, and valine.

Classic MSUD

The first sign is that the patient's cerumen may smell like maple syrup. This may occur as early as on the first day of life.[6]

The newborn with MSUD feeds poorly and is irritable.

Between 4 and 7 days of life, the patient develops lethargy and difficulties with feeding.

The urine begins to smell like maple syrup.

A **progressive encephalopathy** occurs, which may be accompanied by **episodes of apnea, opisthotonic posturing,** or **bicycling or fencing movements**. **Tone fluctuates between hypotonia and hypertonia**.

Then the patient becomes **comatose**. **Seizures** may be seen.

CT/ MRI may show **diffuse edema affecting the white matter**, including the white matter of the cerebellum.

Laboratory findings include: ketoacidosis and **elevated plasma levels of branched chain amino acids (leucine, isoleucine, valine)** and branched chain ketoacids. Elevated plasma **L-alloisoleucine** is diagnostic.

The urine contains ketones and elevated levels of branched chain ketoacids. The dinitrophenylhydrazine test is positive; adding it to urine produces a yellow-white precipitate.

Treatment consists of a special diet that restricts isoleucine, leucine, and valine.

To remember that maple syrup urine disease is due to a defect in metabolism of branched chain amino acids, **think of a maple tree with branches**.

To remember the 3 branched chain amino acids (**Leucine, Isoleucine, and Valine**), which is fair game on the test, just remember that you can't **LIV** without maple syrup.

I ♡ Vermont maple syrup

---

[6] Strauss K, Puffenberger E, Morton D. Holmes. (30 January 2006) Maple Syrup Urine Disease. In: GeneClinics: Medical Genetics Knowledge Base [database online] University of Washington, Seattle. Available at http://www.geneclinics.org.

Intermediate MSUD

This is similar to classic MSUD, but it is less severe. There is **more branched-chain keto-acid dehydrogenase activity.**

Thiamine-Responsive MSUD

This is similar to intermediate MSUD, but it **responds to thiamine.**

Intermittent MSUD

 Patients with intermittent MSUD have **episodes of ataxia and altered mental status as a result of catabolic stress**, such as infection or large protein loads. The urine and cerumen have the odor of maple syrup during acute episodes. Labs are normal between episodes.

Dihydrolipoyl Dehydrogenase-Deficient MSUD

 This form of MSUD is associated with **episodes of ketoacidosis and lactic acidosis in infancy.**

The lactic acidosis occurs because the defective subunit is also needed for pyruvate dehydrogenase and α-ketoglutarate dehydrogenase to function.

McArdle's Disease

Please see muscle phosphorylase deficiency below.

Medium-Chain Acyl-CoA Dehydrogenase (MCAD) Deficiency

MCAD deficiency is the most common disorder of fatty acid oxidation.

MCAD catalyzes the initial reaction in fatty acid β-oxidation for medium chain fatty acids.

MCAD deficiency **presents in the first year of life with episodes of lethargy and vomiting**. Some patients have cardiopulmonary arrest.

It causes **hypoketotic hypoglycemia**. Fasting can result in hypoglycemia that may be fatal.

 It is treated with carnitine and a low-fat diet.

Menkes' Kinky Hair Disease

 Menkes' kinky hair disease is an **X-linked recessive** disorder of copper transport.

Mutations in the **copper-transporting ATPase gene (*ATP7A*)** on Xq12-q13 result in a **failure to absorb copper from the GI tract**.

Menkes' kinky hair disease tends to occur in **men** because it is X-linked recessive.

Hypothermia or hyperbilirubinemia may be seen in neonates with Menkes' disease, but the disease usually **presents at 2 or 3 months of age with hypotonia, seizures, regression**, and **poor feeding**.

Stimulation-induced myoclonic jerks may be seen.

Characteristic features include **cherubic faces** and **depigmented, sparse, "kinky" hair (pili torti)**.

Menkes' kinky hair disease also may be associated with a vasculopathy resulting in **stroke** or **subdural hematomas.**

Bone abnormalities, such as **rib fractures** and **Wormian bones**, may also be present, giving the appearance of child abuse.

Metachromatic Leukodystrophy (MLD)

Like Krabbe's disease, MLD is an autosomal recessive lysosomal storage disease of glycosphingolipid metabolism that results in injury to central and peripheral myelin.

MLD is due to a **deficiency of arylsulfatase A activity**. Decreased activity of arylsulfatase A causes **decreased degradation of galactosylsulfatide** (cerebroside sulfate), a component of myelin. As a result, galactosylsulfatide accumulates, which results in myelin breakdown.

Galactosylsulfatide (cerebroside sulfate) ⟶ Galactosylceramide

arylsulfatase A

MLD is due to deficiency of arylsulfatase A (due to a gene defect on chromosome 22), **deficiency of saposin B** (which activates arylsulfatase A), **or multiple sulfatase deficiency**. (If it is due to multiple sulfatase deficiency, other clinical manifestations are present. See multiple sulfatase deficiency below.)

The name MLD is derived from the color of the **sulfatide deposits** when tissue is stained with cresyl violet or toluidine blue. Deposits are also found in Schwann cell lysosomes and macrophages.

Late-infantile MLD

Late-infantile MLD is the most common form of MLD.

Late-infantile MLD presents at **1 or 2 years of age with falling/gait problems**. Initially, **hypotonia** may be seen.

Patients with MLD regress; they deteriorate intellectually and have a progressive quadriparesis.

As the disease progresses, **mixed upper and lower motor neuron signs occur** because MLD causes **leukodystrophy** and a **demyelinating peripheral neuropathy**. For instance, areflexia with bilateral Babinski signs may be seen.

Late in the course, patients with MLD have decerebrate posturing and are blind.

Labs show an **increased CSF protein. Sulfatide can be detected in the urine**.

MRI shows symmetric demyelination with sparing of the subcortical U-fibers.

Nerve conduction studies show **slowed motor and sensory nerve conduction velocities due to demyelination.**

Bone marrow transplant and hematopoietic stem cell transplant have been used to treat MLD, if detected early.

Juvenile MLD

The onset of juvenile MLD is between age 4 and 14 years of age.

 It presents with **behavior problems and difficulties in school.**

Deterioration is slower than in the late-infantile form.

Adult MLD

The adult form of MLD may present with **dementia or psychiatric symptoms**.

Methylmalonic Acidemia (MMA)

Methylmalonic acidemia is an **organic acidemia**.

A number of defects can result in methylmalonic acidemia. It may be due to vitamin B12 (cobalamin) deficiency (due to defective synthesis, absorption, or transport) or defects in methylmalonyl-CoA mutase.

$$\text{L-methylmalonyl-CoA} \xrightarrow[\text{adenosylcobalamin}]{\text{methylmalonyl-CoA mutase}} \text{succinyl-CoA} \Longrightarrow \text{Kreb's cycle}$$

The classic form of MMA is due to absence of methylmalonyl-CoA mutase and presents in the **neonatal period with vomiting, hypotonia, lethargy, metabolic acidosis, hyperammonemia, and ketotic hyperglycinemia**.

Complications of MMA include **spastic quadriparesis, mental retardation, and basal ganglia injury/stroke** with **movement disorders such as dystonia.**

Labs: methylmalonic acid is increased in the plasma, urine, and CSF. Neutropenia and/or thrombocytopenia may be seen.

MMA is treated with a low-protein diet and carnitine.

A trial of Vitamin B12 supplementation can be given to infants with MMA, but it might not help.

Some patients with MMA due to defective cobalamin synthesis also have homocystinuria due to defective methylcobalamin synthesis. (See the section on homocystinuria above.)

Mitochondrial Encephalopathy, Lactic Acidosis, and Stroke (MELAS)

MELAS presents in childhood with **headaches, vomiting, generalized tonic-clonic seizures, and stroke-like episodes** resulting in transient hemiparesis or blindness.

Patients may have short stature, sensorineural deafness, and exercise intolerance.

MRI shows *multiple infarctions that do not fit a vascular distribution*. Initially they are seen in the occipital lobes.

Labs show **elevated blood and CSF lactate**. Muscle biopsy shows **ragged-red fibers**.

MELAS is frequently due to a mutation in the leucine tRNA gene in mitochondrial DNA.

The treatment for MELAS is carnitine and coenzyme Q10.

To remember the clinical and genetic features associated with MELAS, remember the phrase **"Me lass Lucy GIVES Out $10 at carnivals to children!"**
  · **Me lass Lucy** = **MELAS-Leucine,**
  · **GIVES Out: G**eneralized tonic-clonic seizures, **I**ntolerance to exercise, **V**omiting, **E**levated lactate in blood & CSF, **S**hort stature, **O**ccipital lobe involvement,
  · **$10 at carnivals** = coenzyme Q**10** and **carn**itine = MELAS therapy!
  · **to children** = MELAS presents in childhood.

Mitochondrial Neurogastrointestinal Encephalomyopathy (MNGIE)

 In addition to gastrointestinal symptoms such as **diarrhea** and **episodes of pseudoobstruction**, patients with MNGIE have **weakness, ptosis, progressive external ophthalmoplegia**, and **sensorimotor polyneuropathy**.

MRI shows leukoencephalopathy, but patients do not have CNS dysfunction.

Mucopolysaccharidoses (MPS)

Mucopolysaccharidoses are due to deficiencies of lysosomal enzymes required for degradation of glycosaminoglycans.

Depending on the enzyme, various amounts of dermatan sulfate, heparan sulfate, keratan sulfate, or chondroitin sulfate will be excreted.

Type of MPS	Eponym	Enzyme defect	Mental Retardation (Y/N)
I H	Hurler	α-L-iduronidase	Y
I H/S	Hurler-Scheie	α-L-iduronidase	N
I S	Scheie	α-L-iduronidase	N
II	Hunter	Iduronate sulfatase	Y
III	Sanfilippo	Multiple (Each of the 4 types is due to a different enzyme deficiency.)	Y
IV	Morquio	Galactose-6-sulfatase	N
VI	Maroteaux-Lamy	N-acetylgalactosamine, 4-sulfatase (aryl sulfatase B)	N
VII	Sly	Hyaluronidase	Y

(MPS V is no longer in use.)

Most of these are autosomal recessive. **The exception is Hunter syndrome, which is X-linked.**

Coarse facial features and dysostosis multiplex are characteristic of most of these disorders.

Skeletal deformities at the base of the brain may result in obstructive hydrocephalus or cervical cord compression.

Patients with types IS, IV, and VI have normal intelligence. Types I, II, III, and VII are associated with Mental Retardation.

Hepatomegaly is commonly found in these patients.

Corneal clouding is common; an exception is Hunter syndrome.

Intralysosomal inclusion bodies, called **Zebra bodies,** may be seen in patients with MPS.

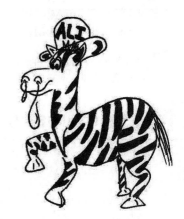

To remember **A-L-I**duronidase is associated with MPS-**1** and Zebra bodies, think about **My Pal'S #1** favorite **Zebra**, named **ALI** who has mucopolysaccharides dripping from his nose.

Some patients with MPS respond to bone marrow transplant or enzyme replacement.

To remember that Hunter syndrome is X-linked: Hunters are usually male and X-linked diseases affect males. In addition if you have corneal clouding you can't hunt; therefore, Hunter syndrome is not associated with corneal clouding.

Multiple Carboxylase Deficiencies

Multiple carboxylase deficiency includes 2 disorders, both of which are **biotin-responsive**.

The first **is holocarboxylase synthase deficiency**, which is also known as early onset multiple carboxylase deficiency.

The second **is biotinidase deficiency**, which is also known as late-onset multiple carboxylase deficiency.

There are **4 biotin-requiring carboxylases**:

> 1. Acetyl-CoA carboxylase (cytosol)
> 2. Methylcrotonyl-CoA carboxylase (mitochondria)
> 3. Pyruvate carboxylase (mitochondria)
> 4. Propionyl-CoA carboxylase (mitochondria)

· Acetyl-CoA carboxylase is important in de novo fatty acid synthesis.

· Methylcrotonyl-CoA carboxylase is involved in leucine metabolism.

· Pyruvate carboxylase converts pyruvate to oxaloacetate, which is an intermediate in the Kreb's cycle and is required for gluconeogenesis.

· Propionyl-CoA carboxylase is discussed in the Propionic Acidemia section below.

Holocarboxylase Synthase Deficiency

As stated above, holocarboxylase synthase deficiency is also known as **early-onset multiple carboxylase deficiency**.

Holocarboxylase synthase catalyzes the binding of biotin to apocarboxylases. Its deficiency leads to impaired function of these enzymes.

This presents in the neonatal period as a metabolic encephalopathy.

Similar to biotinidase deficiency, patients may have alopecia, rash, and ataxia.

It also causes lactic acidosis, ketosis, hyperammonemia, and thrombocytopenia.

Deficiency of the 4 carboxylases listed above causes a characteristic organic aciduria.

Holocarboxylase synthase is treated with biotin.

Biotinidase Deficiency

Biotinidase deficiency is also known as **late-onset multiple carboxylase deficiency**. It is autosomal recessive.

Biotinidase deficiency results in free biotin deficiency, and biotin is required as a cofactor for 4 carboxylases (listed above).

Biotinidase deficiency **presents about 3 months of age with seizures and hypotonia**.

Patients develop **alopecia**, an **erythematous rash**, **ataxia**, **respiratory disturbances**, and **spastic paraparesis**. They may also have hearing and vision loss.

 The association of **epilepsy** with **alopecia** and a **rash** should make you think of biotinidase deficiency.

Labs show *ketosis, lactic acidosis, hyperammonemia*, and a *specific pattern of organic aciduria.*

I own **multiple cars** (multiple carboxylase) but they're all made of **tin** (biotin), and every time I drive them, I lose my hair, have trouble breathing, and get a RASH!

 Biotinidase deficiency is associated with RASH:

    Respiratory disturbances

    Alopecia, **A**cidosis

    Seizures

    Hypotonia, **H**yperammonemia

Biotinidase deficiency is treated with biotin.

Multiple Sulfatase Deficiency

Multiple sulfatase deficiency is a lysosomal storage disorder due mutations in the sulfatase-modifying factor-1 gene (*SUMF1*). This gene encodes an enzyme that is required for formation of the catalytic site of sulfatases.

Patients with multiple sulfatase deficiency have neurologic findings similar to patients with metachromatic leukodystrophy due to deficiency of arylsulfatase A.

Patients also have **skeletal findings** *similar to patients with mucopolysaccharidoses (MPS)* due to iduronate sulfatase deficiency and have **ichthyosis** due to steroid sulfatase deficiency.

Muscle Phosphorylase Deficiency/ McArdle's Disease

 Muscle phosphorylase deficiency is also known as McArdle's disease and Glycogen Storage Disease Type V. This is an autosomal recessive metabolic myopathy that causes fatigue, cramps, and myoglobinuria.

Fifty percent of patients have **myoglobinuria**, which may cause renal failure.

McArdle's disease is associated with a **second-wind phenomenon**.

The **forearm ischemic lactate test is abnormal** in McArdle's disease; these patients *lack a rise in lactate.*

Myoclonic Epilepsy and Ragged Red Fibers (MERRF)

MERRF is a mitochondrial disease. A mutation in the tRNA^{Lys} gene is responsible for most cases.

Patients with MERRF may have **Lipomas, Optic Atrophy, Deafness, short stature, myopathy, neuropathy.**

As with other diseases due to mutations in the **m**itochondrial genome, the condition is **m**aternally inherited, ragged red fibers are seen on muscle biopsy, and lactate and pyruvate are elevated.

To remember the clinical and genetic associations of MERRF, know that **Merve has a LOAD of lice (Lys)**. Poor Merve has **L**ipomas, **O**ptic **A**trophy, **D**eafness, short stature, myopathy, and neuropathy. At least his mother, who passed on her mitochondrial DNA, still loves him.

NARP (Neuropathy, Ataxia, Retinitis Pigmentosa)

NARP is a mitochondrial disease, but patients do <u>not</u> have ragged-red fibers and may not have lactic acidosis.

It is due to a point mutation in the ATPase 6 gene. (This gene mutation is also seen in some cases of Leigh syndrome.)

Also, although they sound alike, NARP is not that clinically or genetically similar to HARP, except for the Retinitis Pigmentosa.

Neuronal Ceroid Lipofuscinoses (NCL)

NCL are a group of autosomal recessive lysosomal storage disorders characterized by accumulation of abnormal amounts of lipopigment.

 They are characterized by **seizures, dementia, and vision loss**.

Electron microscopy on skin, rectal, or conjunctival tissue may show granular osmiophilic deposits, curvilinear bodies, fingerprint profiles, or rectilinear complexes.

To remember that patients have vision loss, remember that **NCL rhymes with not see well**.

NCL also stands for <u>N</u>orwegian <u>C</u>ruise <u>L</u>ines (they paint **NCL** on all their boats).
On a cruise, you'll see:

- as you board, **fingerprint profiles** for security purposes;
- guests in the ship's casino, placing cash **osmiophilic deposits** into **rectilinear complexes** (slot machines);
- on deck, **curvilinear bodies** bathing in the sun;
- **vision loss** if they don't wear their sunglasses; and
- everyone **accumulating lots of lipo-pigment** -- pigment from the sun, and fat (= lipo) at the all-you-can-eat buffet!

Infantile NCL (CLN1)

 Infantile NCL is due to a defect in CLN1 gene at 1p, which codes for **palmitoyl protein thioesterase (PPT1).**

It presents **between 6 months and 2 years**. Patients with infantile NCL have **ataxia, myoclonic seizures, psychomotor regression, progressive vision loss**, and **microcephaly.**

Electron microscopy shows **granular osmiophilic deposits**.

Niemann-Pick Disease

There are multiple types of Niemann-Pick disease, all of which are autosomal recessive lysosomal storage diseases.

Niemann-Pick Disease Type A (NPA)

Niemann-Pick Disease Type A (NPA) is also known as the **classic infantile neuronopathic form**.

In NPA, a mutation in the sphingomyelin phosphodiesterase-1 gene (SMPD1) results in **deficiency of sphingomyelinase**.

NPA causes **persistent neonatal jaundice** but usually presents with **failure to thrive**, **hepatomegaly**, and **developmental delay**. Patients with NPA regress, become rigid, and may develop seizures. Death occurs by age 3-5 years.

Pulmonary infiltrates, lymphadenopathy, and significant **abdominal distention** may be seen.

Some Niemann-Pick patients have **a cherry red spot**, so here's the **cherry-red spot** mnemonic again: Farber Salivates Getting **cherry-picked**, half-off Sales at Sacks Fifth Ave & Nieman Marcus! **(Farber's disease, Sialidosis, GM1-Gangliosidosis, Sandhoff's, Tay-Sachs, and Niemann-Pick type A)**

The liver and bone marrow show **foamy histiocytes** (that contain lipid).

It is more common in Ashkenazi Jewish families than other populations.

Niemann-Pick type **A** is associated with **A**denopathy, **A**bdominal distention, and **A**shkenazi Jewish families.

Niemann-Pick Disease Type B (NPB)

Type B is known as the **visceral form**. Like type A, it is due to sphingomyelinase deficiency.

Niemann-Pick Disease Type C (NPC)

 Most patients with NPC have a mutation in the *NPC1* gene on 18q, which encodes Niemann-Pick C1 protein. NPC is also due to mutations in the *NPC2* gene on 14q.

NPC is associated with **abnormal cholesterol transport**. It causes accumulation of sphingomyelin and cholesterol in lysosomes.

 NP**C** is associated with abnormal **C**holesterol transport.

 NPC can present in **neonates with jaundice and hepatomegaly** or in **infants with hypotonia and developmental delay**.

However, **the classic form of NPC presents later.**

The classic form of NPC presents between ages **3 and 8 years with clumsiness**, which **progresses to ataxia**.

Vertical supranuclear gaze palsy is also characteristic and occurs early in the course. Usually the patients have a problem with downgaze first.

Then **dysarthria, dysphagia, dementia**, and **dystonia** develop.

Also, gelastic **cataplexy**, **choreoathetosis**, and **seizures** may be seen.

 Cataplexy can be seen in NP**C**.

 Skin fibroblasts demonstrate impaired cholesterol esterification in patients with NPC.

Foamy cells are present in the bone marrow, spleen, and liver.

Sea-blue histiocytes can be seen in the bone marrow of patients with advanced disease.

 NP**C** has **C**-blue histiocytes.

Niemann-Pick Disease Type D/ Nova Scotian Type

Type D, like type C1, is due to a mutation in the NPC1 gene. However, type D tends to be found in people from Nova Scotia.

Nonketotic Hyperglycinemia (Glycine Encephalopathy)

Nonketotic hyperglycinemia is an autosomal recessive condition due to a defect in glycine cleavage.

Neonates with nonketotic hyperglycinemia are **lethargic and hypotonic**. They have **Hiccups, Apnea, Multifocal Myoclonus, and seizures with EEG** showing **burst-suppression.**

Mothers have reported noticing hiccups or movements suggestive of myoclonus in utero.

It is diagnosed with an **elevated CSF glycine** and **elevated CSF to plasma glycine ratio**.

To remember the features of NKHG, think of eating a HAMMBurster with extra Glycine.

Treatments have included sodium benzoate, dextromethorphan (NMDA receptor antagonist), and diazepam.

Pelizaeus-Merzbacher Disease

Pelizaeus-Merzbacher is a hypomyelinating leukoencephalopathy.

Classic Form

Classic **Peliz**aeus-Merzbacher Disease presents in infancy with pendular nystagmoids (**roving eye** movements), **head tremor/nodding**, and later, spasticity, ataxia, and **optic atrophy**.

MRI shows **symmetric dysmyelination**. A **tigroid appearance** is due to small regions of normal neurons and myelin in the midst of abnormal white matter.

To remember this, think of the sign at the zoo: **PLEAZ** keep your **EYES** open for the **ROVING TIGER!** Anyone who reads the sign at the zoo will **nod their head** in agreement!"

Death occurs in adolescence or early adulthood.

The classic form is **X-linked recessive**; it is due to a mutation in the *PLP1* gene on Xq21-22, which encodes **proteolipid protein (PLP)**.

X-linked spastic paraplegia type 2 (SPG2) is also due to a mutation in the *PLP1* gene.

Connatal Form

The connatal form of Pelizaeus-Merzbacher disease is autosomal recessive or X-linked. It **presents earlier** and **progresses faster** than the classic form. Patients have less myelin and die younger (in the first decade).

Pompe's Disease

Please see acid maltase deficiency above.

Phenylketonuria (PKU)

Classic PKU is an autosomal recessive condition due to deficiency of **phenylalanine hydroxylase (PAH)**, which converts phenylalanine to tyrosine. As a result, phenylalanine increases in the blood.

$$\text{Phenylalanine} \xrightarrow[\text{Tetrahydrobiopterin (BH}_4)]{\text{Phenylalanine hydroxylase}} \text{Tyrosine}$$

Defects in tetrahydrobiopterin synthesis and regeneration also cause hyperphenylalaninemia.

PKU presents with delayed development, **light pigmentation (blond hair, blue eyes, pale)**, **eczema**, and a **mousy/musty odor**.

If untreated, the patient may develop microcephaly, spasticity, seizures, and mental retardation.

MRI may show **increased signal in the periventricular regions on T2-weighted images due to dysmyelination.**

Phosphofructokinase Deficiency/Tarui's Disease

Phosphofructokinase (PFK) deficiency is also known as Tarui's disease and Glycogen Storage Disease Type VII.

This is an autosomal recessive metabolic myopathy that causes **exercise intolerance** (cramps and fatigue) and **exercise-induced myoglobinuria**. It presents in childhood.

Similar to McArdle disease, **the forearm ischemic lactate test is abnormal in Tarui's disease**; however, there is <u>no</u> second wind phenomenon in Tarui's disease.

Propionic Acidemia

Propionic acidemia is an organic acidemia. It is due to a defect in propionyl-CoA carboxylase.

$$\text{Propionyl-CoA} \xrightarrow[\text{biotin}]{\text{propionyl-CoA carboxylase}} \text{Methylmalonyl-CoA}$$

This enzyme requires biotin and is important in the metabolism of valine, isoleucine, methionine, threonine, cholesterol, and odd-chain fatty acids.

Propionyl-CoA is derived from VOMIT and cholesterol: Valine, Odd-chain fatty acids, Methionine, Isoleucine, Threonine and cholesterol.

Holocarboxylase synthase and biotinidase mutations may also result in deficient activity of this enzyme. See the multiple carboxylase deficiency section above.

Most patients with propionic acidemia present in the **first 3 months of life** with **metabolic decompensation** *i.e. vomiting, dehydration, lethargy, and acidosis.* **Seizures** may occur as well.

Like methylmalonic acidemia, propionic acidemia causes **ketotic hyperglycinemia** and **hyperammonemia. Neutropenia** and **thrombocytopenia** may be seen in either condition as well.

In propionic acidemia, **propionic acid is elevated in urine**.

Patients with propionic acidemia require a protein-restricted diet and carnitine.

Pyridoxine Dependency

Pyridoxine dependency presents in the neonatal period with **refractory seizures** that respond poorly to typical anti-epileptic drugs but respond to pyridoxine.

Some patients with pyridoxine-dependent seizures were found to have mutations in the *ALDH7A1* gene on 5q, which encodes **antiquitin**.[7] Antiquitin is an enzyme involved in catabolism of pipecolic acid. It is an alpha-aminoadipic semialdehyde dehydrogenase that acts on piperideine-6-carboxylate (P6C). **Abolition of antiquitin activity results in accumulation of P6C, which forms a condensation product with pyridoxal 5'-phosphate.**

Pyridoxine (B6) is the cofactor for glutamic acid decarboxylase, which is required for GABA synthesis. Recall that GABA is the major inhibitory neurotransmitter in the CNS.

$$\text{Glutamate} \xrightarrow[\text{Glutamic acid decarboxylase (GAD)}]{\text{B6}} \text{GABA}$$

B6 is also required in GABA metabolism; it is a cofactor for GABA transaminase as well.

$$\text{GABA} \xrightarrow[\text{GABA transaminase}]{\text{B6}} \text{succinic semialdehyde}$$

People with pyridoxine deficiency are never going to quit trying to build the pyramids (pyridoxine) and therefore are anti-Quitting (antiquitin)! They would be sick (vitamin B6) and have seizures (refractory epilepsy) if they were asked to quit in 5 (on chromosome 5q).

---

[7] Mills PB, Struys E, Jakobs C, et al. Mutation in antiquitin in individuals with pyridoxine-dependent seizures. Nat Med 2006; 12:307-309.

Refsum Disease

Childhood Onset (Classic Form)

 The childhood onset form of Refsum disease is due to a defect in the gene that encodes phytanoyl-CoA hydroxylase, which is required for oxidation of phytanic acid. As a result, **phytanic acid accumulates**.

This form presents with **night blindness** in the first or second decade of life.

It causes **retinitis pigmentosa, ataxia, anosmia, deafness, a chronic hypertrophic demyelinating sensorimotor neuropathy** with **onion bulbs**, **ichthyosis**, and **diabetes**.

Skeletal defects, such as epiphyseal dysplasia, are found in some patients.

Cardiac failure may result in death.

CSF protein is very high.

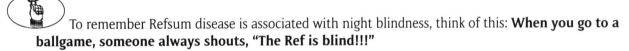 To remember Refsum disease is associated with night blindness, think of this: **When you go to a ballgame, someone always shouts, "The Ref is blind!!!"**

The classic form of childhood onset Refsum disease is treated with a diet low in phytanic acid.

 REFSUM could stand for:

   Rough skin (ichthyosis), **R**etinitis pigmentosa

   Ears-can't hear

   Falls, phytanic acid

   Smell is lost (anosmia)

   Unsteady gait

   Myelin is lost (demyelinating neuropathy)

 It's probably good that patients with Refsum disease can't smell because they have fishy skin (ichthyosis) and onion bulbs.

Since patients with Refsum disease have rough skin (ichthyosis), **think of Refsum disease as Rough skin disease**. Actually, Refsum disease is rough on multiple parts of the body. **The patients can't see, hear, or smell.**

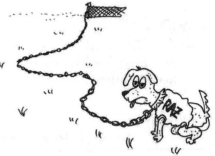

To remember which diseases elevate VLCFA's, think of **RAZ** (**R**efsum disease, **R**hizomelic chondrodysplasia punctata, **A**LD, and **Z**ellweger syndrome), the weak, sickly dog on a **Very Long Chain Far Away**.

Infantile Refsum Disease

Like neonatal adrenoleukodystrophy and Zellweger syndrome, infantile Refsum disease is a disorder of peroxisomal assembly.

Infantile Refsum disease causes **steatorrhea, retinitis pigmentosa, developmental delay**, a **peripheral neuropathy**, and **deafness**.

In addition to phytanic acid, very long chain fatty acids (VLCFA) accumulate, *similar to neonatal ALD and Zellweger syndrome.*

Sandhoff Disease

Sandhoff disease is a neurodegenerative lysosomal storage disease that affects the gray matter. It is classified as a sphingolipidosis.

Specifically, Sandhoff disease is a GM2 gangliosidosis due to **mutations of the beta subunit of hexosaminidase**. This results in **deficiency of hexosaminidase A and B**.

(Hexosaminidase has 2 isoenzymes. Hexosaminidase A consists of α and β subunits. Hexosaminidase B consists of 2 β subunits.)

Sandhoff disease is an autosomal recessive condition that maps to chromosome 5.

Clinically and pathologically, it **resembles Tay-Sachs disease**.

However, **Sandhoff disease is associated with mild hepatosplenomegaly, and Tay-Sachs disease is not.**

Sandhoff disease usually results in death by age 3. Death is often a result of respiratory infection. Sandhoff disease is associated with **coarse granulations in histiocytes in the bone marrow**.

Sandhoff disease causes coarse granulations, like **sand**, in histiocytes in the bone marrow.

Picture someone with a **sandbag under their shirt, making their abdomen bigger**. This may help you remember that patients with Sandhoff disease have hepatosplenomegaly.

What are the major genetic and clinical differences between Tay Sachs and Sandhoff disease?

- **Genetic:** The gene defect in **T**ay **S**achs is *Hexosaminidase A*, and in Sandhoff disease it's both *Hexosaminidase A and B*.
- **Clinical:** Patients with Sandhoff disease have hepatosplenomegaly.

Patients with s**AND**hoff's have an enlarged liver **AND** spleen and have *Hex A* **AND** *Hex B* gene defects!

Both Tay Sachs disease and Sandhoff disease have a cherry-red spot, but here's the **cherry-red spot** mnemonic again anyway: Farber Salivates Getting **cherry-picked**, half-off Sales at Sacks Fifth Ave & Nieman Marcus! **(Farber's disease, Sialidosis, GM1-Gangliosidosis, Sandhoff's, Tay-Sachs, and Niemann-Pick type A)**

Sialidosis

Sialidosis is a lysosomal storage disorder that is due α-**neuraminidase (sialidase) deficiency**. This enzyme cleaves sialic acid from galactose.

Elevated sialyloligosaccharides in urine can help to confirm the diagnosis.

Sialidosis Type I

Patients with Sialidosis type I have **progressive myoclonic epilepsy** (PME).

Funduscopy shows **a cherry-red spot.**

The cherry-red spot mnemonic again: Farber Salivates Getting **cherry-picked**, half-off Sales at Sacks Fifth Ave & Nieman Marcus! **(Farber's disease, Sialidosis, GM1-Gangliosidosis, Sandhoff's, Tay-Sachs, and Niemann-Pick type A).**

Sialidosis Type II (Mucolipidosis Type I)

Sialidosis Type II resembles Hurler syndrome; patients have dysmorphic features and skeletal abnormalities. They also have a **cherry-red spot, hepatosplenomegaly, and developmental delay**.

Sjögren-Larsson Syndrome

Sjögren-Larsson is a leukoencephalopathy due to **decreased activity of fatty aldehyde dehydrogenase**.

It is characterized by a **triad of:**

> 1. **Ichthyosis**
> 2. **Mental retardation**
> 3. **Spastic diplegia or quadriplegia.**

Like patients with Sjögren's disease, patients with Sjögren-Larsson syndrome have dry skin. Alternatively, recall that Gary Larson frequently used fish in his cartoons, and Sjögren-Larsson patients have ichthyosis, which is dry skin resembling fish scales.

Succinic Semialdehyde Dehydrogenase (SSADH) Deficiency

SSADH presents with **developmental delay, childhood-onset hypotonia, ataxia, seizures**, and **behavior disturbances**.

MRI may show **abnormalities in the globus pallidus on T2-weighted images**.

Urine organic acids show the presence of **4-hydroxybutyric aciduria/ gamma-hydroxybutyric aciduria**.

To remember that SSADH is associated with globus pallidus abnormalities: The **SS ADH** sailed around the **globe**.

SSADH deficiency is associated with **S**eizures, **S**assy behavior, **A**taxia, **D**evelopmental delay, and **H**ypotonia (and 4-Hydroxybutyric aciduria).

Normal

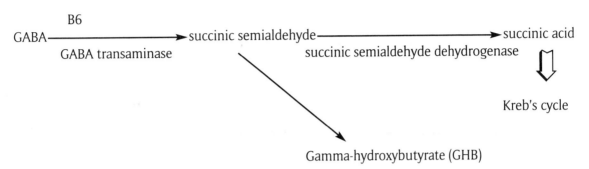

SSADH deficiency:

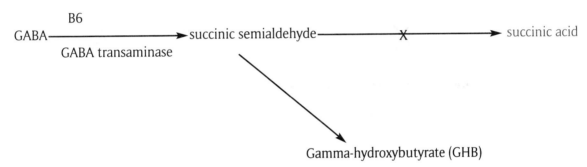

Sulfite Oxidase deficiency

Sulfite oxidase deficiency may be an isolated defect or seen in **molybdenum** cofactor deficiency. It results in abnormal metabolism of sulfated amino acids.

Sulfite Oxidase **(SO)** deficiency causes severe **neonatal seizures, developmental delay, and hypotonia**.

Lack of Sulfite Oxidase **(SO)** leads to the abnormal production of S-sulfocysteine, which leads to ocular **lens dislocation**.

urine sulfite ⊕

That lens is SO Dislocated! It's probably a result of all of Molly's severe seizures.

Tangier Disease

Tangier disease is due to **deficiency of alpha-lipoprotein**.

It is associated with a mutation in the **ATP-binding-cassette-1 gene** (ABCA1) on 9q.

Recall that adrenoleukodystrophy is also associated with defects in an ATP-binding casette protein.

Patients with Tangier disease have **large orange tonsils**, **lymphadenopathy**, and **splenomegaly**.

They also have a primarily **sensory neuropathy affecting distal upper extremities** and **atrophy of the intrinsic muscles of the hand.**

Laboratory findings in Tangier disease include: decreased cholesterol and LDL, very low HDL.

Remember: You hold a tangerine in your hand, which is where the atrophy occurs. When you take the tangerine from your hand and put it into your mouth, it turns your tonsils orange.

Tarui's Disease

Please see phosphofructokinase deficiency above.

Tay-Sachs Disease

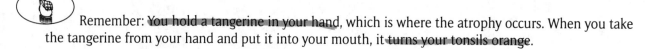

Tay-Sachs disease is a neurodegenerative lysosomal storage disease that affects the gray matter.

Tay rhymes with gray. Therefore, Tay-Sachs is a **gray matter disease**.

Tay-Sachs disease is a GM-2 gangliosidosis, like Sandhoff disease. However, Tay-Sachs disease is due to mutations in the alpha subunit of the hexosaminidase A gene, which results in hexosaminidase A deficiency. It is an autosomal recessive condition that maps to chromosome 15. There is an **increased**

---

8 Please see the Movement Disorders chapter for more information.

frequency of Tay-Sachs disease in **patients with Ashkenazi Jewish ancestry**. (Sandhoff disease is panethnic.)

 The onset of Tay-Sachs disease is in the **first few months of life**.

It presents with irritability and **sensitivity to noise (hyperacusis)** with an **increased startle response.**

Patients have **progressive weakness** and are **hypotonic with hyperreflexia**.

Patients develop **seizures, blindness, and megalencephaly.**

A **cherry-red spot** can be seen on funduscopic exam, so again here's the **cherry-red spot** mnemonic: Farber Salivates Getting **cherry-picked**, half-off Sales at Sacks Fifth Ave & Nieman Marcus! **(Farber's disease, Sialidosis, GM1-Gangliosidosis, Sandhoff's, Tay-Sachs, and Niemann-Pick type A).**

At age 2, patients continue to worsen. Posturing is seen. Then they become unresponsive.

Death occurs by 5 years of life.

 You have to tie sacks to the Tay-Sachs patients' limbs to prevent them from hitting ceiling after a noise.

 The liver is NOT enlarged in Tay Sachs disease.

On microscopy, **ballooned neurons with foamy cytoplasm** are seen in the CNS of patients with Tay-Sachs disease.

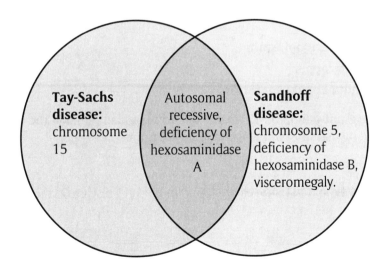

Tyrosine Hydroxylase Deficiency

Tyrosine hydroxylase deficiency is one cause of **dopa-responsive dystonia**.[8] It is due to a mutation in the tyrosine hydroxylase gene on 11p and is autosomal recessive.

Tyrosine hydroxylase catalyzes the rate-limiting step of dopamine synthesis, the conversion of tyrosine to levodopa. Tyrosine hydroxylase requires tetrahydrobiopterin (BH_4) as a cofactor in this reaction.

$$\text{Tyrosine} \xrightarrow[\text{BH}_4]{\text{Tyrosine hydroxylase}} \text{levodopa}$$

Wilson's Disease

Wilson's disease is an autosomal recessive neurodegenerative disorder due to a defect in copper metabolism. It is due to mutations in the **ATP7B gene on chromosome 13q**. This gene codes for **copper transporting adenosine triphosphatase, which transports copper from the hepatocyte into the bile.**

Patients less than 10 years of age present with **liver failure**.

Over 10 years, patients tend to have **neurologic or psychiatric symptoms**.

Characteristic features of Wilson's disease include a **wing-beating tremor**, **Kayser-Fleischer rings**, **sunflower cataracts**, and **risus sardonicus**.

Patients with Wilson's disease have:

- **Decreased serum ceruloplasmin**
- **Decreased serum copper**
- **Increased 24-hour copper excretion**.

MRI may show **face of the giant panda** on T2 images due to decreased signal in the superior colliculi and increased signal in the medial substantia nigra and tegmentum.

Alzheimer type I and type II astrocytes are found in Wilson's disease. Alzheimer type I astrocytes are more common.

Wilson's disease is treated with **Chelation**. D-penicillamine, ammonium tetrathiomolybdate, zinc, and triethylene tetramine dihydrochloride have been used.

 To remember how to treat Wilson's, **TRI DAZ Chelation**:

> **TRI**ethylene tetramine dihydrochloride,
>
> **D**-penicillamine,
>
> **A**mmonium tetrathiomolybdate,
>
> **Z**inc.
>
> **Chelation**

Menkes' Kinky Hair Disease versus Wilson's Disease

 Both Menkes' Disease and Wilson's Disease involve copper-transporting ATPase.
- In **Menkes' disease**, the **alpha** subunit is involved.
- In **Wilson's disease**, the **beta** subunit is involved.

- In Menkes' kinky hair disease, the **a**lpha subunit is defective, and there's an **a**bsorption problem in the GI tract/**a**bdomen.
- In Wilson's disease, the **b**eta subunit is defective, and there's a **b**ile problem.

	Menkes' Kinky Hair Disease	Wilson's Disease
Subunit involved	Alpha	Beta
Serum copper	Low	Low
Serum ceruloplasmin	Low	Low
Liver copper	Low	High
Treatment	Copper	**TRI DAZ Chelation**

Wolman Disease

Wolman disease is a lysosomal disease due to **acid lipase deficiency**, which results in xanthomatous changes in multiple organs due to the accumulation of cholesteryl esters.

Symptoms of Wolman disease begin in infancy. Patients have **jaundice, vomiting, diarrhea, malabsorption, poor weight gain, adrenal insufficiency**, and **hepatosplenomegaly.**

The primary neurologic symptoms are *hypotonia and developmental delay.*

Calcified adrenals are seen in Wolman disease.

To remember that Wolman disease causes vomiting and adrenal insufficiency: If I saw the Wolfman, I'd vomit and my adrenals would be affected.

Zellweger Syndrome (Cerebro-Hepato-Renal Syndrome)

Zellweger syndrome is an autosomal recessive disorder of peroxisome biogenesis.

It is similar to neonatal adrenoleukodystrophy, which is also a disorder of peroxisomal assembly associated with deficiency of multiple peroxisomal enzymes. However, Zellweger syndrome is more severe.

Multiple genes affecting peroxisome biosynthesis can cause this syndrome.

Patients with Zellweger syndrome have a characteristic appearance: they have a **prominent forehead, epicanthal folds**, and a **large fontanelle. Cataracts** or **Brushfield spots** (which are usually seen in Down syndrome) may be present. **Renal cysts** and **hepatomegaly** are seen. X-rays show **calcific stippling** of the patellae and hips.

Patients are **weak** and **hypotonic.**

Development is delayed, and these patients have impaired vision and hearing.

Seizures may occur.

Migration defects e.g. polymicrogyria, heterotopia, pachygyria may be seen on MRI.

Periventricular pseudocysts

Deficiency of myelin is seen, but it is less severe than in adrenoleukodystrophy.

Labs show an *increased bilirubin, iron, CSF protein, and very long-chain fatty acids (VLCFA).*

To remember which diseases elevate VLCFA's, think of **RAZ** (**R**efsum disease, **R**hizomelic chondrodysplasia punctata, **A**LD, and **Z**ellweger syndrome), the weak, sickly dog on a **Very Long Chain Far Away**.

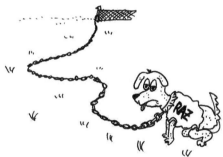

The Most

Ornithine transcarbamylase (OTC) deficiency is the most common urea cycle defect.

Medium-chain acyl-CoA dehydrogenase (MCAD) deficiency is the most common fatty acid oxidation disorder.

CPT2 deficiency is the most common metabolic etiology of recurrent myoglobinuria.

The Only

Fabry's disease is the only X-linked sphingolipidosis.

Metabolic Diseases Quiz

(Answers on page 739)

1. Which of the following diseases is associated with a cherry-red spot?

    A. Abetalipoproteinemia

    B. Canavan disease

    C. Cerebrotendinous xanthomatosis

    D. Fabry's disease

    E. Farber's disease

2. Match the enzyme defect with the disease

    1). Canavan disease   A. Aspartoacylase deficiency

    2). Gamma-hydroxybutyric acidemia   B. Galactocerebrosidase deficiency

    3). Gaucher's disease   C. Glucocerebrosidase deficiency

    4). Krabbe disease   D. Succinic acid dehydrogenase deficiency

3. Match the odor with the disease

    1) Glutaric acidemia type II   A. Maple syrup

    2) Isovaleric acidemia   B. Musty

    3) Maple syrup urine disease   C. Like sweaty feet

    4) Phenylketonuria

4. Some patients with this disease respond to _____.

    1) Ethylmalonic-adipicaciduria   A. B12

    2) Maple syrup urine disease   B. Pyridoxine (B6)

    3) Methylmalonic acidemia   C. Riboflavin

                                  D. Thiamine

5. Ichthyosis is found in which of these conditions?

    A. Multiple sulfatase deficiency

    B. Refsum disease

    C. Sjögren-Larsson syndrome

    D. All of the above

6. Pyridoxine dependency has been found to be due to a defect in which gene?
   A. ABCD1
   B. Antiquitin
   C. PLP1
   D. SUMF1

7. Multiple carboxylase deficiencies respond to which of the following?
   A. Biotin
   B. B12
   C. Pyridoxine

8. Choose whether each disease primarily affects the gray or the white matter.
   1) Alexander disease   A. Gray
   2) Canavan disease   B. White
   3) Krabbe disease
   4) Pelizaeus-Merzbacher disease
   5) Sandhoff disease
   6) Tay-Sachs disease

Chapter 6

Movement Disorders

Anatomy of the Basal Ganglia

Components of the Basal Ganglia

The basal ganglia include these structures:
- Caudate
- Globus pallidus
- Putamen
- Substantia Nigra
- Subthalamic Nucleus

The term *striatum* refers to the *caudate* and *putamen*.

If someone is truly **strong** then they are both **courageous** and **potent**. **(striatum = caudate + putamen)**

Recall from the Pediatric Neurology chapter that the striatum is derived from the telencephalon.

The globus pallidus, substantia nigra, and subthalamus originate from the diencephalon.

Blood Supply

Most of the blood supply to the caudate, putamen, and globus pallidus is from the lenticulostriate branches of the middle cerebral artery (MCA).

Exceptions:

The medial globus pallidus is supplied by the anterior choroidal artery off of the internal carotid artery.

The caudate head, anterior putamen, and a portion of the outer segment of the globus pallidus are supplied by the recurrent artery of Heubner off of the anterior cerebral artery.

Recurrently, A.C.A. **Heubner** hits the **Head** (of the caudate), before traveling the **Outer Globe** with his **Aunt Putamena**.

Pathways

The major input to the basal ganglia is from the cortex. The cortex provides excitatory input to the basal ganglia using the neurotransmitter glutamate.

Most input to the basal ganglia arrives via the caudate and putamen, which together form the **Striatum**.

 If someone is truly ***strong*** then they are both ***courageous*** and ***potent***. *(striatum = caudate + putamen)*

Information from the somatosensory cortex, primary motor cortex, and premotor cortex project to the putamen.

The substantia nigra pars compacta also provides input to the striatum via the nigrostriatal pathway, which uses dopamine. This input can be excitatory or inhibitory.

Other sources of input to the striatum include the intralaminar nuclei of the thalamus, especially the centromedian (CM) and parafascicular nuclei, and the brainstem raphe nuclei.

In summary, the following structures provide input to the striatum:

- Cortex (excitatory, glutamate)
- Substantia nigra pars compacta (excitatory or inhibitory, dopamine)
- Raphe nuclei (modulatory, serotonin)
- Intralaminar nuclei of the thalamus (excitatory, glutamate)

Outputs leave the basal ganglia via the internal segment of the globus pallidus (GPi) and the substantia nigra pars reticulata (SNr), which are similar structurally and functionally. Output from these regions is inhibitory; GABA is the neurotransmitter.

One of the major pathways from the GPi/SNr is to the ventral thalamic nuclei (ventral anterior [VA] and ventral lateral [VL]).

GPi/SNr ——————————→ ventral thalamic nuclei (VA and VL)
                GABA

There are **excitatory connections from the ventral anterior and ventrolateral thalamic nuclei to the cortex.** Thalamocortical fibers travel to the premotor cortex, supplementary motor area, and primary motor cortex for motor control.

The cortex and globus pallidus are like a divorced couple. They don't talk to each other directly. The cortex talks to the striatum (caudate and putamen), which in turn talks to the globus pallidus internal segment and substantia nigra pars reticulata. These structures send messages back to the cortex via the thalamus.

The GPi/SNr project to the reticular formation, which affects the reticulospinal tract, and to the pedunculopontine nucleus in the brainstem.

Gait abnormalities in Parkinson's disease have been correlated with loss of neurons in the pedunculopontine nucleus (PPN).

Also, the GPi projects to the centromedian nucleus of the thalamus.

In addition, the SNr projects to the superior colliculus. It affects control of eye movements by influencing the tectospinal pathways. The SNr also projects to the mediodorsal thalamic nuclei, which is part of the limbic system.

Basal Ganglia Anatomy

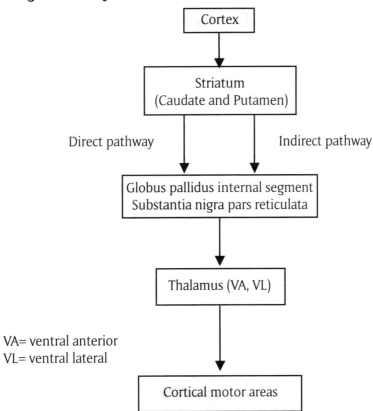

Excitatory and Inhibitory Relationships

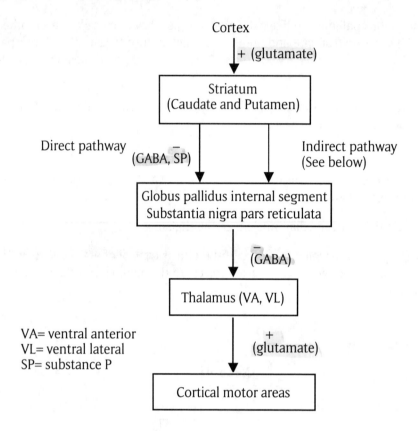

Direct Pathway

The direct pathway is from the striatum to the substantia nigra pars reticulata (SNr) and the internal segment of the globus pallidus (GPi).

Striatum ⟶ GPi/SNr

The striatum provides inhibitory input (GABA and substance P) to the GPi/SNr.

Striatum ⟶ GPi/SNr
GABA, substance P

Since the striatum provides inhibitory input to the GPi/SNr, which provide inhibitory input to the thalamus, the direct pathway results in excitation of the thalamus. By disinhibiting the thalamus, **the direct pathway facilitates the thalamocortical pathway**, which is excitatory. Therefore it ultimately **results in increased activity of the motor cortex**.

To remember that the direct pathway results in excitation of the thalamus (and ultimately the cortex), remember that the **D**irect pathway **D**rives the thalamus, causing cortical **D**isinhibition.

Indirect Pathway

The indirect pathway is from the striatum to the external segment of the globus pallidus (GPe). Then the pathway goes to the subthalamic nucleus (STN). Like the direct pathway, it ends at the substantia nigra pars reticulata and the internal segment of the globus pallidus.

Striatum ⟶ GPe ⟶ STN ⟶ GPi/SNr

The striatum provides inhibitory input to the external segment of the globus pallidus (GABA and enkephalin).

The GPe provides inhibitory input to the subthalamic nucleus. The subthalamus, like the thalamus, has excitatory output (glutamate); it provides excitatory projections to the GPi/SNr.

```
        GABA, enkephalin              GABA                  Glutamate
Striatum ─────────────────→ GPe ─────────────────→ STN ─────────────────→ GPi/SNr
              −                        −                        +
```

By providing excitation to the GPi/SNr, which is inhibitory to the thalamus, the indirect pathway causes inhibition of the thalamocortical pathway. This leads to cortical inhibition.

In summary, **increased activity in the indirect pathway causes cortical inhibiton**.

Comparison of the Direct and Indirect Pathways

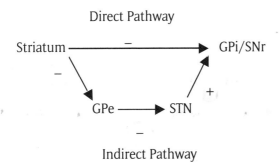

The direct pathway results in cortical excitation, and the indirect pathway results in cortical inhibition.

Pallidothalamic Connections

There are multiple routes by which information travels from the globus pallidus to the thalamus.

 The **ansa lenticularis** takes a winding route from the ventral aspect of the internal segment of the globus pallidus to the thalamus. It goes around the internal capsule.

The **lenticularis fasciculus,** also known as **Forel Field H2,** goes from the medial aspect of the internal segment of the globus pallidus through the internal capsule.

The ansa lenticularis and the lenticularis fasciculus meet in the **H fields of Forel** to enter the thalamus together. When they join, it is called the **thalamic fasciculus**, which is also called **Forel Field H1**.

 Imagine that the ansa lenticularis and lenticularis fasciculus are secret lovers. The ansa lenticularis sneaks out the back and takes the long way. The lenticularis fasciculus takes the short cut through the internal capsule. They meet in the H fields of Forel. It is there that the 2 become 1. Their new name is thalamic fasciculus or Forel Field H1.

Basal Ganglia Toxins

Carbon Monoxide poisoning causes necrosis of the globus pallidus.

 Carbon Monoxide Can **M**urder everyone on the **globe**.

Methanol damages the putamen.

 When you drink **methanol**, you **meth** up your **putamen** – **al**l of it.

MPTP causes parkinsonism.[1]

 MPTP: Might **P**rovoke **T**errible **P**arkinsonism!

Manganese toxicity can deplete dopamine in the caudate and putamen and deposit in the substantia nigra. In turn, this can decrease spontaneous motor activity and look like Parkinson's disease as well.

 When you hear of manganese toxicity, think of the man who cannot move with ease anymore.

---

[1] MPTP is a contaminant produced during synthesis of MPPP, a meperidine (Demerol®) analogue.

Specific Movement Disorders

Abetalipoproteinemia/ Bassen-Kornzweig Syndrome

Abetalipoproteinemia, which is also known as Bassen Kornzweig syndrome, causes a progressive ataxia due to vitamin E deficiency that can look like Friedreich's ataxia. However, retinitis pigmentosa, steatorrhea, acanthocytosis, and low triglyceride and cholesterol levels are seen in abetalipoproteinemia.[2] Also, patients with this condition do **not** have cardiomyopathy, which can be seen in Friedreich's ataxia.

Abetalipoproteinemia is just one cause of vitamin E deficiency that causes a phenotype similar to Friedreich's ataxia. See the section on ataxia with isolated vitamin E deficiency (AVED) below.

Alternating Hemiplegia

Alternating hemiplegia of childhood, which **presents at less than 18 months of age**, causes **episodes of paralysis**. The patient may have monoparesis, hemiparesis, diparesis, or quadriparesis. Involuntary movements such as dystonia and choreoathetosis may be seen. Also, ophthalmoparesis, bulbar paralysis, and autonomic changes such as hyperpnea may be seen. The episodes last minutes to days. Progressive cognitive impairment occurs.

Alternating hemiplegia of childhood is due to a mutation in the ***ATP1A2* (sodium-potassium-ATPase, alpha-2 polypeptide)** gene on 1q. Recall from the Pediatric Neurology chapter that this is also the gene responsible for familial hemiplegic migraine-2 (FHM2). See below.

Alternating hemiplegia has been treated with flunarizine.

Ataxia with Isolated Vitamin E Deficiency (AVED)

Ataxia with isolated vitamin E deficiency is also known as **Friedreich-like ataxia** because the phenotype is similar to Friedreich's ataxia. Ataxia with isolated vitamin E deficiency is due to a mutation in the gene that encodes **alpha-tocopherol transfer protein (ATTP)** on chromosome 8q.

---

[2] Please see the Metabolic Diseases chapter for more information about abetalipoproteinemia.

Symptoms of AVED usually begin in puberty. Patients have a progressive ataxia, loss of proprioception, areflexia, and upgoing toes. Some patients have titubation, deafness, tendon xanthomas, or retinitis pigmentosa.

Vitamin E prevents progression and may reverse some deficits.

AVED can be used to remember the characteristics of this disease:

Ataxia, **A**reflexia

Vitamin E deficiency

Eye findings (retinitis pigmentosa)

Deafness

AVED looks like Fred (Friedreich's ataxia) but Fred has a heart problem.

Ataxia-Telangiectasia (AT)

Ataxia-telangiectasia is a neurodegenerative and neurocutaneous syndrome.

It is an autosomal recessive condition.

AT is due to a defect in the **ATM gene** (Ataxia Telangiectasia Mutant gene), which is on chromosome **11q**. The ATM protein coordinates the responses to the double-stranded DNA break. Patients with ataxia-telangiectasia have a defect in DNA repair.

The presenting symptoms:

· Mainly **truncal ataxia** is seen. Patients with AT present with ataxia when they start to walk around one year of age.

· **Eye telangiectasias** appear at 3-5 years of age.

· **Skin telangiectasias** may appear on the ears, nose, cheeks, neck, and creases of forearms between ages 3-7 years.

· **Recurrent sinopulmonary infections** present around age 5 years.

Abnormal movements associated with AT include:

· **A**thetosis

· **T**remor.

· **M**yoclonic jerks

Think of **A** **T**remulous **M**an with **A**thetosis, **T**remor, and **M**yoclonic jerks, who requests **$11** (chromosome 11) from an **ATM** (the ATM gene), but the bank's ATM is **defective** and needs **repair** (**defect** in DNA **repair**).

Patients with AT can develop a polyneuropathy.

Reflexes are decreased or absent after age 7 or 8 years.

Usually children lose the ability to walk independently by age 12 years and are wheelchair dependent.

Bassen-Kornzweig Syndrome

Bassen-Kornzweig syndrome is also known as abetalipoproteinemia. (See above.)

Patients with **Bassen**-Kornzweig may need a **basin** due to steatorrhea.

Chorea Gravidarum

Chorea gravidarum is chorea associated with pregnancy.

Patients should be worked up for rheumatic fever, antiphospholipid antibody syndrome, and systemic lupus erythematosus.

To remember the work up for chorea gravidarum think of **RAPS** (**R**heumatic fever, **A**nti-**P**hospholipid antibody syndrome, and **S**ystemic lupus), and pregnant women with chorea dancing raps and starring in a rap video.

Corticobasal Ganglionic Degeneration (CBGD)

CBGD is a tauopathy that starts around 60 years of age.

The name says it all. Patients have cortical atrophy and extrapyramidal signs.

Patients with CBGD have an array of movement disorders: **myoclonus, dystonia, tremor, and rigidity**. **Parkinsonism** is seen in CBGD, but it is asymmetric and **unresponsive to levodopa**.

Symptoms usually start in one limb, usually an arm.

Patients with CBGD also have pyramidal signs and contractures.

The letters in CBGD can be used to remember the features of the disease:

Cortical sensory loss, **C**oiled bodies of tau in oligodendrocytes

Ballooned neurons, **B**alance impaired

Gee, why is my arm doing that? (alien limb phenomenon)

Dystonia, **D**ysphasia, **D**ysarthria, **D**egeneration of the substantia nigra and striatum

Dementia with Lewy Bodies (DLB)

Dementia with Lewy Bodies is a degenerative dementia associated with **parkinsonian features, visual hallucinations, sensitivity to neuroleptics, and fluctuating levels of alertness.**

Parkinsonism in DLB usually begins after the onset of dementia or <u>shortly</u> before. Patients with DLB may have bradykinesia, masked facies, rigidity, a stooped posture, and a shuffling gait.

DLB patients may also have tremor or myoclonus.

Patients with DLB have visual hallucinations, but neuroleptics can worsen their motor symptoms.

Patients with <u>DLB</u> absolutely <u>D</u>on't <u>L</u>ike <u>B</u>rain-o-leptic medications.

Patients with DLB may have REM sleep behavior disorder.

In Dementia with Lewy Bodies, Lewy bodies are widespread in the cortex, in addition to being found in the brainstem.

Dentatorubral-pallidoluysian Atrophy (DRPLA)

DRPLA is an autosomal dominant ataxia that is found primarily in Japan.

It is due to an expansion of a CAG repeat in *ATN1*, the gene encoding atrophin-1, on chromosome 12.

The same genetic mutation was found in an African-American family in North Carolina. In these patients the disease was called Haw River Syndrome, which has a slightly different phenotype. See below.

There are multiple forms of DRPLA.

A progressive myoclonic epilepsy phenotype is seen in patients with onset less than 20 years of age.

 Patients who develop DRPLA after 20 years of age have ataxia, choreoathetosis, dementia, and psychosis.

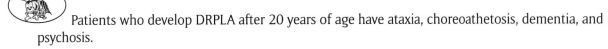 Think of DRPLA as DRoP Lots, because you drop lots due to ataxia and chorea.

Adults with DRPLA, which is due to an expanded CAG repeat in *ATN1*, have problems with:

C horeoathetosis

A taxia

G oofiness (psychotic)

The major global concentration/locations for DRPLA also can be remembered with CAG:

C arolina (NC)

A nd

G apan (Japan, but hey it's close!)

Adult-onset DRPLA and Huntington disease are clinically similar.

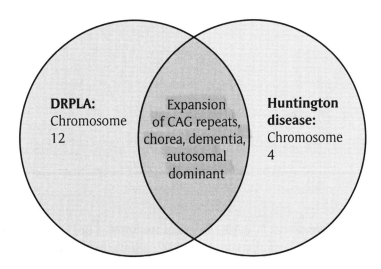

DRPLA: Chromosome 12

Expansion of CAG repeats, chorea, dementia, autosomal dominant

Huntington disease: Chromosome 4

As one might expect by the name, there is degeneration of the dentatorubral and pallidoluysian systems in DRPLA. The dentate nucleus and globus pallidus are particularly affected.

On autopsy, patients have intranuclear neuronal inclusions that stain positive for ubiquitin and atrophin-1.

Dyssynergia Cerebellaris Myoclonica

See Ramsay Hunt syndrome below.

Dystonia

Dystonia is an abnormal posture or repetitive movement that is due to simultaneous contraction of agonist and antagonist muscles. It occurs in a consistent direction and often worsens with voluntary movement. It also is exacerbated by stress and fatigue and improves with sleep. Some patients have a **sensory trick**, which is a maneuver used to improve the dystonia.

Dystonia is classified by age of onset, location, or etiology.
- · Dystonia that begins in **childhood** tends to involve the **lower extremities and may spread**.
- · Dystonia that begins in **adulthood** tends to occur in the **upper body and does not usually spread**.

KIDS KICK THE DYSTONIA FROM THE **LEGS** ON UPWARDS.

Cervical dystonia is the most common focal dystonia.

DYT1

DYT1 dystonia is also known as Oppenheim's torsion dystonia or Dystonia Musculorum Deformans. This is an autosomal dominant disease due to a GAG deletion in the *TOR1A* gene on 9q that encodes torsin A, which is an ATP-binding protein. DYT1 dystonia has an increased prevalence in Ashkenazi Jews.

Inversion of the foot is the first sign of DYT1. It occurs around 10 years of age. The dystonia gradually progresses to a generalized dystonia.

 DYT1 has been treated with pallidal deep brain stimulation.

 To remember features of DYT1, ask yourself:

Did **Y**ou **T**each **one** (**DYT-1**) the **TORAH (TOR1A** = old testament) to **C**hildren **A**nd **G**randparents (CAG deletion)? Even a **10-year-old boy** (age of onset) wouldn't **invert his foot** (foot inversion is the first sign) from his **Jewish** duty!

DYT5 (Dopa-Responsive Dystonia)

 Dopa-responsive dystonia presents as **gait dysfunction in childhood**. The symptoms have **diurnal variation**; they worsen as the day goes on. They improve after a nap.

 Do **Y**ou **T**olerate a **5**-minute **nap**??? DYT5 improves with an afternoon siesta!

Patients with dopa-responsive dystonia may also have parkinsonism, increased tone, and hyperreflexia.

Dopa-responsive dystonia can be diagnosed by sending CSF for neurotransmitters.

 As the name suggests, dopa-responsive dystonia is treated with levodopa.

There are multiple causes of dopa-responsive dystonia.

GTP Cyclohydrolase 1 Deficiency

Mutations in the *GCH1* gene, which encodes **guanosine triphosphate cyclohydrolase 1 (GTP cyclohydrolase 1)**, are the most common cause of dopa-responsive dystonia. The *GCH1* gene is located at 14q. This form of dopa-responsive dystonia is **autosomal dominant**.

GTP cyclohydrolase catalyzes the rate-limiting step in tetrahydrobiopterin (BH_4) synthesis.

Tyrosine Hydroxylase Deficiency

Tyrosine hydroxylase deficiency also results in dopa-responsive dystonia. It is **autosomal recessive**. It is due to a mutation in the TH gene on 11p, which encodes tyrosine hydroxylase.

Tyrosine hydroxylase catalyzes the rate-limiting step of dopamine synthesis, the conversion of tyrosine to levodopa. Tyrosine hydroxylase requires BH_4 as a cofactor in this reaction.

$$\text{Tyrosine} \xrightarrow[BH_4]{\text{Tyrosine hydroxylase}} \text{levodopa}$$

DYT8

DYT8 is paroxysmal nonkinesigenic dyskinesia, which is due to a mutation at 2q. See below.

DYT10

DYT 10 is paroxysmal kinesigenic dyskinesia, which is due to a mutation at 16p. See below.

DYT11 (Myoclonus-Dystonia)

Myoclonus-dystonia is autosomal dominant. It is due to a mutation in the **epsilon-sarcoglycan gene** on chromosome 7q.

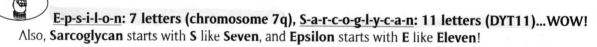

E-p-s-i-l-o-n: 7 letters (chromosome 7q), S-a-r-c-o-g-l-y-c-a-n: 11 letters (DYT11)...WOW! Also, **Sarcoglycan** starts with **S** like **Seven**, and **Epsilon** starts with **E** like **Eleven**!

Myoclonus-dystonia presents in childhood. As the name implies, patients have **myoclonic jerks** associated with dystonia. The myoclonus occurs primarily in the neck, trunk, and arms. The dystonia usually involves the arm or neck (torticollis).

Myoclonus associated with DYT11 may improve with **alcohol** consumption.

So, think of this: At the **SEVEN-ELEVEN**, those **myoclonic jerks** will serve you alcohol!

DYT 12 (Rapid Onset Dystonia-Parkinsonism)

As the name implies, patients with DYT12 develop dystonia and parkinsonism over a short time (days to weeks). This is due to a mutation in the alpha-3 subunit of the Na+/K+-ATPase (*ATP1A3*) gene on 19q.

HOT TIP

Recall that alternating hemiplegia and familial hemiplegic migraine-2 are due to mutations in *ATP1A2*.

Episodic Ataxia

Episodic Ataxia-1 (EA-1)/ Episodic Ataxia with Myokymia

Episodic ataxia-1 is also known as **episodic ataxia with myokymia**.

EA-1 is due to a mutation in the gene *KCNA1* on chromosome 12, which causes a **potassium channel defect**.

BUZZ WORDS

EA-1 is characterized by periods of ataxia lasting seconds to minutes beginning in childhood. They may be spontaneous or provoked by sudden movement, exercise, illness, or stress. They can occur multiple times per day.

Patients with EA-1 also have **myokymia**, which is a writhing/rippling movement of muscle, particularly around the eyes and in the hand. This can be seen between attacks as well.

Episodic Ataxia-2 (EA-2)

EA-2 is associated with a **calcium channel defect**. Specifically, it is due to mutations in the gene *CACNA1A* (voltage-dependent P/Q-type calcium channel alpha-1A) on 19p.

HOT TIP

Mutations in this gene also cause Familial Hemiplegic Migraine 1 (FHM1) and spinocerebellar ataxia-6 (SCA 6).

MNEMONIC

To remember that gene *CACNA1A* on chromosome 19p causes FHM1, EA2, and SCA6, think of this:

Have a FEAST on route A1A for 19 people!

The disorders in this mnemonic are in order: FHM-**1**, EA-**2**, and SCA-**6**. Route *A1A*=CACN*A1A*; 19 people = 19p.

EA-2 is characterized by intermittent ataxia and dysarthria that begins in childhood or adolescence. The attacks range in duration from minutes to a few days. Other symptoms such as vertigo, nausea, weakness, diplopia, or headache may also be present during the attack. Nystagmus and mild ataxia can be seen between attacks.

EA-2 responds to acetazolamide.

EA-1 versus EA-2

Disease	Chromosome	Gene	Channel defect	Clinical findings	Duration of attack
EA-1	12	**K**CNA1	**K** 1^+	Myo**K**ymia	Minutes
EA-2	19	**CA**CNA1A	**Ca** 2^+	Nystagmus, acetazolamide-responsive	Hours

Episodic ataxia-**1** is associated with a potassium channel defect. Potassium has **1** positive charge. Episodic ataxia-**2** is associated with a calcium channel defect. Calcium has **2** positive charges.

To remember that EA-2 is the type of episodic ataxia associated with nystagmus, remember that people have 2 eyes.

To remember that EA-2 is treatable with acetazolamide, think of its trade name Diamox (Di = two)!

In a nutshell, to remember that EA-2 is treatable, lasts hours, is associated with nystagmus and calcium, remember that **T**wo (EA-2, Ca+2, 2 eyes), **T**reatable, and **T**oo long-lasting all start with **T**.

Essential Tremor (ET)

ET is the most common tremor and probably the most common movement disorder.

Essential tremor is a 4 to 12 Hz postural tremor that usually affects the hands or forearms. It may also be seen during voluntary movement.

ET may involve the head or vocal cords.

ET improves with alcohol and worsens with stress, caffeine, and fatigue.

ET may be sporadic or familial. A couple of genes have been identified: 3p (FET1) and 2p (ETM2).

 In 2011, the AAN updated its 2005 guidelines for treatment of ET.[3]

Level of Evidence	Effectiveness	Intervention (medical or surgical)
A	Strong	primidone, propranolol
B	Probable	alprazolam, atenolol, gabapentin, sotalol, topiramate, levetiracetam and 3,4-diaminopyridine
C	Possible	nadolol, nimodipine, clonazepam, botulinum toxin A, flunarizine, deep brain stimulation, and thalamotomy
U	Insufficient evidence	gamma knife thalamotomy, pregabalin, zonisamide, or clozapine

Not all patients improve on or tolerate propranolol or primidone; 30% to 50% of patients will not respond to either agent.

 Essential Tremor (ET) improves with EThanol. 🍸

Fahr's Disease

 Fahr's disease is characterized by **idiopathic bilateral calcification of the basal ganglia.**

It causes subcortical dementia and parkinsonism. It can also cause psychiatric symptoms, chorea, and dysarthria.

There are familial (autosomal dominant or recessive) and sporadic forms.

Familial Hemiplegic Migraine

See Hemiplegic Migraine below.

---

3 Zesiewicz TA, Elble RJ, Louis ED, Gronseth GS, Ondo WG, Dewey RB Jr, Okun MS, Sullivan KL, Weiner WJ. Evidence-based guideline update: Treatment of essential tremor: Report of the Quality Standards Subcommittee of the American Academy of Neurology. Neurology. 2011 Nov 8;77(19):1752-5.

Fragile X-associated Tremor/Ataxia Syndrome (FXTAS)

FXTAS is a neurodegenerative syndrome characterized by **intention tremor and gait ataxia later in life**. Cognitive dysfunction, particularly affecting executive functions, may be present.

MRI may show white matter lesions in the **middle cerebellar peduncles** or brainstem.

FXTAS is found in males carrying a premutation in the fragile X mental retardation-1 (FMR1) gene. These patients have an **increased number of CGG repeats**, but not sufficient to cause Fragile X. The patient's grandson is at high risk for Fragile X, however.

Friedrich-like Ataxia

Please see the section on Ataxia with isolated vitamin E deficiency (AVED) above.

Friedreich's Ataxia

no cardiac involvement

Friedreich's ataxia is an autosomal recessive neurodegenerative disease that affects the spinocerebellar tracts, corticospinal tracts, posterior columns, dorsal root ganglia, and the axons of large myelinated peripheral nerves.

Friedreich's ataxia is due to a **GAA expansion in the *FXN* gene on chromosome 9q, which encodes frataxin**. Frataxin is a mitochondrial protein.

Patients with Friedreich's ataxia begin having **symptoms in puberty**. They often present with **gait ataxia**.

Patients with Friedreich's ataxia develop **dysarthria, hyporeflexia, upgoing toes, scoliosis**, and **pes cavus**. They **lose proprioception**. Patients are eventually wheelchair bound.

Cardiomyopathy, arrhythmias, and cardiac failure occur.

Diabetes may also be seen.

GAA, the expanded repeat in Friedreich's ataxia, could stand for **Gait Ataxia** and **Arrhythmia**.

	Friedreich's ataxia	Ataxia-telangiectasia
Onset	Around 13 years	Early childhood
Chromosome	9, Autosomal Recessive	11, Autosomal Recessive
Defective gene	FRDA	ATM
Systemic	Cardiomyopathy, diabetes, scoliosis	Prone to infection, malignancy such as lymphoma

Atypical Friedreich's Ataxia

There are multiple atypical forms of Friedreich's ataxia:

· Late onset Friedreich ataxia (onset over 25 years of age)

· Very late onset Friedreich's ataxia (onset over 40 years of age)

· Friedreich ataxia with retained reflexes

· Spastic paraparesis with mild ataxic features

Glutaric Acidemia Type I

Glutaric acidemia type 1 is an autosomal recessive condition due to deficiency of glutaryl-coenzyme A dehydrogenase that causes an extrapyramidal syndrome in infancy.[4]

Patients with glutaric acidemia type 1 have **dystonia, dyskinesias,** and **developmental delay.** They may also have **hypotonia** or **opisthotonus.**

MRI shows **frontotemporal atrophy** with prominent Sylvian fissures. This results in a **bat wing** appearance.

Infants with **glu**taric acidemia type 1 may wish that they could be **glu**ed to the crib due to dystonia, dyskinesias, and opisthotonus, which must make them **batty.**

HARP Syndrome

HARP syndrome is characterized by **hypobetalipoproteinemia, acanthocytosis, retinitis pigmentosa,** and **pallidal degeneration.**

---

4 See the Metabolic Diseases chapter for more information.

Some patients with HARP syndrome have a mutation in the *PANK2* gene, which is responsible for pantothenate kinase-associated neurodegeneration.

When you see HARP, think of a **pink harp**. This may remind you that it is associated with the *PANK2* **gene**.

Haw River Syndrome

An African-American family in North Carolina was found to have the same genetic mutation as is found in DRPLA (expanded CAG repeat in the *ATN1* gene on chromosome 12p). In this family, the disease was called Haw River syndrome.

Patients with Haw River syndrome have ataxia, dementia, choreiform movements, and generalized seizures.

Unlike patients with DRPLA, patients with **Haw River syndrome** lack myoclonus and **have basal ganglia calcifications (in the globus pallidus)**. They also tend to have demyelination in the centrum semiovale and neuroaxonal dystrophy of the posterior columns.

Hemiballismus

Hemiballismus, which is characterized by a **sudden violent flinging movement of the extremity**, is due to a lesion of the contralateral subthalamic nucleus.

Hemifacial Spasm

Hemifacial spasm is characterized by twitching of one side of the face.

It most commonly involves the orbicularis oculi muscle.

Hemifacial spasm may be due to compression of the facial nerve by an aberrant artery and can be treated with botulinum toxin or decompressive surgery.

Hemiplegic Migraine

 This is a type of migraine with aura. Patients with hemiplegic migraine have a **transient hemiparesis followed by a headache.** Hemisensory changes, visual field defects, and aphasia may accompany the weakness.

There are sporadic and familial forms.

Familial Hemiplegic Migraine-1 (FHM1)

FHM1 is due to a mutation in the *CACNA1A* gene on 19p.

To remember that gene *CACNA1A* on chromosome 19p causes FHM1, EA2, and SCA6, think of this:

Have a FEAST on route A1A for 19 people!

The disorders in this mnemonic are in order: FHM-**1**, EA-**2**, and SCA-**6**. Route ***A1A***=CACN***A1A***; 19 people = 19p.

Familial Hemiplegic Migraine-2 (FHM2)

FHM2 is due to a mutation in the *ATP1A2* (sodium-potassium-ATPase, alpha-2 polypeptide) gene on 1q.

Mutations in this gene also cause alternating hemiplegia of childhood, which shares clinical features with FHM. See above.

Familial Hemiplegic Migraine-3 (FHM3)

FHM3 is due to a mutation in the *SCN1A* gene.

Recall that mutations in the *SCN1A* gene also cause generalized epilepsy with febrile seizures plus.

Familial Hemiplegic Migraine-4 (FHM4)

FHM4 is due to a mutation on 1q.

Huntington Disease (HD)

Huntington disease is an autosomal dominant neurodegenerative disease that is due to an expanded CAG triplet repeat in the *HD* gene on chromosome 4p, which encodes huntingtin.

 Hunters **C**apture **A**nimal **G**ame and Huntington patients have an **expanded CAG repeat**.

 Hunters hunt **for** animals, Huntington disease is due to a mutation on chromosome **four**.

The age of onset of Huntington disease is usually in the late thirties, but it depends on the length of the CAG triplet repeat.

Most patients present with motor signs, but some present with behavior changes. Some patients present with both.

The first sign may be a change in **saccadic eye movements**.

Clumsiness and fidgeting are seen followed by chorea. Later bradykinesia and difficulty maintaining movement is seen. Dystonic movements appear. Ultimately, patients are forced to use wheelchairs due to falls.

Irritability and mood changes are a frequent finding.

Patients may anger easily or be violent. Apathy is seen later in the course of the disease.

Patients with HD have an increased risk for suicide.

Executive dysfunction is seen followed later by subcortical dementia.

Imaging shows atrophy of the caudate and putamen, as well as generalized cerebral atrophy.

Histology shows loss of GABA-synthesizing neurons, primarily in the striatum.

(Loss of GABAergic neurons in the striatum leads to decreased inhibition of the substantia nigra. This leads to increased dopamine production by nigrostriatal neurons. As a result, chorea is seen.)

In 2008, tetrabenazine became the first drug approved by the FDA to treat Huntington Disease chorea.

Tetrabenazine (TBZ) is a VMAT2-inhibitor, which causes early metabolic degradation of monoamines, like dopamine, and decreases involuntary, hyperkinetic, limb movements.

Side effects include **P**arkinsonism, **A**kathisia and **D**epression. It can also potentially prolong the QT interval and cause neuroleptic malignant syndrome. Genotyping for CYP2D6, which metabolizes TBZ, is recommended in the prescribing information. (CYP2D6 also metabolizes fluoxetine and paroxetine.)

MNEMONIC

If a patient with 4-limb chorea doesn't want 4-point limb restraints, then take the pill 4-benazine (**tetra**benazine), which will slam him on the **V**ictory **MAT** (which has a **PAD** so it won't hurt).

Evidence-based guidelines support using tetrabenazine, amantadine, or riluzole for chorea in patients with HD.[5] They recommend monitoring for depression and parkinsonism in patients who take tetrabenazine and liver monitoring if patients take riluzole. The guidelines state that there is not enough evidence to comment upon using neuroleptics for treatment of chorea.

Westphal Variant

Westphal variant is an akinetic, dystonic form of Huntington disease.

These patients have dementia and may have seizures.

Increased T2 signal is seen in the striatum.

Juvenile Huntington Disease

Juvenile Huntington disease is characterized by dystonia and parkinsonism. These are more prominent than chorea. Myoclonus and seizures may also be seen.

Hyperekplexia

Hyperekplexia is characterized by an exaggerated startle beginning in infancy. Infants may have apnea during the episodes. They also are stiff, with hypertonic shoulder-girdle muscles that relax in sleep.

When older, muscle tone improves, but the patient may **fall** when **startled**.

Hyperekplexia is due to mutations in the **glycine receptor** on chromosome **5q**.

MNEMONIC

To remember the features of Hyperekplexia, think about what happened when someone spilled **5** quarts of **glycine**:

The baby slipped and **fell** and was **startled**, screaming, "**Ek**!" (for hyper**Ek**plexia).

---

[5] Armstrong MJ, Miyaskaki JM. Evidence-based guideline: Pharmacologic treatment of chorea in Huntington disease. Neurology 2012;79:597-603.

Lance-Adams Syndrome

See Posthypoxic Myoclonus below.

Marinesco-Sjögren Syndrome

Marinesco-Sjögren syndrome is characterized by cerebellar ataxia with cerebellar atrophy, cataracts, and mental retardation.

Infants tend to have hypotonia. Weakness is seen later.

Patients with Marinesco-Sjögren syndrome may also have primary gonadal failure and scoliosis.

Marinesco sounds like Maraschino, as in **Maraschino cherries**. Imagine a person with *Maraschino cherries instead of eyes*. Like cataracts, these would prevent patients from seeing, which would make them more likely to trip.

McLeod Syndrome

McLeod syndrome is an X-linked recessive form of neuroacanthocytosis.

It is due to mutations in XK gene.

It is has a later age of onset than the autosomal recessive form of neuroacanthocytosis; McLeod syndrome begins around age 50.

It is associated with facial tics and an axonal peripheral neuropathy.

To remember McLeod Syndrome, think of a dark, ominous **cloud** with the letters **XK** on it, causing people to have **facial** tics due to the impending storm!

Meige Syndrome

Meige syndrome is characterized by oromandibular dystonia with blepharospasm.

The letters in MEIGE can be used to remember the symptoms:

> **M**andibular dystonia
> **E**yelid muscle spasm
> **I**nvoluntary eyelid closure
> **G**ee, here's another reason to use Botox
> **E**xcessive blinking

It can be treated with botulinum toxin.

Multiple System Atrophy (MSA)

MSA is a neurodegenerative disease that usually presents in sixth decade.

Clinical Findings

MSA is associated with varying degrees of autonomic and urinary dysfunction, parkinsonism, cerebellar, and corticospinal tract dysfunction.[6]

Examples of **autonomic dysfunction** include orthostatic hypotension, urinary incontinence, incomplete bladder emptying, and erectile dysfunction.

Parkinsonian features seen include bradykinesia, rigidity, postural instability, and postural tremor.

Cerebellar findings include gait ataxia, dysarthria, limb ataxia, and nystagmus.

Corticospinal tract findings include hyperreflexia and extensor plantar responses.

---

[6] Gilman S, Low PA, Quinn N, et al. Consensus statement on the diagnosis of multiple system atrophy. Journal of the Neurological Sciences 1999;163:94-98.

Pathology

Varying degrees of neuronal loss and gliosis are found in the cerebellum, intermediolateral cell column, inferior olive, locus ceruleus, middle cerebellar peduncles, Onuf's nucleus in the sacral cord, pontine nuclei, striatum, and substantia nigra.

Recall from the Neuropathology chapter that MSA is an alpha-synucleinopathy.

To remember that Multiple system atrophy (**MSA**) is an alpha-synucleinopathy, remember that MSA could also stand for **M**ade of **S**ynuclein-**A**lpha (alpha-synuclein).

It's important to differentiate the "*alpha-Synucleinopathies*" from the "*Tao-opathies*". So, to remember the *alpha-Synucleinopathies*, think of "**PALM Synday**".

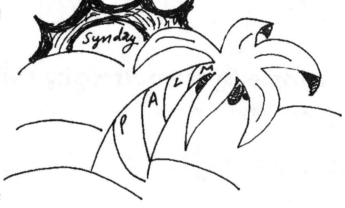

P is for **P**arkinson's disease,

A is for **A**lzheimer's disease (but trickily, Alzheimer's can be both an "*alpha-Synucleinopathy*" and/or "*Tao-opathy*"),

L is for **L**ewy Body dementia, and

M is for **M**ultiple Systems Atrophy.

Synday is for Synucleinopathy.

The best thing about this mnemonic is that you don't need to recall all the *Tao-opathies* – if they're not there on **PALM Synday**, they're Tao!

Also, recall that **glial cytoplasmic inclusions (GCIs)** are found in oligodendrocytes of patients with MSA.

Olivopontocerebellar atrophy may be seen in patients with MSA-C.

MRI Findings

MSA is associated with the **hot-cross bun sign** on MRI due to degeneration of pontocerebellar fibers.

Putaminal atrophy may be seen. Sometimes decreased signal is seen in the putamen with an area of increased signal lateral to it on T2-weighted images.

---

[7] Gilman S, Low PA, Quinn N, et al. Consensus statement on the diagnosis of multiple system atrophy. Journal of the Neurological Sciences 1999;163:94-98.

Old MSA Nomenclature

In the past, MSA was said to include sporadic olivopontocerebellar atrophy [OPCA], Shy-Drager syndrome, and striatonigral degeneration. A consensus statement from 1999 recommended changing the nomenclature.[7]

Olivopontocerebellar Atrophy (OPCA) – also known as Olivopontocerebellar Degeneration (OPCD)

Some patients with sporadic OPCA have a type of MSA.

 They have dysarthria and ataxia.

Atrophy occurs in the pons, middle cerebellar peduncles, inferior olives, and cerebellum.

Originally there were many types of OPCA but reclassification into SCA by genetic testing has determined only 2 remain as true OPCA:

| OPCA type 1 | Fickler-Winkler Syndrome: ataxia, dysarthria, head tremor, scanning speech, lack of involuntary movements, albinism autosomal recessive | autosomal recessive |
| OPCA type 2 | dementia and extrapyramidal signs autosomal dominant | autosomal dominant |

Shy-Drager Syndrome

Patients with Shy-Drager syndrome have parkinsonism and dysautonomia.

Dysautonomia is manifested by impotence in men, orthostatic hypotension, decreased sweating, and difficulties with urination.

Cell loss in the intermediolateral cell column of the thoracic cord leads to orthostatic hypotension.

Cell loss is also seen in the putamen, substantia nigra, locus ceruleus, and Onuf's nucleus.

(Onuf's nucleus is located at in the spinal cord at S2-4 and controls urethral and anal sphincters.)

Striatonigral Degeneration (SND)

Striatonigral degeneration is a form of MSA in which patients have parkinsonism and laryngeal stridor.

Striatonigral degeneration causes **stri**dor.

New MSA Nomenclature

MSA-P

The term MSA-P has replaced Striatonigral degeneration. It is used **if parkinsonism is the major finding**.

MSA-C

The term MSA-C has replaced sporadic OPCA. This is used **if cerebellar signs/symptoms are the major findings.**

Neuroacanthocytosis

Neuroacanthocytosis has also been called chorea acanthocytosis (CHAC).

It is a movement disorder associated with behavior and cognitive changes.

Neuroacanthocytosis presents around age 30 years.

Abnormal movements such as chorea, dystonia, and tics occur. Late in the course, parkinsonism may be seen.

Orofacial dystonia interferes with eating. The tongue protrudes and food is expelled.

Also, patients accidently bite their tongue and lips. Dysarthria also is seen.

The autosomal recessive form is due to mutations in the gene on chromosome 9 that encodes chorein.

(McLeod syndrome is the X-linked form of neuroacanthocytosis.)

Patients with Neuroacanthocytosis have chewed up lips and chewed up red blood cells (acanthocytes).

*Causes of **Acant**hocytosis – think of someone studying so hard for the boards that they must stop playing the Harp!*

ACAN'T WAVE Bye At My HARP!

· Neuro**acant**hocytosis

· **W**olman disease (acid lipase deficiency).
· **A**betalipoproteinemia
· **V**itamin **E** deficiency

· **B**assen-Kornzweig syndrome

· **At**axia-telangiectasia

· **M**cLeod syndrome
· **HARP** syndrome

Opsoclonus-Myoclonus Syndrome (Dancing Eyes-Dancing Feet Syndrome)

Opsoclonus-myoclonus syndrome is characterized by irregular, multidirectional eye movements and myoclonus.

There are multiple etiologies.

In **children**, opsoclonus-myoclonus may be associated with **neuroblastoma**, which is a tumor that tends to arise from the sympathetic chain or adrenal gland. This can be detected with imaging. Also, urine catecholamines may be elevated (homovanillic acid or vanillylmandelic acid) in patients with neuroblastoma.

Neuroblastoma makes patients look like they are having a blast. It causes dancing eyes-dancing feet syndrome (opsoclonus-myoclonus).

Opsoclonus-myoclonus syndrome can also be seen in **adults**. It is associated with breast, gynecologic, and lung cancers. Patients with opsoclonus-myoclonus syndrome may have antibodies to Ri (ANNA-2).

Orthostatic Tremor

Orthostatic tremor is a 13-18 Hz tremor of the legs when standing. The calves cramp, and the thighs shake.

It causes a sense of unsteadiness.

It is relieved by sitting or walking.

Palatal Myoclonus/ Palatal Tremor

Palatal myoclonus is now referred to as **palatal tremor**.

It is divided into 2 categories.

1. **Essential palatal tremor**, which has no etiology
2. **Symptomatic palatal tremor**, which is associated with a structural lesion of the brainstem or cerebellum. (See below.)

Essential Palatal Tremor

Essential palatal tremor is characterized by a **clicking sound in the ear that resolves during sleep**. This is due to contractions of the tensor veli palatini, which result in movement of the palate.

Patients with **e**ssential palatal tremor have an **e**ar click that makes them <u>tense</u> due to the <u>tensor</u> veli palatini. Luckily, it **eases in sleep**.

Symptomatic Palatal Tremor

Unlike essential palatal myoclonus, symptomatic palatal myoclonus is due to contractions of the levator veli palatini. This causes the edges of the soft palate to move. It **continues in sleep**.

Symptomatic palatal tremor may be associated with oscillopsia, limb tremor, or tremor of other regions.

Since symptomatic palatal tremor is due to a **fixed lesion**, you can understand why it **continues in sleep.** Because the levator muscle is involved, the patient may be kept up awake (levated) all night!

Sometimes hypertrophy of the superior olive is seen on MRI in patients with symptomatic palatal tremor.

Palatal tremor may be seen with lesions in the **Triangle of Guillain-Mollaret**, which connects the dentate nucleus, contralateral red nucleus, and inferior olive.[8]

Pantothenate Kinase-associated Neurodegeneration (PKAN) (Hallervorden-Spatz)

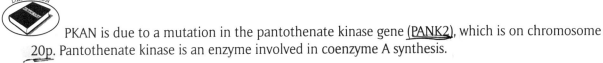

PKAN is one of the disorders associated with **neurodegeneration with brain iron accumulation**.

PKAN is due to a mutation in the pantothenate kinase gene (PANK2), which is on chromosome 20p. Pantothenate kinase is an enzyme involved in coenzyme A synthesis.

PKAN starts in childhood.

First rigidity is seen in the foot producing an **equinovarus deformity**. Then it is seen in the **hand**.

Patients also have **dysarthria, rigidity**, and **choreoathetosis**.

Some patients have **pigmentary retinopathy**.

Patients develop dementia and die in early childhood.

On MRI, decreased signal is seen in the globus pallidus due to iron deposition. It surrounds an area of hyperintensity. This results in "**the eye of the tiger**" sign.

Pathology also shows iron in the SNr and GPi. Spheroid bodies are seen in the cortex and basal ganglia.

Pantothenate **sounds like panther**, which is a jungle cat like a tiger. This may help you remember that pantothenate kinase-degeneration is associated with the **eye of the tiger sign**.

---

[8] See the Anatomy chapter for more information about the Triangle of Guillain-Mollaret.

Parkinson's Disease Versus Parkinsonian Features

If you see a patient with parkinsonian features, remember to look at the medications. Medications such as dopamine blockers or dopamine-depleting agents can cause parkinsonian symptoms. See the section on medication-induced movement disorders below.

Parkinson's Disease

Clinical Features of PD

Parkinson's disease is characterized by **resting tremor (4-6Hz), bradykinesia, rigidity**, and late **postural instability**. The mean age of onset is in the sixth decade.

Tremor in one hand, which is described as a **pill-rolling tremor**, is often the presenting symptom.

As the disease progresses, the patient with PD walks with elbows and knees flexed, **decreased arm swing**, and a **shuffling gait**.

Later in the course, patients **lose postural reflexes** and demonstrate **freezing**.

Masked facies and **micrographia** are also characteristic features of PD.

Eventually, **cognitive changes** may occur. **Dementia** can be seen later.

Also, **sleep disturbances** such as **REM-sleep behavior disorder** may occur in PD.

Pathology of PD

In PD, there is a loss of neuromelanin-containing neurons in the substantia nigra and locus ceruleus and a loss of pigmentation of these structures. The neurons in these regions contain **Lewy bodies**, which are eosinophilic cytoplasmic inclusions. (Lewy bodies are also found in aging and Dementia with Lewy Bodies.)

The loss of dopaminergic neurons that project to the striatum leads to a decrease in dopamine in the caudate and putamen. This ultimately leads to increased inhibition of thalamocortical neurons. (See above.)

Recall from the Neuropathology chapter that Lewy bodies contain alpha-synuclein (α-synuclein), and Parkinson's disease is considered a synucleinopathy like MSA and dementia with Lewy bodies.

Gait abnormalities in Parkinson's disease have been correlated with loss of neurons in the pedunculopontine nucleus (PPN).

Genetics of PD

There are multiple types of inherited PD. Luckily, there are fewer than types of SCA.

PARK 1

PARK 1 is due to mutations in the *SNCA* (alpha-synuclein) gene on 4q, which encodes **α-synuclein**. It is autosomal dominant.

It is associated with **early-onset Parkinson's disease**.

The protein α-synuclein is cleared through the ubiquitin proteasome pathway. Mutations in this protein interfere with its degradation and result in protein aggregation.

PARK 2

PARK 2 is associated with mutations in **parkin** on chromosome 6q. It is autosomal recessive. + hyperreflexia

Patients with PARK 2 tend to have **dystonia**. It is associated with juvenile-onset parkinsonism with slow progression. **Diurnal variation** and **improvement with sleep are seen in some patients**.

Parkin is an ubiquitin-protein ligase involved in protein degradation. A form of α-synuclein is a substrate for this enzyme.

PARK 4

The locus for PARK 4 is the same as PARK 1. PARK 4 is thought to be due to a triplication of the gene.

PARK 5

PARK 5 is associated with a mutation in the gene that encodes **ubiquitin carboxy-terminal hydrolase L1 (UCH-L1)**, which is on chromosome 4p.

PARK 6

PARK 6 is associated with mutations in *PINK1* on 1p , which encodes serine/threonine-protein kinase PINK1 (PTEN-induced kinase 1). This is an autosomal recessive form of early-onset parkinsonism.

---

9 PARK 3 was intentionally omitted.

PARK 7

PARK 7 is associated with a mutation in the *DJ-1* gene. Similar to PARK 6, this is an autosomal recessive early-onset form of parkinsonism and is due to a mutation on 1p.

Both DJ-1 and PINK1 are mitochondrial proteins.

PARK 8

PARK 8 is associated with a mutation in the *LRRK2* gene, which encodes leucine-rich repeat serine/threonine-protein kinase 2.

The G2019S mutation in the *LRRK2* gene is the most common mutation found in PD.[10]

PARK 8 causes a phenotype like idiopathic Parkinson's disease.

Treatment of PD

Medical Treatments of PD

Treatments for Parkinson's Disease

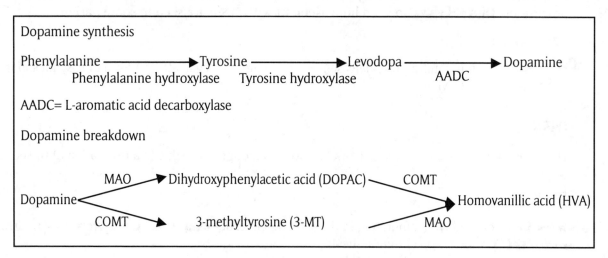

MAO = monoamine oxidase, COMT = catechol-O-methyltransferase

---

[10] Shapira, A. Etiology of Parkinson's disease. Neurology 2006;66:S10-23.

Types of agents used to treat PD:

- **Levodopa (L-dopa):** Carbidopa is combined with L-dopa in Sinemet. Carbidopa inhibits aromatic acid decarboxylase and prevents peripheral metabolism of L-dopa. There are multiple forms of Sinemet®, including an oral disintegrating form (Parcopa®).
- **Dopamine agonists:** bromocriptine (Parlodel®), pergolide (Permax®), pramipexole (Mirapex®), ropinirole (Requip®), apomorphine (Apokyn®)
- **Monamine oxidase B (MAOB) inhibitors:** selegiline (Eldepryl®, Emsam®, Zelapar®), rasagiline (Azilect®)

- **Indirect dopamine agonist:** amantadine (Symmetrel®)
- **Catecholamine-o-methyl transferase (COMT) inhibitors:** tol**capone** (Tasmar®), enta**capone** (Comtan®) – **THE CAPONE BROTHERS!!! They always said, "COM To Papa!"**
- **Anticholinergics:** trihexyphenidyl (Artane®) and benztropine (Cogentin®)
- **Combo pills:** Stalevo® combines carbidopa, levodopa, and entacapone.

Side Effects

- *Dopamine agonists* are associated with *sudden attacks of sleepiness.*
- Dopamine agonists that are *ergot derivatives* (pergolide and bromocriptine) may cause *pulmonary fibrosis, hallucinations, seizures, syncope,* or *erythromelalgia.*
- Amantadine can cause CHF, cardiac arrhythmias, and even bone marrow toxicity.
- *Tolcapone* is associated with *liver toxicity.* **Ol' Tol Capone got his Life into Trouble with Liver Toxicity.**
- *Anticholinergics* improve tremor and rigidity but may cause *confusion, constipation,* and *urinary retention.*

Surgery for PD

Targets of **surgery** and deep brain stimulation (DBS) for PD have included the ventral intermediate (VIM) nucleus of the thalamus, the internal segment of the globus pallidus (GPi), and the subthalamic nucleus (STN).

Thalamic DBS and thalamotomy primarily improve tremor.

The subthalamic nucleus is the most common target for DBS; this improves all motor symptoms.

Parkinson-Dementia-ALS Complex of Guam

Parkinson-dementia-ALS complex of Guam is found in Chamorro Indians.

 It may be related to ingestion of the ~~cycad nut.~~

Patients have symptoms of all disorders in the name: ~~parkinsonism, dementia, and motor neuron disease.~~

~~Neurofibrillary tangles~~ are seen.

Paroxysmal Dyskinesias

 Paroxysmal dyskinesias refer to conditions that are characterized by **intermittent athetosis, ballismus, chorea**, or **dystonia**. Each condition has different triggers.

Paroxysmal Kinesigenic Dyskinesia (PKD)

Attacks are **triggered by sudden movement** or **startle in patients with PKD**.

The attacks may occur multiple times per day. They are brief (seconds to minutes) and may *respond to phenytoin or carbamazepine.*

Paroxysmal Nonkinesigenic Dyskinesia (PNKD)

In PNKD, attacks start in childhood. They are **triggered by fatigue**, **alcohol, caffeine**, or **excitement** but <u>not</u> by exercise.

The attacks are longer (minutes to a few hours) than in PKD but are less frequent.

Paroxysmal Exertion-induced Dyskinesia

As one might expect, this is *due to exertion.*

Paroxysmal Hypnogenic Dyskinesia

In paroxysmal hypnogenic dyskinesia, **attacks occur in sleep**.

Pediatric Autoimmune Neuropsychiatric Disorder Associated with Streptococcal Infection (PANDAS)

PANDAS refers to a syndrome in children with a **RAPID ONSET** of tics, obsessive-compulsive behavior, (OCD), Tourette's Syndrome and other behavioral disturbances thought to be due to a recent infection with Group A -hemolytic *Streptococcus* *(such as Strep throat or Scarlet fever)*.

Onset is before puberty. Symptoms appear suddenly and/or are episodic. The neurologic symptoms should have a temporal association with the infection. PANDAS is thought to involve autoimmunity to the basal ganglia.

Pelizaeus-Merzbacher Disease

Pelizaeus-Merzbacher is a hypomyelinating leukoencephalopathy.

Classic Form

Classic **Peliz**aeus-Merzbacher disease presents in infancy with **abnormal eye movements**, such as **pendular nystagmus** or **roving eye movements**. Patients also have **head tremor/nodding**.

Later spasticity, ataxia, and **optic atrophy** are seen.

MRI shows **symmetric dysmyelination**. A **tigroid appearance** is due to small regions of normal neurons and myelin in the midst of abnormal white matter.

To remember this, think of the sign at the zoo: **PLEAZ** keep your **EYES** open for the **ROVING TIGER**! Anyone who reads the sign at the zoo will **nod their head** in agreement!

Death occurs in adolescence or early adulthood.

The classic form is **X-linked recessive**; it is due to a mutation in the *PLP1* gene on Xq, which encodes **proteolipid protein (PLP)**.

X-linked spastic paraplegia type 2 (SPG2) is also due to a mutation in the *PLP1* gene.

Connatal Form

The connatal form of Pelizaeus-Merzbacher disease, which is associated with absence of myelin, presents earlier and progresses faster than the classic form. It is autosomal recessive or X-linked.

Symptoms begin soon after birth.

Hypotonia, stridor, feeding difficulties, and extrapyramidal signs are seen.

Later, spasticity is seen. Development is delayed.

Patients die in the first decade.

Periodic Limb Movement Disorder

Periodic limb movement disorder is a sleep disorder diagnosed with polysomnography.

Patients with PLMD have daytime sleepiness or insomnia and excessive periodic limb movements (PLMS). Specifically, patients with PLMD have greater than 5 PLMS per hour of sleep.

Periodic limb movements (PLMS) are involuntary, stereotyped movements that meet specific criteria on polysomnography. They usually involve the legs and resemble a triple flexion response. They tend to last 0.5 – 10 seconds[11] and occur in a cluster of at least four movements separated by 5 to 90 seconds (usually 20 to 40 seconds).[12]

Periodic limb movements of sleep occur in **light sleep**.

Limbs with PLMS move in light sleep.

There are primary and secondary forms of PLMD.

Causes of secondary PLMD include uremia; diabetes; spinal cord injury; and abnormalities of iron, calcium, potassium, or magnesium.

To remember the causes of secondary PLMD, think about your Dear Uncle Stu who has this disease and Can't Move, Kick, or Feel his legs: Diabetes, Uremia, Spinal cord injury, calcium, magnesium, potassium (K+), and iron (Fe+++).

Antidepressants and caffeine can worsen PLMD.

---

[11] The old criteria used 5 seconds as the maximum.

[12] Zucconi M, Ferri R, Allen R, et al. The official World Association of Sleep Medicine (WASM) standards for recording and scoring periodic leg movements in sleep (PLMS) and wakefulness (PLMW) developed in collaboration with a task force from the International Restless Legs Syndrome Study Group (IRLSSG). Sleep Medicine 2006;7:175-183.

Treatments for primary PLMD include pramipexole, pergolide, Sinemet, clonazepam, carbamazepine, clonidine, and opiates.

Posthypoxic Myoclonus (Lance-Adams Syndrome)

This is myoclonus seen in a patient who has suffered a hypoxic injury.

Progressive Supranuclear Palsy (PSP)

PSP is one of the atypical parkinsonian disorders/Parkinsonism-plus syndromes.

Clinical Features of PSP

 Slow vertical saccades and square-wave jerks of the eyes are early eye findings in PSP.

Patients develop supranuclear ophthalmoplegia. **Downgaze is lost first.**

These patients have a **wide-eyed appearance** and tend to **hyperextend the neck**.

Patients with PSP have **postural instability** and **tend to fall backward**.

Like Parkinson's patients, these patients have **bradykinesia, rigidity,** and **dementia**. *axial rigidity*

Progressive supranuclear palsy patients also may have **pseudobulbar palsy**.

 Postural instability is more prominent in PSP than in Parkinson's disease, and patients with PSP lack tremor.

PSP could stand for

    Postural
    Stability is
    Poor.

If you stand on a precipice (**Pre<u>Si</u>Pice**), don't **gaze down**! Your **wide-eyed appearance** will cause you to **fall backwards**!

Neuropathologic changes are seen in the globus pallidus, subthalamic nucleus, hippocampus, entorhinal cortex, and the dentate nucleus of the cerebellum, in addition to the midbrain (superior colliculus, periaqueductal gray, red nucleus, and substantia nigra) and pons (locus ceruleus).

PSP is a tauopathy. As in CBGD, tau is found in glia and neurons. **Tau is found in oligodendrocytes as coiled bodies and as neurofibrillary tangles in neurons.**

rounded vs. flame shaped in AD

Patients with **CBGD** have **astrocyte plaques**.

Patients with **PSP** have **astrocytic tufts** (tuft-shaped astrocytes), which are tau-immunoreactive lesions.

Neuroimaging/Neuropathologic Findings of PSP

MRI shows **atrophy of the pons and midbrain in PSP**.

Ramsay Hunt Cerebellar Syndrome (Dyssynergia Cerebellaris Myoclonica)

Ramsay Hunt syndrome is also known as **progressive myoclonic ataxia**.

Patients with Ramsay Hunt syndrome have action and intention myoclonus, rare generalized tonic-clonic seizures, and cerebellar ataxia.

Patients with **Ramsay** Hunt syndrome may accidentally **ram** into things due to ataxia and myoclonus.

Ramsay Hunt syndrome also has been used to refer to an infection of the geniculate ganglion with varicella-zoster virus. This syndrome is now called Herpes zoster oticus. Ramsay Hunt syndrome can also refer to a third, albeit much less commonly referenced condition, an occupational-provoked deep-palmar-branch ulnar neuropathy, also called artisan's palsy.

Refsum Disease

Please see page 205-206 for info about Refsum disease.

Restless Leg Syndrome

Patients with restless leg syndrome (RLS) have an unpleasant sensation in the limbs, such as a crawling feeling, resulting in the desire to move them. Sensations are worse in the evening and when sitting or lying down. They are relieved by leg movement.

Patients with RLS may also have **periodic limb movement disorder**, which is a distinct condition that is diagnosed with objective testing. RLS may be primary (idiopathic) or secondary. Causes of **secondary RLS** include *pregnancy, kidney failure* (ARF), *and abnormalities of iron* (Fe+++), *calcium* (Ca++), *potassium* (K+), or *magnesium* (Mg++).

To remember the causes of secondary RLS, think about your father (Pa) who suffers from this disease:

PA Can't Move, Kick, or Feel his legs!
Pregnancy, ARF, Ca++, Mg++, K+, Fe+++

Treatments for primary RLS include dopaminergic medications (ropinirole, pramipexole, pergolide, bromocriptine, Sinemet); benzodiazepines such as clonazepam; and opiates.

Spasmus Nutans

Spasmus nutans is characterized by a triad:

1) Titubation / nodding of head

2) Nystagmus

3) Torticollis / neck in weird position

Patients with spasmus nutans present at 4 to 12 months of age. Symptoms usually resolve within one or two years.

A mass lesion of the optic chiasm or third ventricle is in the differential diagnosis.

To remember that spasmus nutans is associated with **T**itubation, **N**ystagmus, and **T**orticollis, remember the phrase: I would spaz if I saw T.N.T. **in my grandma's cellar!** (suprasellar glioma = grandma's super cellar)

There's a **Spasm of N's** with spasmus nutans:

Nystagmus

Nodding of head / titubation

Neck in weird position / torticollis

Spinocerebellar Ataxia (SCA)

SCA is a group of autosomal dominant ataxias associated with cerebellar atrophy.

There are many[13] forms of SCA.

SCA1, 2, 3, and 6 are the most common dominantly inherited ataxias.

Many SCAs are associated with an expanded triplet repeat. For instance, types 1, 2, 3, 6, 7, 12, and 17 are associated with CAG repeats. Recall the Huntington's disease and DRPLA are also associated with CAG repeats.

---

[13] About a kajillion.

SCA 1

SCA 1 is due to an expanded CAG repeat in the gene *ATXN1* on chromosome 6p, which conveniently encodes Ataxin1.

The age of onset is in the 30s. Patients have ataxia and spasticity. Pontocerebellar atrophy is seen on imaging.

SCA 2

SCA 2 is due to an expanded CAG repeat in the gene *ATXN2* on chromosome 12q, which encodes for Ataxin-2.

SCA 2 also presents in the thirties. It is associated with ataxia and early **slowing of saccades**. Patients with SCA 2 may have **ophthalmoplegia.**

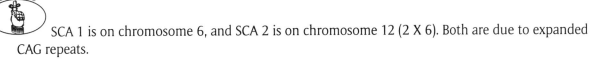 SCA 1 is on chromosome 6, and SCA 2 is on chromosome 12 (2 X 6). Both are due to expanded CAG repeats.

 People have 2 eyes, so eye findings (abnormal saccades and ophthalmoplegia) are found in SCA 2.

SCA 3/ Machado-Joseph Disease

SCA 3 is due to an expanded CAG repeat in the *ATXN3* gene on chromosome 14q.

SCA3 causes a progressive ataxia with additional features that vary.

There is a dystonic-rigid form; a parkinsonian form, which may be dopa-responsive; and a form with dystonia and peripheral neuropathy.

 Bulging eyes, ophthalmoplegia, tongue atrophy, facial fasciculations, and amyotrophy can be seen. Some patients have restless leg syndrome.

SCA 3 is the most common autosomal dominantly inherited ataxia in the US.

To remember the features of SCA 3/ Machado-Joseph Disease, think of this mnemonic: **Joseph's macho** three (3) **C**hildren **A**nd **G**randparents (CAG repeat) were told **REPEATEDLY** not to eat the bad nuts, but they **A**te **T**he **X**tra **N**uts (ATXN3) and now have **tongue atrophy, bulging eyes, and facial fasciculations**!

Dopa-responsive dystonia due to mutations in GTP cyclohydrolase 1 deficiency and Machado-Joseph disease, which has can cause parkinsonism that may be dopa-responsive or dystonia, are both due to mutations on 14q.

SCA 6

SCA 6 is due to an expanded CAG repeat in the *CACNA1A* gene on chromosome 19p, which encodes voltage-dependent P/Q-type calcium channel alpha-1A.

The age of onset is later for SCA 6. Patients have progressive cerebellar ataxia, dysarthria, and nystagmus. Imaging shows **pure (isolated) cerebellar atrophy**.

To remember that gene *CACNA1A* on chromosome 19p causes FHM1, EA2, and SCA6, think of this:

Have a **FEAST** on route **A1A** for **19** people!

The disorders in this mnemonic <u>are in order</u>: FHM-**1**, EA-**2**, and SCA-**6**. Route **_A1A_**=CACN*A1A*; 19 people = 19p.

Recall that mutations in this gene are also responsible for episodic ataxia type 2 (EA-2) and Familial Hemiplegic Migraine-1 (FHM1).

SCA 7

SCA 7 is associated with **retinal degeneration** and **vision loss**.

To remember that SCA 7 is associated with retinal degeneration, note that there are 7 letters in retinal.

SCA 8

TSCA 8 is associated with a CTG repeat. **CTG** repeat also may stand for **C**lutch **T**he **G**uardrail.

Anticipation is greater with maternal transmission in SCA8; whereas, the other SCAs have greater anticipation with paternal transmission.

Like myotonic dystrophy, SCA 8 is associated with a CTG repeat and has greater anticipation with maternal transmission.

To remember the triplet repeat and maternal transmission: If you have ataxia from SCA 8 or are unsteady when you skate (SCa8), think of your mother's advice to **C**lutch **T**he **G**uardrail.

SCA 10

Seizures are found in SCA 10. It is associated with an ATTCT repeat.

SCA-10 patients have **10 repeated ATTACKS** (ATTCT) of **seizures**.

Stereotypy

A stereotypy is a purposeless, patterned movement that a child performs repetitively, especially when excited. The child may be unaware of the behavior. An example is hand flapping.

Stiff Person Syndrome

Stiff person syndrome is a progressive disorder that results in symmetric stiffness and rigidity of the axial and proximal muscles. This is considered normal for people working in the undertaking/mortuary profession.

Patients with stiff person syndrome have a prominent lumbar lordosis and paraspinal hypertrophy.

They may also have painful spasms that can be due to startle or emotion.

— GABA neurons + pancreatic B cells

Anti-GAD (glutamic acid decarboxylase) antibodies are found in many patients with stiff person syndrome.

Stiff person syndrome may be a paraneoplastic condition; it may be seen with breast or small cell lung cancer.

To remember that stiff person syndrome is associated with anti-GAD antibodies: A patient with stiff person syndrome may think, "eGAD I'm stiff".

EMG shows continuous motor unit activity. *without neuromyotonia, pyramidal sx, EPS, spinal cord focal dxn*

Sydenham Chorea

Sydenham Chorea is a sign of rheumatic fever; it occurs 1-2 months after infection with Group A β-hemolytic *Streptococcus*.

Patients have chorea and may have emotional lability and obsessive-compulsive behavior.

Patients need treatment and then prophylaxis with penicillin.

Sydenham chorea is the number one cause of acquired chorea in childhood.

Torticollis

Torticollis is a focal dystonia.

There are multiple causes of torticollis.

If the **head is in a fixed position**, a **structural lesion** should be suspected.

If it occurs **episodically in an infant**, it may be **benign paroxysmal torticollis**, which is a *migraine variant.*

Recall that it is also seen in spasmus nutans.

Tourette's Syndrome

Tourette's syndrome criteria in brief:

· Onset less than 18 years.
· Tics for at least one year with no breaks greater than 3 months.
· At least one vocal and multiple motor tics.

Patients do not necessarily have coprolalia in Tourette's syndrome.

Look for **co-morbidities** such as **ADHD** and **OCD** in patients with Tourette's syndrome. Often these can be found in family members as well. *tx- guanfacin - α2 agonist*

To remember this trio of diseases, think of **OAT**s: an **O**CD patient **organizing** his morning **O**ATs, an **A**DHD patient **hyperactively** eating his O**A**Ts, and a Tourette patient repeatedly shouting, "OA**T**s!"

Whipple's Disease

Whipple's disease is due to *Tropheryma whippelii*, which is a gram-positive PAS-positive bacillus.

Diagnostic **triad** for Whipple's disease:

1) **Dementia**
2) **Supranuclear gaze palsy**
3) **Myoclonus**

Oculomasticatory and skeletal myorhythmias are pathognomonic for Whipple's disease.

Patients with Whipple's disease also may have **convergence-divergence nystagmus**.

Symptoms of Whipple's Disease *(triad first: My Super Duodenum)*

My Super Duodenum Smells Like We Can't Digest Nothing!

Myoclonus-**Supra**nuclear palsy-**D**ementia, **S**teatorrhea, **L**ymphadenopathy, **W**eight loss, **C**onvergence/**D**ivergence-**N**ystagmus!

Patients have systemic symptoms such as **lymphadenopathy, steatorrhea,** and **weight loss**.

 It may look like you are dancing and singing "Whip it" by Devo if you have Whipple's disease, due to the oculomasticatory and skeletal myorhythmias.

Wilson's Disease (Hepatolenticular Degeneration)

Wilson's disease is an autosomal recessive neurodegenerative disorder due to a defect in copper metabolism.

It is due to mutations in the ***ATP7B* gene on chromosome 13q**. This gene codes for **copper transporting adenosine triphosphatase, which transports copper from the hepatocyte into the bile**.

Patients **less than 10 years** of age present with **liver failure**.

Over 10 years, patients tend to have **neurologic** or **psychiatric symptoms**.

Patients with Wilson's disease have **dysarthria, dystonia, dysdiadochokinesia**, and sometimes **drooling**.

Other characteristic features of Wilson's disease include a **wing-beating tremor, Kayser-Fleischer rings, sunflower cataracts**, and **risus sardonicus (a rigid, devilish smile)**.

A **Kayser-Fleischer ring** is an abnormality of the cornea due to copper deposition in Descemet's membrane. It can be detected with a slit-lamp.

Bulbar dystonia causes dysarthria and risus sardonicus and may result in a whining noise upon inspiration.

Other movement disorders can also be seen in Wilson's disease such as ataxia, parkinsonism, and chorea.

Patients with Wilson's disease have decreased serum ceruloplasmin, decreased serum copper, and increased urinary copper excretion.

Due to changes in signal in the midbrain, T2-weighted MRI images may show **face of the giant panda**.

Alzheimer type I and type II astrocytes are found in Wilson's disease. Alzheimer type I astrocytes are more common.

Wilson's disease is treated with **Chelation**. *D-penicillamine, ammonium tetrathiomolybdate, zinc, and triethylene tetramine dihydrochloride* have been used.

To remember how to treat Wilson's, **TRI DAZ Chelation**:

TRIethylene tetramine dihydrochloride,

D-penicillamine,

Ammonium tetrathiomolybdate,

Zinc.

Chelation

Menkes' Kinky Hair Disease versus Wilson's Disease

Both Menkes' Disease and Wilson's Disease involve copper-transporting ATPase.

· In **Menkes' disease**, the **alpha** subunit is involved.

· In **Wilson's disease**, the **beta** subunit is involved.

· In Menkes' kinky hair disease, the **a**lpha subunit is defective, and there's an **a**bsorption problem in the GI tract/**a**bdomen.

· In Wilson's disease, the **b**eta subunit is defective, and there's a **b**ile problem.

	Menkes' Kinky Hair Disease	Wilson's Disease
Subunit involved	Alpha	Beta
Serum copper	Low	Low
Serum ceruloplasmin	Low	Low
Liver copper	Low	High
Treatment	Copper	**TRI DAZ Chelation**

Medication-induced Movement Disorders

Acute Dystonic Reaction

An acute dystonic reaction may cause **opisthotonus**, an **oculogyric crisis**, or affect the neck or face.

It is seen with dopamine receptor blockers (especially the D2 receptor), such as **neuroleptics**.

Antiemetics such as *metoclopramide* (Reglan®), *prochlorperazine* (Compazine®), and *promethazine* (Phenergan®) can also cause an acute dystonic reaction.

Acute dystonic reaction is treated with *anticholinergics* such as Benadryl® (diphenhydramine) and cogentin.

Chorea

Many medications can cause chorea. Examples include: *lithium, amphetamines, theophylline, birth control pills*, some *antiepileptic medications* (phenytoin, carbamazepine, and valproate), and some *antidepressants*.

Patients with Parkinson's disease may develop chorea secondary to dopaminergic agents.

Cocaine can cause chorea.

Poisoning with carbon monoxide, mercury, or organophosphates can also cause chorea.

Neuroleptic Malignant Syndrome (NMS)

NMS is a reaction to medications that block specific dopamine receptors (D2 receptors).

It is characterized by *muscle rigidity* and *hyperthermia*.

Autonomic dysfunction, altered mental status, leukocytosis, and an elevated creatine kinase also tend to be present in NMS.

NMS can also occur with rapid withdrawal of dopaminergic agents.

 NMS is treated with dopaminergic agents such as bromocriptine or dantrolene.

Parkinsonism

Drug-induced parkinsonism is usually due to D2 receptor blockade or a dopamine-depleting agents such as alpha-methyldopa or reserpine.

 MPTP, manganese, and carbon monoxide are toxins that cause parkinsonism.
   MPTP: **M**ight **P**rovoke **T**errible **P**arkinsonism! (Substantia Nigra)

Carbon Monoxide Can Murder everyone on the **globe** (necrosis of the globus pallidus).

Manganese toxicity can deplete dopamine in the caudate and putamen and deposit in the substantia nigra.   \GP

methanol → putamen damage

 When you hear of manganese toxicity, think of the man who gannot move with ease anymore.

In turn, this can decrease spontaneous motor activity and look like Parkinson's disease as well.

Serotonin Syndrome

Serotonin Syndrome is due to toxic levels of serotonin.

First **D**iarrhea is seen. This is followed by **R**estlessness.

Then, **A**ltered **M**entation, autonomic **I**nstability, **R**igidity, and **T**emperature elevation are seen, similar to NMS.

   Ser DR. -- AM I Rigid? MY TEMP Elevated?

In the final stages, serotonin syndrome can cause coma, status epilepticus, and cardiovascular collapse resulting in death.

However, unlike NMS, Serotonin Syndrome **may cause MYoclonus**.

Patients with Parkinson's disease who are taking MAO-B inhibitors, such as selegiline (Eldepryl) or rasagiline (Azilect), are at risk for Serotonin Syndrome, if they are placed on a SSRI.

Tardive Dyskinesia

Tardive dyskinesias are medication-induced movements associated with chronic use of dopamine receptor blockers, particularly D2 receptor antagonists. Commonly, masticatory movements are seen.

Tardive dyskinesia is **less likely to be seen with quetiapine** and **clozapine** than other neuroleptics.

However, **clozapine** is associated with **agranulocytosis** and **lowers the seizure threshold**.

List of Mosts

Essential tremor is the **most common tremor**.

Sydenham chorea is the most common cause of **acquired chorea in childhood**.

SCA 3 (Machado-Joseph disease) is the most common **autosomal dominantly inherited ataxia in the US**.

Movement Disorders Quiz

(Answers on page 741)

1. Match the disease with the triplet repeat with which it is associated.

    1) DRPLA   A. CAG

    2) Friedreich's ataxia   B. CTG

    3) Huntington disease   C. GAA

    4) SCA 3 (Machado-Joseph disease)

    5) SCA 8

2. Deficiency of which vitamin causes a phenotype similar to Friedreich's ataxia?

    A. Vitamin A

    B. Vitamin B12

    C. Vitamin C

    D. Vitamin E

3. Match the imaging finding with the disease.

    1) Batwing   A. Glutaric acidemia type 1

    2) Eye of the tiger   B. MSA

    3) Face of the giant panda   C. PKAN

    4) Hot cross bun   D. Wilson's disease

4. Which of the following is not associated with Corticobasal Ganglionic Degeneration (CBGD)?

    A. Astrocytic plaques

    B. Astrocytic tufts

    C. Ballooned neurons

    D. Coiled bodies of tau in oligodendrocytes

    E. Degeneration of the substantia nigra and striatum

5. Match the eye findings with the disease. Answers may be used more than once. There may be more than one correct answer.

1) Abetalipoproteinemia (Bassen-Kornzweig syndrome)   A. Kayser-Fleischer rings

2) Ataxia with isolated vitamin E deficiency (AVED)   B. Pendular eye movements

3) HARP syndrome   C. Retinitis pigmentosa

4) Pelizaeus-Merzbacher disease   D. Sunflower cataracts

5) Whipple's disease   E. Supranuclear gaze palsy

6) Wilson's disease

Chapter 7

Neurocutaneous Disorders
(Also known as Phakomatoses)

Ataxia-Telangiectasia (AT)

Genetics of AT

Ataxia-telangiectasia is an autosomal recessive condition due to a defect is in the ATM gene (Ataxia Telangiectasia Mutant gene), which is on chromosome 11q. The ATM protein coordinates the responses to the double-stranded DNA break.

Patients with ataxia-telangiectasia have a defect in DNA repair.

Other neurological conditions associated with **defective DNA repair** include **Cockayne syndrome** and **xeroderma pigmentosa**. See below.

Clinical Features of AT

Clinical Course

Patients with AT present with ataxia when they start to walk around one year of age.

The presenting symptoms of AT:

- Mainly **truncal ataxia** is seen.
- **Eye telangiectasias** appear at 3-5 years of age.
- **Skin telangiectasias** may appear on the ears, nose, cheeks, neck, and creases of forearms between ages 3-7 years.

At around 5 years of age, children with AT develop **recurrent sinopulmonary infections**.

Abnormal movements associated with AT include:

- **A**thetosis
- **T**remor.
- **M**yoclonic jerks

Think of **A T**remulous **M**an with **A**thetosis, **T**remor, and **M**yoclonic jerks, who requests $**11** (chromosome 11) from an **ATM** (the ATM gene), but the bank's ATM is **defective** and needs **repair** (**defect** in DNA **repair**).

 Patients with AT can develop a polyneuropathy.

Reflexes are <u>decreased or absent</u> after age 7 or 8 years.

Usually children lose the ability to walk independently by age 12 years and are wheelchair dependent.

Other Clinical Findings

Eyes

 In addition to eye telangiectasias, children with AT also have **oculomotor apraxia**.

Skin

Dermatological manifestations of AT could include:

- Progeric skin
- Hair changes
- Café-au-lait patches.

Neurologic

Patients with AT are often dysarthric and can develop a polyneuropathy.

Abnormal movements associated with AT include:

- Choreoathetosis
- Myoclonic jerks
- Tremor.

Reflexes are decreased or absent after age 7 or 8 years.

Oncologic

Children with ataxia-telangiectasia are at A ONE HUNDRED FOLD *increased risk for malignancy*, especially **L**ymphoma and **L**eukemia (L&L). Mothers of children with ataxia-telangiectasia are at increased risk for breast cancer.[1]

Laboratory/Pathology of AT

Laboratory findings in AT include:

Increased	Decreased
AFP and CEA	Ig**A**, Ig**G**, Ig**E** (AGE)

To remember the specific low Immunoglobulins. Remember that AT affects patients of a young (low) AGE!

Cells are hypersensitive to radiation in vitro due to defective DNA repair.

MRI shows *cerebellar atrophy.*

Additional findings include degeneration of the posterior columns and loss of cells from the dorsal root ganglia and anterior horn cells.

Of course, the **ATM** should produce **CASH**:

    Cancer - especially **L**ymphoma and **L**eukemia (L&L), *cerebellar atrophy*

    Ataxia, oculomotor **A**praxia, **A**FP elevated, and **A**GE decreased
    (low Immunoglobulins IgA, IgG, and IgE)

    Sinopulmonary infections

    Hypersensitivity to radiation

---

[1] Chenevix-Trench G, Spurdle A, Gatei M, et al. Dominant negative ATM mutations in breast cancer families. Journal of the National Cancer Institute 2002; 94:205-215.

Cockayne Syndrome

Cockayne syndrome is a disorder of DNA repair.

 Patients with Cockayne syndrome have **progeria, cataracts, photosensitive skin, and short stature**. They **lack adipose tissue**.

Neurologic problems include mental retardation, ataxia, basal ganglia calcifications, patchy demyelination, and peripheral neuropathy. They also develop pigmentary retinopathy, sensorineural deafness, and contractures.

Patients with **Cockayne** syndrome are very thin and look older than they are, like someone who spends all their money on **cocaine**.

Hypomelanosis of Ito

Genetics of Hypomelanosis of Ito

The inheritance of Hypomelanosis of Ito is usually sporadic. However, there are some links to chromosomes X, 12 and 18. The incidence of Ito is 1/8,000.

Clinical Features of Hypomelanosis of Ito

Skin

Skin findings include *hypopigmented whorls* and *streaks*, usually following *Blaschko's lines*.

Neurologic

The most common neurologic findings in Hypomelanosis of Ito are **seizures** and **mental retardation**. **Infantile spasms** are seen in about 10% of patients.

Patients may have *gray matter heterotopias, macrocephaly, hemimegalencephaly,* or *autistic features*.

Musculoskeletal

The most common musculoskeletal abnormality in Hypomelanosis of Ito is **hemihypertrophy**.

Incontinentia Pigmenti (IP)

Genetics of IP

 Incontinentia Pigmenti (IP) is X-linked **dominant**.

> The following are other X-linked dominant disorders in addition to Incontinentia Pigmenti:
>
> Rett syndrome
>
> Aicardi syndrome
>
> Periventricular Nodular Heterotopia[2]

Incontinentia Pigmenti is caused by a mutation at Xq in the NF-kappa-B essential modulator gene (NEMO).

 Incontinentia Pigmenti is associated with NEMO. To remember this, think of water when you see **incontinent** in **Incontinent**ia and recall that NEMO swims in water. The film "Finding Nemo" dominated the bo**X** offices and that's how you can remember that incontinentia pigmenti is an X-linked dominant disorder.

Clinical Features of IP

IP often involves the *eyes, skin, teeth*, and *CNS*.

Neurologic Manifestations

Seizures are the most common neurologic finding and begin in the first few weeks of life. Mental retardation and spasticity are also seen.

Dermatologic Manifestations

Skin findings go through 4 stages:

    1) Vesicular = <u>BULLAE</u>

    2) Verrucous = <u>W</u>ARTS

---

[2] Due to a defect in the filamin A gene.

3) Hyperpigmented = "<u>MARBLECAKE</u>" TRUNK

4) Atrophic/Hypopigmented = <u>LINEAR ALOPECIA</u>

Patients may have pegged/conical teeth or lack teeth.

NEMO went through **4 stages** of life yet still has **NO teeth** because he ate **Black & White Marblecakes in a Line!**

Eye Manifestations

Multiple ophthalmological findings can be seen in IP including:

- Microphthalmos
- Keratitis
- Cataracts
- Optic atrophy
- Retinal anomalies.

Klippel-Trenaunay-Weber Syndrome

Like patients with Sturge-Weber syndrome (see below), patients with Klippel-Trenaunay-Weber syndrome have a <u>port-wine stain/hemangioma</u>.

In **Klippel-Trenaunay-Weber syndrome**, the skin lesion(s) may involve the face, trunk, or extremities. To remember **KTW** syndrome: **eKstremities-Trunk-Wine face**

In **Sturge-Weber syndrome**, the port-wine stain tends to occur in the V1 or V2 distribution of the face.

Patients with Klippel-Trenaunay-Weber syndrome also have <u>venous varicosities</u> and **unilateral limb hypertrophy** due to bone and/or soft tissue enlargement.

Possible neurologic findings include: macrocephaly, an intracranial angioma, or a spinal arteriovenous malformation.

Linear Sebaceous Nevus Syndrome

Linear sebaceous nevus syndrome is a form of epidermal nevus syndrome characterized by a **linear nevus** usually on the **face** or **scalp**. **Hemihypertrophy** and/or **hemimegalencephaly** *ipsilateral* to the nevus can occur.

Mental retardation and seizures may be present. EEG abnormalities, if seen, are ipsilateral to the nevus.

Neurofibromatosis (NF)

· Neurofibromatosis type 1 is the most common neurocutaneous syndrome. The 2nd most common is Tuberous Sclerosis.

· Both Neurofibromatosis type 1 and Neurofibromatosis type 2 are autosomal dominant and result from mutations in tumor suppressor genes.

Neurofibromatosis Type I (NF1)

NF1 is due to mutations in the *NF1* gene at 17q.

The protein encoded by this gene, **neurofibromin**, plays a role in the negative regulation of the RAS proto-oncogene.

Neurofibromin facilitates the conversion of guanosine triphosphate (GTP)-bound RAS, which is active, to guanosine diphosphate (GDP)-bound RAS, which is inactive. In NF1, absence of neurofibromin leads to more active RAS, which leads to increased cell growth and tumor formation.

The word neurofibromatosis has 17 letters and it is due to a mutation in a gene on chromosome 17. The eponym for this disease is Von Recklinghausen syndrome, which also has 17 letters, ironically!!!

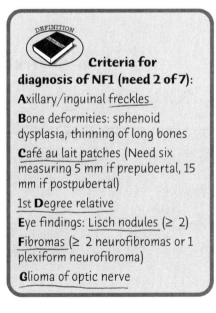

Criteria for diagnosis of NF1 (need 2 of 7):

Axillary/inguinal freckles

Bone deformities: sphenoid dysplasia, thinning of long bones

Café au lait patches (Need six measuring 5 mm if prepubertal, 15 mm if postpubertal)

1st **D**egree relative

Eye findings: Lisch nodules (≥ 2)

Fibromas (≥ 2 neurofibromas or 1 plexiform neurofibroma)

Glioma of optic nerve

Normal

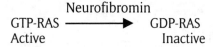

GTP-RAS   Neurofibromin   →   GDP-RAS
Active   Inactive

NF-1

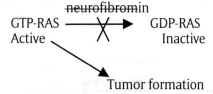

GTP-RAS ——✗——→ GDP-RAS
Active   ~~neurofibrom~~in   Inactive

Tumor formation

The most common CNS tumor in NF1 is optic nerve glioma.

In addition to the conditions above, patients with NF1 can have **ADHD** and **learning disabilities**.

Compression of the renal artery, renal artery stenosis, or pheochromocytoma can cause hypertension.

Neurofibromatosis Type 2 (NF2)

Diagnostic Criteria

Bilateral acoustic nerve tumor

OR

A unilateral eighth nerve tumor and a first degree relative with NF2

OR

Any two of the following and a first degree relative with NF2:

    1. Neurofibroma

    2. Meningioma

    3. Glioma

    4. Schwannoma

    5. Juvenile posterior subcapsular lenticular opacity.

Clinical Features

NF2 is associated with fewer or no skin lesions compared to NF1.

Progressive deafness occurs in NF2.

Genetics

NF2 is due to mutations in **merlin.** Chromosomal locus: 22q.

It's somewhat magical that NF2 is due to a gene defect on chromosome 22 and is associated with 2 (**bi**lateral) vestibular schwannomas. No wonder the gene is called merlin.

The severity of NF2 depends on the type of merlin mutation: **M**issense mutations tend to cause **M**ild disease. However nonsense or frame-shift mutations in merlin cause severe disease! Severity also depends on the splice site.

	NF1	NF2
Chromosome	17	**22**
Protein	Neurofibromin	**Merlin**

> ### Heading up to Number 17
>
> **Big Heads**
>
> **NF1, Alexander's disease,** and **Canavan's disease** (aspartoacylase deficiency) all cause **macrocephaly** and are found on **chromosome** 17.
>
> **Little Heads**
>
> On the other hand, **lissencephaly** due to LIS1 and **Miller-Diecker** are associated with **microcephaly** and are also found on **chromosome 17.**
>
> **After drinking 17 Miller beakers (Miller-Diecker) Lisa has a Little (micro) LISp.**

Osler-Weber-Rendu Syndrome
(Also known as Hereditary Hemorrhagic Telangiectasia = HHT)

Clinical Features of HHT

Patients with Osler-Weber-Rendu syndrome have **skin** **angiomas** and **angiomas in the gastrointestinal** and **genitourinary tracts, nose, lung, and CNS**.

Recurrent epistaxis is frequently the first symptom, often presenting around *age 12.*

Gastrointestinal bleeding (hematochezia/melena) is also a common symptom.

When you see Osler-Weber-Rendu think, *"Will you hand me a tissue?"* These patients can frequently present with recurrent epistaxis.

Neurologic complications:

- AVMs in the lung can lead to brain abscesses and embolic strokes.
- Brain AVMs can cause intracranial hemorrhage and subarachnoid hemorrhage.
- Paraparesis may occur if a spinal AVM bleeds.

Genetics of HHT

HHT is autosomal dominant.

HHT 1

Hereditary Hemorrhagic Telangiectasia type 1 (HHT1) is caused by mutations in the **endoglin gene (ENG) at 9q**. Endoglin is a component of transforming growth factor beta (TGF-beta) receptor complex.

Recall that TSC1 (Tuberous Sclerosis Complex 1) and DYT1 also have gene loci at 9q.

HHT 2

Hereditary Hemorrhagic Telangiectasia type 2 is due to a mutation in ACVRL1 (at 12q). ACVRL1 encodes the activin receptor-like kinase 1, a receptor for the TGF superfamily of ligands.

To remember the differences between HH1 and HH2, think of this:

Highschool part 1 (9th grade **ENG**lish class: a transforming growth field (TGF) in your life.)

and

Highschool part 2 (12th grade **A**nte-**C**ollege **V**ery **R**elaxed **L**ife to spend more time with your superfamily.)

PHACES Syndrome

PHACES syndrome is characterized by **P**osterior fossa malformations, **H**emangiomas of the face, **A**rterial anomalies, **C**oarctation of the aorta and other cardiac defects, **E**ye abnormalities, and **S**ternal clefting or **S**upraumbilical raphe.

 Cases of PHACES syndrome have been mistaken for Sturge-Weber syndrome.

Dandy-Walker syndrome can be seen as part of PHACES syndrome.[3]

Sturge-Weber Syndrome (SWS)
(Also known as **encephalotrigeminal angiomatosis**)

 However, we'll call it **S**tained-**W**ine **S**yndrome.

Genetics of SWS

SWS occurs sporadically with no inheritance pattern.

Clinical Features of SWS

Clinical features of Sturge-Weber syndrome include a **facial port-wine nevus** and **ipsilateral Lepto-Meningeal Angioma**, usually over the *Occipital region.*

Just think when someone spills wine on your face you'll text your friends:
LMAO !! for **Lepto-Meningeal Angioma**, over the **O**ccipital region.

Skin

The **port wine stain** typically occurs in the ophthalmic (V1) and maxillary (V2) distributions of the trigeminal nerve.

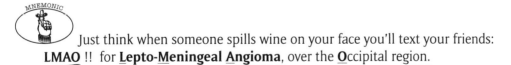

---

[3] Additional information can be found in the Pediatric Neurology chapter.

Eye

Glaucoma is the primary ophthalmologic problem. **Buphthalmos** (eye enlarges and protrudes out of its socket) can be seen.

Neurologic

Neurologic manifestations of SWS include **hemiparesis** contralateral to the facial lesion, **seizures**, **intellectual impairment**, and **possibly hemianopia**. Episodes of **transient hemiplegia** can occur; some are associated with **migraine-type headaches**.

Hemispherectomy is sometimes necessary due to intractable seizures.

Imaging of SWS

Gyral calcification can be seen on CT. Classically, x-**rays showed "trolley-track" / "tram-track" cal-cifications** over the occipital or parieto-occipital regions.

Tuberous Sclerosis (TS)
(Also known as Bourneville's Disease)

TS is characterized by Vogt's triad and spells out SAM:

1) **S**eizures/Epilepsy
2) **A**denoma **S**ebaceum
3) **M**ental retardation/Stupid

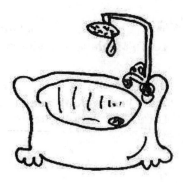

To remember Vogt's triad, think of your friend **SAM** in your **Tub**! Only about 33% of all TS patients have the full triad. And, of course, **SAM** would never use your **Tub** without your permission.

Clinical Features of TS

Skin

Cutaneous lesions in TS:

- **Ash-leaf spots**-hypopigmented macules. (A Wood's lamp may help to find these.)
- **Adenoma sebaceum** on face usually by age 4
- **Shagreen patch**-rough area of skin usually over the lumbosacral region
- Café au lait patches
- **Fingernail or toenail fibromas**
  SAM was cutting his **toenails** and drinking a **Café au lait in your Tub.** How rude!

Eyes

- Hamartomas of the retina or optic nerve
- **Mulberry tumor** of the optic disc

Systemic

- Renal hamartoma, cysts, carcinoma, Renal angiomyolipoma
- Pulmonary hamartoma, Lymphangiomyomatosis, spontaneous pneumothorax
- Cardiac rhabdomyoma

To remember the systemic features of TS, think of "**MY, MY, MY**!" which is what you said when you saw **SAM** in your **Tub**!

CNS

- **Subependymal nodules** on lateral ventricles
- **Cortical tubers**   *SEGA, seizures, stupid*
- Infantile spasms
- Mental retardation
- **S**ub**E**pendymal **G**iant cell **A**strocytoma—SEGA—**now SAM is playing SEGA in your Tub!**

The FDA approved everolimus (Afinitor), which is a mTOR inhibitor, to treat SEGA in TS patients. **Vigabatrin** is the drug of choice to treat infantile spasms in patients with TS.

Diagnostic Criteria for TS

Revised Diagnostic Criteria for Tuberous Sclerosis Complex (TSC)

Definite TSC: Either 2 major features or 1 major with 2 minor features.
Probable TSC: One major feature and one minor feature.
Possible TSC: Either 1 major feature or 2 or more minor features.

Major Features

1. Facial angiofibromas or forehead plaque
2. Ungual or periungual fibroma—cut SAM's nails
3. Hypomelanotic macules (> 3)
4. Shagreen patch
5. Multiple retinal nodular hamartomas
6. Cortical tuber
7. Subependymal nodule
8. **S**ub**E**pendymal **G**iant cell **A**strocytoma—SEGA
9. Cardiac rhabdomyoma-**MY**
10. Lymphangiomyomatosis-**MY**
11. Renal angiomyolipoma-**MY**

Minor Features

1. Multiple pits in dental enamel
2. Hamartomatous rectal polyps
3. Bone cysts
4. Cerebral white matter radial migration lines
5. Gingival fibromas
6. Non-renal hamartoma
7. Retinal achromic patch
8. Confetti skin lesions
9. Multiple renal cysts

To make things even more confusing:

· When cortical dysplasia and cerebral white matter migration tracts are both present, they should be counted as one feature.
· When both lymphangiomyomatosis and renal angiomyolipomas are present, other features are needed for definitive diagnosis.

Genetics of TS

Disease	Gene Product	Genetic locus
TS-1	Hamartin	9q
TS-2	Tuberin	16p

 This is one situation in which the gene defects are in **alphabetical order** and the chromosomal defects are in numerical order.

Both TS-1 and TS-2 are autosomal dominant. Likewise, NF1 and NF2 are autosomal dominant.

Von Hippel-Lindau Disease (VHL)

Genetics of VHL

VHL is autosomal dominant. It is due to mutations in the VHL tumor suppressor gene located on chromosome 3p.

VHL has 3 letters and is on chromosome 3. Also, remember that VHS tapes were played on channel 3.

Clinical Features of VHL

Patients with VHL may have:

- **Retinal hemangioblastomas**
- **CNS hemangioblastomas**
- **Pancreatic cysts**
- **Hepatic cysts**
- **Renal tumors**
- **Pheochromocytoma**.

Recall that pheochromocytomas are also seen in NF. If you see a cerebellar hemangioblastoma in an adult, think of Von Hippel-Lindau disease (VHL).

Think of VHL as **V**on **H**emangioblastoma.

Xeroderma Pigmentosa (XP)

Xeroderma pigmentosa is a neurodegenerative disease associated with defective DNA repair.

Patients with xeroderma pigmentosa have photosensitive skin from infancy and are at a ONE-THOUSAND FOLD increased risk for skin cancer and an increased risk for ocular melanoma.

Patients with XP must avoid the sun!!

Premature cutaneous ageing results in easy freckling, sunburns, and blisters.

Neurologic symptoms that may be seen in XP include **acquired microcephaly, dementia, sensorineural hearing loss, ataxia,** and **peripheral neuropathy**.

To remember XP features, think of XP standing for:

    X - e**X**tra small head, e**X**tremely confused, e**X**tremely deaf, and ata**X**ic

    P - **P**eripheral neuropathy, **P**remature cutaneous ageing, **P**hotosensitive skin

Cerebro-Tendonous Xanthomatosis (CTX)
(also known as Van Bogaert-Scherer-Epstein syndrome)

Patients with CTX have excess **cholestanol** (a form of cholesterol) deposit in their brain and other tissues.

"Lipid nodules" especially collect in the cerebellum, Achilles' tendons, and eyes.

Clinical Features of CTX

 Symptoms include tendineous or tuberous xanthomas, juvenile cataracts, and progressive cerebellar ataxia (beginning after puberty).

And oh yeah, chronic diarrhea.

Genetics of CTX

CTX is an autosomal recessive disorder associated with mutations in the CYP27A1 gene, located on chromosome 2q.

Patients are treated with chenodeoxycholic acid (CDCA) and a statin for elevated cholesterol (although LDL is usually normal).

Pseudo-Xanthoma Elasticum (PXE)
(also known as Grönblad–Strandberg syndrome)

PXE causes fragmentation and mineralization of elastic fibers in the skin, eyes, and blood vessels (premature atherosclerosis).

Clinical Features of PXE

Yellow Skin: Cutaneous laxity/redundancy; small, yellow, papules in the neck, axillae, groin, and flexural creases.

 "Oblique mental creases" can form, with diagonal grooves in the chin.

Orange Eyes: Dimpling of the Bruch membrane (which separates the retina's blood vessel layer from its pigment layer), called peau d'orange (French for "skin of an orange").

"Angioid streaks" develop from elastic fiber mineralization, and provoke retinal hemorrhages and loss of central vision.

Red Legs: Premature atherosclerosis causes intermittent claudication (leg pain during walking, resolves at rest), but also coronary artery disease (angina/MI) and stroke.

Genetics of PXE

PXE is caused by autosomal recessive mutations in the *ABCC6* gene on chromosome 16p.

Wyburn-Mason Syndrome (WMS)
(also known as Bonnet-Dechaumme-Blanc syndrome)

Clinical Features of WMS

 WMS is characterized by arteriovenous malformations (AVMs) in the retina of one eye and in the CNS.

Larger AVMs causing visual or neurologic impairment are usually diagnosed earlier, and smaller AVMs can go undiagnosed for years, making the presentation quite diverse.

Besides variations in CNS lesion size, different AVM locations and configurations also may provoke anything from mental changes to headaches to seizures to hemiparesis to cranial nerve palsies.

- Orbital involvement can present with proptosis, which may be pulsatile with a bruit. So listen to your patient's eyeball!

Other AVMs may be present elsewhere in the body, including facial skin, eyelids, cheeks, forehead, oronasopharnyx, orbit, lung, and bone.

Genetics of WMS

This condition is thought to be congenital, nonhereditary, and without sex or race predilection.

Neurocutaneous Disorders Quiz

(Answers on page 743)

1. Match the inheritance pattern to the disease.

     1) Ataxia-telangiectasia

     2) Neurofibromatosis type 1 (NF1)

     3) Neurofibromatosis type 2 (NF2)

     4) Osler-Weber-Rendu

     5) Sturge-Weber Syndrome

     6) Tuberous Sclerosis Complex-1 (TSC-1)

     7) Tuberous Sclerosis Complex-2 (TSC-2)

     8) Incontinentia Pigmenti

     A. Sporadic

     B. Autosomal dominant

     C. Autosomal recessive

     D. X-linked dominant

     E. X-linked recessive

2. Match the genetic locus with the disease.

     1) 3p

     2) 9q

     3) 9q

     4) 16p

     5) 17q

     6) 22q

     A. Hereditary Hemorrhagic Telangiectasia Type 1

     B. Neurofibromatosis type 1

     C. Neurofibromatosis type 2

     D. Tuberous Sclerosis

     E. Von Hippel-Lindau

3. Match the gene product with the disease.

      1) Activin receptor-like kinase 1

      2) Endoglin

      3) Hamartin

      4) Merlin

      5) Neurofibromin

      6) Tuberin

      A. HHT1

      B. HHT2

      C. NF1

      D. NF2

      E. TSC-1

      F. TSC-2

4. Match the tumor with the disease with which it tends to be associated.

      1) Bilateral acoustic nerve tumor

      2) Cardiac rhabdomyoma

      3) Hemangioblastoma

      4) Lymphoma

      5) Leukemia

      6) Mulberry tumor of the optic disc

      7) Optic glioma

      8) Pheochromocytoma

      9) Pulmonary hamartoma

      10) Renal hamartoma

      11) Subependymal Giant Cell Astrocytoma

      A. Ataxia-Telangiectasia

      B. NF1

      C. NF2

      D. Tuberous Sclerosis

      E. Von Hippel-Lindau

Chapter 8

Neurodegenerative Diseases

Alzheimer's Disease (AD)

Alzheimer's disease is the most common dementia in the U.S.

Clinical Findings

AD causes a cortical dementia.

Memory loss is the main complaint initially. Patients have difficulty retaining new information. **Remote memory is intact until later**.

Speech declines. Patients initially have **difficult naming**. Later, they become almost mute.

In addition to aphasia, **apraxias** occur in Alzheimer's disease and other cortical dementias.

Agnosias, such as **prosopagnosia** and **anosognosia**, are also seen in Alzheimer's disease.

Alzheimer's disease is associated with **a**praxia, **a**nomia, and **a**gnosia.[1]

Patients with Alzheimer's disease may suffer from depression or paranoid delusions.

Pathology

Grossly, Alzheimer's disease is characterized by **generalized cortical atrophy**.

The **hippocampus is involved early**.

Alzheimer's disease is a **tauopathy**.[2]

> **Pathology of Alzheimer's disease:**
> - Amyloid deposition
> - Granulovacuolar degeneration
> - Hirano bodies
> - Neuritic plaques
> - Neurofibrillary tangles

---

[1] See the Behavioral Neurology chapter for definitions of these terms.

[2] Please see the Neuropathology chapter for more details.

Recall that corticobasal ganglionic degeneration, frontotemporal dementia with parkinsonism, Pick's disease, and progressive supranuclear palsy are also considered tauopathies.

Amyloid Deposition

In Alzheimer's disease, amyloid is deposited in the brain as plaques.

- This amyloid is composed of Aβ peptide, which is derived from breaking down amyloid precursor protein.
    - The **gene for amyloid β-precursor protein is on chromosome 21**.
    - The 42-residue form of β-amyloid (Aβ), also known as Aβ1-42, is the most toxic form of β-amyloid.

Granulovacuolar Degeneration (of Simchowitz)

Vacuoles containing a granule are seen in the cytoplasm of pyramidal neurons in the hippocampus of patients with Alzheimer's disease.

Hirano Bodies

Hirano bodies are eosinophilic inclusions found in the cytoplasm of hippocampal neurons with age. They are more abundant in patients with Alzheimer's disease.

Neuritic Plaques

When amyloid plaques are associated with degenerating nerve endings, the plaque is called a neuritic plaque.

Neurofibrillary Tangles

Neurofibrillary tangles, which are found in neurons, are composed of paired helical filaments. These paired helical filaments are composed of hyperphosphorylated tau.

Tau is a **microtubule-associated protein** encoded by a gene on **chromosome 17**.

ApoE, a protein that has a role in cholesterol transport, is found in neurofibrillary tangles and neuritic plaques.

To remember the pathology findings in Alzheimer's disease:

Think of granulovacuolar degeneration as **Granny-vacuolar** degeneration because Grannies often get Alzheimer's disease.

Hirano sounds a little like "How would I know?". When you see **Hirano bodies** think of the phrase "**How would I know**? I have Alzheimer's dementia."

Patients with Alzheimer's dementia are **plagued** by confusion and have **neuritic plaques**.

Genetics

Most familial forms of Alzheimer's disease (AD) are autosomal dominant (AD).

 Alzheimer's Disease is usually Autosomal Dominant.

The Genetics of Alzheimer's Disease

Defect	Chromosome
Amyloid precursor protein (APP)	21
ApoE	19
Presenilin 1	14
Presenilin 2	1
Superoxide dismutase (SOD1)	21

} gamma secretase

The E4 allele for apolipoprotein E is associated with Alzheimer's at an earlier age, especially if one is homozygous for E4.

 The **E4 allele** for apolipoprotein E means you're **in for (4) Early Alzheimer's** before your peers. Alternatively, the E4 allele for apolipoprotein E means you're in for Alzheimer's B4 (before) your peers.

 It's pretty silly (presenilin) that Presenilin 1 is on chromosome 14 and Presenilin 2 is on chromosome 1.

Familial ALS (FALS) is due to a defect in SOD1 on chromosome 21.

 When you get drunk at age 21, you often **fall (FALS) on the grass/SOD.**

Neurochemistry

A number of neurotransmitters are reduced in the brains of patients with Alzheimer's disease.

Acetylcholine and **choline acetyltransferase** are thought to be reduced primarily due to **loss of neurons in the basal forebrain from the nucleus basalis of Meynert**.

Treatment

The AAN practice parameters[3] recommend considering **cholinesterase inhibitors** in mild to moderate AD patients and recommend **vitamin E to slow the progression of AD**.

Cholinesterase inhibitors used to treat Alzheimer's disease include:

- Donepezil (Aricept®)
- Galantamine (Reminyl®)
- Rivastigmine (Exelon®) – available in a transdermal patch formulation
- Tacrine (Cognex®) – this was the 1st Alzheimer's drug on the market, but has limited use now due to its 4-times daily dosing and considerable adverse drug reactions

Memantine (Namenda®), an NMDA receptor antagonist, is the newest drug to be used in Alzheimer's patients.

When excess glutamate builds up in the brain due to its release by cells, it attaches to cell surface NMDA receptors, permitting calcium to flow into the cell.

Chronic overexposure to calcium speeds up cell damage, but Memantine prevents this by partially blocking the NMDA receptors.

Antipsychotics can be used to treat agitation and psychosis in AD if changing the environment fails.

---

[3] AAN practice parameters regarding dementia: Neurology 2001;56:1133-1142, Neurology 2001;56:1143-1153, Neurology 2001;56:1154-1156, Neurology 2000;55:2205-2211.

Amyotrophic Lateral Sclerosis (ALS)

ALS is a degenerative disease involving the anterior horn cells and corticospinal tracts.[4]

Upper and lower motor neuron signs are seen.

 Sensation and continence are relatively preserved.

A recent study showed that about half of patients with ALS have **cognitive impairment**.

Most often, **executive dysfunction** is seen. For example, ALS patients had **problems with concentration**. When more severe impairment occurred, patients had features seen in **frontotemporal dementia** (FTD).[5]

Corticobasal Ganglionic Degeneration (CBGD)

CBGD is a **tauopathy** that starts around 60 years of age.

 The name says it all. Patients with CBGD have cortical atrophy and extrapyramidal signs.

Clinical Findings

As far as cortical signs, patients with CBGD have **apraxia, cortical sensory loss, sensory or visual neglect, and the alien limb phenomenon**.

Patients with CBGD have an array of movement disorders: myoclonus, dystonia, tremor, and rigidity.

Parkinsonism is unresponsive to levodopa. Symptoms start in one limb, usually an arm.

Patients with CBGD also have pyramidal signs and contractures.

Dysarthria is common.

---

[4] Please see the Neuromuscular Diseases chapter for more information.
[5] Ringholz GM, Appel SH, Bradshaw M, et al. Prevalence and patterns of cognitive impairment in sporadic ALS. Neurology 2005;65:586-590.

Imaging

MRI shows **asymmetric parietal lobe atrophy** in CBGD.

Pathology

Pathologic findings of CBGD:

Astrocytic plaques, which are astrocytic lesions that are immunoreactive for tau.

Ballooned neurons, which are swollen neurons, are seen. They are also seen in Pick's disease.

Coiled bodies of tau in oligodendrocytes.

Cortical atrophy, especially of the parietal and frontal lobes.

Degeneration of the **substantia nigra and striatum**.

ABCD can be used to remember the pathologic findings of CBGD:

   Astrocytic plaques that are immunoreactive for tau.

   Ballooned neurons

   Cortical atrophy, especially of the parietal and frontal lobes and **C**oiled bodies of tau in oligodendrocytes.

   Degeneration of the substantia nigra and striatum.

CBGD can be used to remember some of the findings in corticobasal ganglionic degeneration:

   Cortical sensory loss

   Ballooned neurons

   Gee, why is my arm doing that? (alien limb phenomenon)

   Dystonia, **D**ysarthria

Dementia with Lewy Bodies (DLB)

Clinical Findings

Patients with DLB have **cognitive dysfunction, psychiatric symptoms, parkinsonian features**, and **autonomic dysfunction.**

Cognitive Dysfunction

DLB causes a mixed cortical-subcortical dementia.

Patients have **executive dysfunction**, may lose their train of thought, and may have memory impairment. They may be **apathetic** and **bradyphrenic**.

One characteristic feature of dementia with Lewy bodies is that patients have **fluctuating levels of alertness and lucidness.** Sometimes patients are alert and cognitively near normal, and at other times patients are confused or hypersomnolent.

Patients also may get **lost in familiar environments** and have **difficulty copying drawings**.

Psychiatric Symptoms

Visual hallucinations are another characteristic finding in DLB.

Patients may see animals or humans.

Patients with Dementia with Lewy Bodies may see **D**ogs, **L**ions, or **B**ears (animals), or **D**avid, **L**ouie, or **B**ob (humans).

Patients with DLB may have delusions, depression, or anxiety.

Capgras' syndrome can be seen with DLB. This is the delusion that imposters have replaced people around you.

Extrapyramidal Signs

Patients with DLB are parkinsonian. They may have bradykinesia, masked facies, rigidity, a stooped posture, and a shuffling gait.

DLB patients may have tremor or myoclonus.

Autonomic Dysfunction

Patients with DLB may have postural hypotension, constipation, impotence, or urinary incontinence.

Sleep Disturbance

Patients with DLB may have REM sleep behavior disorder or excessive daytime somnolence.

Pathology

In Dementia with Lewy Bodies, Lewy bodies are widespread in the cortex, in addition to being found in the brainstem.

To remember the **alpha-Synucleopathies**, think of **"PALM Synday"** –

P for Parkinson's disease,

A for Alzheimer's disease (but trickily, Alzheimer's can be both an "*alpha-Synucleopathy*" and/or "*Tao-opathy*"),

L for Lewy Body dementia, and

M for Multiple Systems Atrophy.

Synday is for **Synucleopathy**.

The best thing about this mnemonic is that you don't need to recall all the *Tao-opathies* – if they're not there on **PALM Synday**, they're Tao!

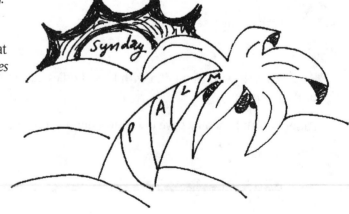

Fahr's Disease

Fahr's disease is characterized by **idiopathic bilateral calcification of the basal ganglia**.

Patients with Fahr's disease have **subcortical dementia and parkinsonism.** They can also have psychiatric symptoms, chorea, and dysarthria.

There are familial (autosomal dominant or recessive) and sporadic forms.

Friedreich's Ataxia

Friedreich's ataxia is an autosomal recessive progressive ataxia due a triplet repeat (GAA).[6]

Clinical Findings

Friedreich's ataxia begins before adolescence and may cause death before age 40.

It usually presents with **gait ataxia.** Later incoordination of the arms is seen.

Patients **lose position sense and vibration** due to damage to the posterior columns; as a result, they develop a **positive Romberg.**

They also develop **weakness in the distal limbs** and **foot deformities** such as **talipes equinovarus** and **pes cavus.**

Lower extremity reflexes are lost, but **extensor plantar responses are seen.**

Patients also develop **dysarthria, nystagmus,** and late in the course have **swallowing difficulties.**

Patients may also have **diabetes, scoliosis,** and **hypertrophic cardiomyopathy.** They may die from heart failure.

---

6 Please also see the Movement Disorders chapter.

Genetics

Friedreich's ataxia is due to an expansion of a GAA triplet repeat in the gene that encodes frataxin on chromosome 9.

 Friedreich's ataxia is associated with a triplet repeat in **GAA**, which could stand for **Gait Ataxia and Arrhythmia**.

Pathology

Primarily the spinal cord is affected. Cell loss occurs in the posterior columns, corticospinal tracts, spinocerebellar tracts, and Clarke's column.

 Cell loss is also seen in the nuclei of cranial nerves VIII, X, and XII; dentate nuclei; superior vermis; and superior cerebellar peduncle.

Frontotemporal Dementia (FTD)

Clinical Findings

Patients with FTD present at 45-65 years of age with behavioral changes.

The onset is gradual.

Patients with FTD have executive dysfunction.

Patients may have **echolalia**.

There is a **decline in social skills and ability to interpret facial expression**. Patients may lose the ability to empathize and sympathize with others.

Personal hygiene deteriorates.

Unlike patients with Alzheimer's disease, **FTD patients have preservation of spatial skills.**

Patients with **FTD** may be **FeTiD (fetid),** because they have **poor hygiene**.

 Patients with frontotemporal dementia (FTD) <u>could</u> drive FTD® flower delivery trucks because they have spatial skills. Smelling more like flowers wouldn't be a bad thing.

Pathology

As expected from the name, frontal and anterior temporal atrophy are seen in FTD.

 FTD causes gliosis in cortical layer 2, neuronal loss, and **microvacuolation**.

Some cases do not have other histological findings. These are called dementia lacking distinctive histological features.

The FTLD-ubiquitinated (FTLD-U) type is characterized by ubiquitinated intraneuronal inclusions as well as the typical features of FTD.

There are also types of FTD that are tauopathies.

Frontotemporal Dementia with Motor Neuron Disease (FTD-MND)

The course of FTD-MND is more rapid than other forms of FTD due to dysphagia and respiratory failure.

Frontotemporal Dementia with Parkinsonism (FTDP-17)

FTDP-17 is an autosomal dominant form of FTD that is associated with parkinsonism.

Most of the cases are due to **mutations in microtubule-associated protein tau on 17q**.

Pick's Disease

Pick's disease is a type of FTD with specific pathological features.

Patients with **Pick's** disease may end up **picking their nose** because they **lack inhibition**, like other patients with FTD.

Due to atrophy of the frontal and anterior temporal lobes, patients with Pick's disease have **knife edge gyri**.

When you see Pick in Pick's disease, think of an **ice pick**, which is **sharp like a knife**. This should help you remember that patient's with Pick's disease have **knife-edge gyri**.

Pick's disease is a tauopathy like FTDP-17, progressive supranuclear palsy, corticobasal degeneration, and Alzheimer's disease.

Recall from the Neuropathology chapter that patients with Pick's disease have **ballooned neurons** and **Pick bodies**.

· Pick bodies are spherical intracytoplasmic inclusions found in neurons in patients with Pick's disease. They are slightly basophilic, tau-positive, and can be seen well with silver staining.

· Ballooned neurons are swollen neurons that are achromatic.

Hopefully a patient with Pick's Disease won't **pick their nose** with a **knife-like ice pick**, because then they would wind up in the hospital and get **balloons** from friends wishing them to get well soon.

Huntington Disease (HD)

Huntington disease is an autosomal dominant disease that is due to **expanded CAG triplet repeats in the huntingtin gene on chromosome 4**.

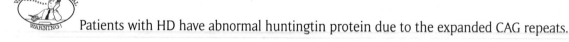

Patients with HD have abnormal huntingtin protein due to the expanded CAG repeats.

This mutant huntingtin protein is not degraded normally during proteolysis. Products of this process form aggregates in the cytoplasm. These are translocated into the nucleus and intranuclear aggregates form. These aggregates may interfere with cell function.

Hunters **C**apture **A**nimal **G**ame and Huntington patients have expanded CAG repeats.

The onset of Huntington disease is usually in the late thirties.

The first sign may be a **change in saccadic eye movements**, but patients present with motor and/or behavior symptoms.

Clumsiness is seen **followed by chorea**.

Later bradykinesia and dystonia appear.

Irritability and mood changes are followed by executive dysfunction and **subcortical dementia**.

Atrophy of the caudate and putamen is seen, as well as generalized cerebral atrophy.

Loss of GABA-synthesizing neurons occurs, **primarily in the striatum**.

Westphal Variant

Westphal variant is an **akinetic, dystonic form of Huntington's disease**.

It is seen in patients with **juvenile-onset HD**.

These patients have **dementia** and may have **seizures**.

Increased T2 signal is seen in the striatum.

Marchiafava-Bignami Disease

Marchiafava-Bignami disease is characterized by **demyelination of the corpus callosum** and is found in middle-aged alcoholics. It can present with dementia.

Marchiafava-Bignami disease was initially found in **Italians who drank red wine excessively**.

To remember that Marchiafava-Bignami is associated with alcoholism: Hannibal Lecter from "Silence of the Lambs" could have developed Marchia**fava**-Bignami if he drank too much Chianti with fava beans.

Multi-infarct Dementia

Please see Vascular Dementia section below.

Multiple Sclerosis (MS)

MS is a CNS demyelinating disease, the pathogenesis of which is still being determined. Evidence suggests that it is a T-cell mediated autoimmune disease; the T cells are directed against myelin antigens.

Epidemiology

MS most commonly presents in women, ages 20 to 40 years. However, it has been described in young children and in people over 60 years of age.

MS becomes more common the further from the equator (in either direction) that an individual is raised. If one moves before age 15 to an area of lesser risk, one acquires a risk similar to one's neighbors.

There is a genetic component. MS is more common in monozygotic than in dizygotic twins. ^3% ^6%

The **HLA-DR2 (DR1501) haplotype** is associated with an increased risk for MS.

Clinical Features

Optic neuritis (ON) is one of the most common presentations of MS.

In the Optic Neuritis Treatment Trial (ONTT), mild-to-severe eye pain was present in 92% of patients.[7]

Corticospinal tract involvement results in weakness, clonus, and spasticity.

Sensory symptoms are common. Patients may complain of numbness or tingling, which does not necessarily follow an anatomic distribution. Vibratory loss is commonly found on examination.

Nystagmus, when seen, tends to be horizontal.

Dysarthria is common.

---

[7] Optic Neuritis Study Group. The clinical profile of optic neuritis. Experience of the Optic Neuritis Treatment Trial. *Arch Ophthalmol.* Dec 1991;109(12):1673-8.

Dysmetria and intention tremor are common findings in patients with MS.

Transverse myelitis can be seen. ↑risk for MS: incomplete TM, asym. S/M findings, abnormal CSF/MRI, MRI spine with limited nonconfluent intramedullary lesions, alone multimodality evoked potentials

MS is associated with lots of signs[8]:

· Marcus Gunn pupil   relative APD
· Internuclear ophthalmoplegia (INO)
· Uhthoff's sign
· Lhermitte sign

Bilateral trigeminal neuralgia, bilateral INO, and bilateral ON are suggestive of MS but can be seen in other conditions.

Patients also have fatigue, cognitive dysfunction, depression, sexual dysfunction, and bowel and bladder dysfunction.

Clinically Isolated Syndrome (CIS)

As per the National MS Society: CIS is the "first neurologic episode that lasts at least 24 hours, and is caused by inflammation/demyelination in one or more sites in the CNS."

CIS is monofocal or multifocal:

· **Monofocal episode:** 1 neurologic sign or symptom (ie., ON) caused by a lesion in 1 location.
· **Multifocal episode:** >1 sign or symptom (ie., ON accompanied by hemibody weakness) caused by lesions in > 1 location.

CIS may or may not progress to MS based on risk:

Higher Risk: CIS *with* MRI brain lesions similar to those in MS

Lower Risk: CIS *without* MRI lesions similar to those in MS (risk of developing MS over the same time period is less).

Diagnosis

Patients with MS have CNS white matter lesions, which are separated in time and space.

The Revised McDonald-Criteria are used for diagnosis.

MRI, evoked potentials, and CSF findings can aid with diagnosis.

---

[8] Please see the appendix for a description of these signs.

CSF may reveal an elevated IgG synthesis rate, elevated IgG index, or oligoclonal bands.

Cell counts, glucose, and protein are usually normal. CSF protein that is mildly elevated is common, but >100mg/dL is distinctly unusual.

The CSF may have a mild pleocytosis with predominantly mononuclear cells. During the first weeks of an exacerbation, myelin basic protein will be high. However, this is a non-specific finding.

Visual evoked potentials are the most useful evoked potentials for diagnosis; they may be prolonged, with a normal appearing P100 waveform.

Neuropathology/Neuroimaging

The pathologic hallmark of MS is the plaque.

Plaques are frequently found in the corpus callosum, periventricular region (lateral ventricles), cerebellar peduncles, medial longitudinal fasciculi, optic nerves, and cervical cord.

Plaques are characterized by myelin loss, which tends to occur around small veins and venules.

The appearance of a plaque depends on its age.

- Active plaques are pink grossly. They contain lymphocytes (mainly T-cells, but sometimes also B cells and plasma cells) and macrophages.
- Inactive plaques are well-demarcated gray lesions on gross inspection. Microscopically, they are hypocellular areas of gliosis that lack oligodendrocytes. Some axonal loss occurs as well.

Shadow plaques are plaques where demyelination is incomplete/partial remyelination has occurred.

On MRI, plaques are hypointense or isointense on T1 and hyperintense on T2-weighted images. Active lesions enhance, sometimes in a ring pattern.

Dawson fingers are perivascular, ovoid/linear ares of demyelination that are perpendicular to the long axis of the lateral ventricles. **They are a classic finding in MS.**

Tumefactive MS is associated with lesions that cause mass effect. These are associated with **incomplete rings of enhancement**.

Disease Course

10% benign MS

There are multiple clinical courses possible:

Relapsing-remitting MS (RRMS) *2:1 F:M*

Secondary progressive MS (SPMS)

Primary progressive MS (PPMS) *slow UMN pattern - legs*

Progressive relapsing MS (PRMS).

more severe course
male
frequent relapses in 1st 2 yrs
progressive course
early motor/cerebellar
OCB in CSF
older age @ onset
incomplete remission p̄ 1st relapses

Most patients present with RRMS. About half of these patients will evolve into SPMS.

PPMS occurs in 10-15% of all MS patients, and PRMS occurs in less than 5%.

RRMS is usually found in young women. PPMS is equally common in men and women. The mean onset of PPMS is about 10 years later than RRMS.

clinical disability α axonal loss (atrophy)

MS has undergone a revolution in new therapies over the past few years, especially in prevention.

Exacerbation

Corticosteroids, such as methylprednisolone, are used during acute MS exacerbations to hasten recovery. This may be followed by a prednisone taper.

There is no firm evidence that corticosteroid treatment alters the *long-term* course of disease.

In 1991, the landmark **Optic Neuritis Treatment Trial (ONTT)**[9] randomized patients within 8 days of symptom onset into 1 of 3 groups: oral prednisone (1 mg/kg/d for 14 d), IV MethylPrednisolone (250 mg every 6 h for 3 d followed by an oral taper) or placebo. The oral group demonstrated an ***increased*** incidence of recurrent optic neuritis, but ***all groups*** had visual recovery over time. Yet IV steroids increased the rate of recovery of optic neuritis and decreased the incidence of the development of MS over a 2 year period, but no longer than that.

---

[9] Optic Neuritis Study Group. The clinical profile of optic neuritis. Experience of the Optic Neuritis Treatment Trial. *Arch Ophthalmol.* Dec 1991;109(12):1673-8.

Prevention

The orals

Fampridine/4-aminopyridine (Neurelan® / Ampyra®)

Fampridine is indicated for use in MS to improve walking in patients who are moderately disabled already. It is a potassium channel blocker and prolongs channel repolarization. This can lead to improved neurological function in demyelinated axons by enhancing action potential formation.

Fingolimod (Gilena®)

In 2010, fingolimod became the first FDA-approved, oral, disease-modifying drug for MS. It is thought to work by sequestering lymphocytes in lymph nodes, thereby preventing them from moving into the CNS and causing auto-immune MS attacks. Adverse medication reactions include basal cell carcinoma, bradycardia, and a case of focal hemorrhagic encephalitis.

Cladribine (Litak® /Movectro®)

Used in the treatment of hairy cell leukemia, Cladribine (like fingolimod) received much attention as a new oral MS drug. In 2010, a large clinical trial documented significant reduction in MS relapse rates with use of cladribine. However, the FDA did not approve it and the drug manufacturer withdrew it among concerns of bone marrow suppression, cancer, and infection.

Dimethyl Fumarate or BG12 (Tecfidera®)

Unknown therapeutic effect but its metabolite, monomethyl fumarate (MMF), activates the Nuclear factor (erythroid-derived 2)-like 2 (Nrf2) pathway, which is involved in the cellular response to oxidative stress. Side effects include flushing and GI problems.

Teriflunomide (Aubagio®)

Another oral MS possibility, Teriflunomide blocks pyrimidine synthesis and thus inhibits rapidly dividing cells, like activated T cells in MS. Teriflunomide may have less infection risk compared to chemotherapy-like drugs because of less immunosuppression, and thus may get FDA approval soon.

The injectables

Glatiramer Acetate (Copolymer-1/Copaxone®)

Copaxone is a copolymer that was designed to resemble myelin basic protein. It consists of four amino acids in random association: L-glutamic acid, L-lysine, L-alanine, and L-tyrosine (which spell out glat as in glatiramer acetate).

Interferon β-1a (Avonex®)

The CHAMPS study was a double-blinded, randomized controlled trial that showed that Avonex delays clinically definite MS following an initial single CNS demyelinating event with subclinical MRI findings.

Interferon β-1a (Rebif®)

The PRISMS study showed that Rebif is better than placebo at preventing relapse in patients with RRMS.

In the EVIDENCE study, Rebif was better than Avonex at preventing active MRI lesions in patients with RRMS.

Interferonβ-1b (Betaseron®)

This was the first medication approved by the FDA for the treatment of RRMS.

Avonex, Rebif, and Betaseron can cause flu-like symptoms as a side effect.

Interferon β-1a and Interferon β-1b have been associated with neutralizing antibodies.

Mitoxantrone

Mitoxantrone (Novantrone®) was the first medication approved for secondary progressive MS.

Cardiotoxicity is a concern. There is also a risk of development of treatment-induced leukemia.

The infusions

Natalizumab (Tysabri®)[10,11]

Natalizumab is an intravenous infusion treatment for RR MS and is given every 28 days.

It is a recombinant monoclonal antibody that binds to **α4 integrin**; this will prevent migration of leukocytes into the brain.

It was developed to block the adhesion of activated T cells to endothelial cells and hence decrease inflammatory multiple sclerosis plaques.

It increases the risk of progressive multifocal leukoencephalopathy (PML).*

* In the 2006 AFFIRM trial, patients with MS were randomly given Tysabri or placebo every 4 weeks for 2 years. Tysabri reduced annual MS relapse rates by 68% versus placebo.

** The SENTINEL trial, also in 2006, gave MS patients who were already on interferon beta-1a treatment either Tysabri or placebo, randomly. It was stopped early because 2 patients developed PML, however Tysabri again reduced MS relapses, this time by 54% over 1 year.

Alemtuzumab (Lemtrada® or Campath®)

In 2011, the CARE-MS I study showed that 78% of MS patients on alemtuzumab remained relapse-free for 2 years, compared to only 59% of Rebif-treated patients.

Like Tysabri, Alemtuzumab is also a monoclonal antibody but is humanized and targets CD52 on mature lymphocytes. It is currently approved for treatment of CLL but soon may gain approval for MS treatment also.**

Daclizumab (Zenapax®)

Zenapax is an IgG1 monoclonal antibody (90% human and 10% mouse) that binds to the alpha subunit of the IL-2 receptor expressed on the surface of activated lymphocytes. Side effects with immunosuppressants can include risk of developing certain types of cancer (like lymphoma) and infection (like CMV).

Symptomatic

amantadine (DA) , modafanil
4-AMP (K⁺ ant.)

Spasticity, depression, fatigue, sexual dysfunction, bowel and bladder dysfunction may need treatment as well.

baclofen GABA agonist , dantrolene
tizanidine α2 agonist (sympathetic) , cyproheptadine

[10] AFFIRM Investigators. A randomized, placebo-controlled trial of natalizumab for relapsing multiple sclerosis. N Engl J Med. 2006 Mar 2;354(9):899-910.

[11] SENTINEL Investigators. Natalizumab plus interferon beta-1a for relapsing multiple sclerosis. N Engl J Med. 2006 Mar;354(9):911-23.

MS Variants

MS variants:

> · Devic Syndrome (Neuromyelitis Optica)
>
> · Malignant MS (Marburg Disease)
>
> · Baló's Concentric Sclerosis
>
> · Relapsing transverse myelitis
>
> · Relapsing optic neuritis

Baló's Concentric Sclerosis

Baló's Concentric Sclerosis is an acute, progressive form of MS in which concentric areas of demyelination are seen alternating with normal brain.

Devic's Disease/Neuromyelitis Optica (NMO)

NMO/Devic's disease is a demyelinating disease which causes **transverse myelitis and optic neuritis**.

On spinal MRI, cord lesions typically extend 3 or more segments during acute attacks.

CSF pleocytosis and the absence of oligoclonal bands help to distinguish this from MS. Unlike MS, NMO is associated with other autoimmune disorders.

Also, patients with Devic's disease have seropositivity for **NMO-IgG**. This autoantibody targets aquaporin-4, and is not found in MS patients.[12]

The female to male ratio is >4:1.

Onset of NMO varies, with two peaks, one in childhood and the other in adults in their 40s.

Treatment with Rituxan (rituximab, a monoclonal antibody against CD20 on B-cells) may reduce frequency of NMO attacks, and stabilize or improve disability.

---

[12] Wingerchuk DM, Lennon VA, Pittock SJ et al. Revised diagnostic criteria for neuromyelitis optica. Neurology 2006;66:1485-1489.

Malignant MS (Marburg Disease)

Malignant MS is a rapidly progressive form of MS, which can cause **coma** and may lead to death from brainstem injury or mass effect.

 In addition to demyelination, tissue necrosis and significant axonal loss occur.

Multiple System Atrophy

MSA is a neurodegenerative disease that usually **presents in the sixth decade**.

 It is associated with varying degrees of **autonomic and urinary dysfunction**, **parkinsonism**, **cerebellar**, and **corticospinal tract dysfunction**.[13]

In MSA, varying degrees of neuronal loss and gliosis are found in the cerebellum, intermediolateral cell column, inferior olive, locus ceruleus, middle cerebellar peduncles, Onuf's nucleus in the sacral cord, pontine nuclei, striatum, and substantia nigra.

Recall from the Neuropathology chapter that MSA is an **alpha-synucleinopathy**.

To remember that multiple system atrophy (**MSA**) is an alpha-synucleinopathy, remember that MSA could also stand for **M**ade of **S**ynuclein-**A**lpha (alpha-synuclein).

Glial cell inclusions (GCIs) are found in **oligodendrocytes** of patients with MSA.

GCIs are flame/sickle-shaped inclusions detected with silver stain that are **immunoreactive for alpha-synuclein**.

---

[13] Please also see the Movement Disorders chapter.

Normal Pressure Hydrocephalus (NPH)

 NPH is characterized by a triad

1) Ataxic gait: **"magnetic"** in which the feet appear to be stuck to the floor
2) Urinary incontinence: spastic hyperreflexic, increased urgency
3) **Subcortical** Dementia: manifested as apathy, forgetfulness, inertia, inattention, slow thinking (bradyphrenia)

NPH presents over 60 years of age.

NPH can be idiopathic (no known cause) or "secondary" – due to a subarachnoid hemorrhage (SAH), head trauma, tumor, abscess, or a complication of brain surgery.

 Some patients with NPH respond to shunting.

Parkinson's Disease

Parkinson's disease is characterized by **resting tremor**, **rigidity**, **akinesia**, and **postural instability** (which develops later in the course of the disease).[14]

Eventually, cognitive changes occur in most patients.

Initially, cognitive slowing may be seen.

Patients may also have impaired attention, problems with memory retrieval, and visual spatial difficulties.

Later, dementia can be seen.

---

[14] Please see the Movement Disorders chapter for more information.

Parkinsonism-Dementia-ALS Complex of Guam

 Parkinsonism-Dementia-ALS Complex of Guam is found among the **Chammorros Indians in Guam.**

It may be related to ingestion of the **cycad nut**.

Patients have symptoms of all disorders in the name: parkinsonism, dementia, and motor neuron disease.

Neurofibrillary tangles are seen.

Pick's Disease

Please see the frontotemporal dementia (FTD) section above.

Prion Diseases

Please see the Infectious Diseases chapter.

Progressive Supranuclear Palsy (PSP)

PSP is one of the atypical parkinsonian disorders/Parkinsonism-plus syndromes.

Clinical Findings

Slow **vertical saccades** and **square-wave jerks of the eyes** are early eye findings.

Patients develop **supranuclear ophthalmoplegia. Downgaze is lost first.**

These patients have a **wide-eyed appearance** and tend to **hyperextend the neck.**

Like Parkinson's patients, these patients have **bradykinesia, rigidity, and dementia**.

However, **postural instability is more prominent in PSP** than in Parkinson's disease, and PSP patients lack tremor.

PSP could stand for **P**ostural **S**tability is **P**oor.

Patients with PSP have behavioral changes.

Apathy is very common.

Pseudobulbar affect is also seen.

If you stand on a precipice (**P**re**S**i**P**ice), don't **gaze down**! Your **wide-eyed appearance** will cause you to **fall backwards**!

Despite the fact that patients tend to have a surprised or worried appearance and may cry due to pseudobulbar affect, patients with PSP are often apathetic.

Neuroimaging/Neuropathologic Findings

Patients with PSP have **atrophy of the pons and midbrain**. *hummingbird sign*

Neuropathologic changes are seen in the globus pallidus, subthalamic nucleus, hippocampus, entorhinal cortex, and the dentate nucleus of the cerebellum, in addition to the midbrain (superior colliculus, periaqueductal gray, red nucleus, and substantia nigra) and pons (locus ceruleus).

PSP is a **tauopathy**.

As in CBGD, 4-repeat tau is found in glia and neurons.

Tau is found in oligodendrocytes as **coiled bodies** and as **neurofibrillary tangles** in neurons.

Patients with CBGD have **astrocyte plaques**.

Patients with PSP have **astrocytic tufts** (tuft-shaped astrocytes), which are tau-immunoreactive lesions.

Spinocerebellar Ataxia

Please see the Movement Disorders chapter.

Vascular Dementia

Patients with vascular dementia do not have a specific neuropsychological profile.

Stroke patterns that can cause vascular dementia[15]:

· Single infarcts in key locations

 CHIRP Mt. = **C**audate, **H**ippocampus, **R**ight **P**arietal lobe, **M**edial **t**halamus

· Multiple large infarcts

· Multiple lacunar infarcts

· Subcortical white matter infarcts

· Various infarcts with Alzheimer's disease.

Most definitions of vascular dementia include these points:

· Dementia is temporally related to a stroke.

· There are bilateral infarcts in the cortex of the frontal, temporal, or parietal lobes; basal ganglia; or thalamus.

· Signs of stroke are present on physical examination.

 Vascular Dementia is measured on the *Hachinski* ischemic score, which includes:

V - **Vascular Dementia**

A – **A**cute onset

S – **S**tepwise decline in abilities

C – **CHIRP Mt.**

U – **U**nstable emotions (emotional lability)

L – **L**acunar disease on neuroimaging

A – **A**lzheimer's Disease previously diagnosed

R – **R**isk factors, like hypertension, hyperlipidemia, and prior stroke

---

[15] Knopman D. Vascular Dementia. Continuum Lifelong Learning in Neurol 2004;10(1):113-134.

Neurodegenerative Diseases Quiz

(Answers on page 745)

1. Which mitochondrial disease is not associated with ragged-red fibers?

    A. KSS

    B. MELAS

    C. MERRF

    D. MNGIE

    E. NARP

2. Which pathologic finding is not found in Alzheimer's disease?

    A. Amyloid deposition

    B. Astrocytic tufts

    C. Granulovacuolar degeneration

    D. Hirano bodies

    E. Neuritic plaques

    F. Neurofibrillary tangles

3. Which is not a tauopathy?

    A. Alzheimer's disease

    B. CBGD

    C. FTDP-17

    D. MSA

    E. Pick's disease

    F. PSP

4. Knife-edge gyri are associated with which disease?

    A. Alzheimer's disease

    B. CBGD

    C. OPCA

    D. Pick's disease

    E. PSP

Chapter 9

Neuromuscular Diseases

Anatomy

There are 31 pairs of spinal nerves: 8 cervical, 12 thoracic, 5 lumbar, 5 sacral, and 1 coccygeal.

Pre-Brachial Plexus

The **dorsal scapular nerve** and the **long thoracic nerve** originate proximal to the brachial plexus.

 The dorsal scapular and long thoracic nerves are like me, they try to avoid the brachial plexus.

The dorsal scapular and long thoracic nerves head out the door to escape (dorsal scapular) and are long (long thoracic) gone before the brachial plexus arrives.

Evidence of injury to the dorsal scapular or long thoracic nerve indicates that the lesion is <u>proximal</u> to the plexus.

The Dorsal Scapular Nerve

The dorsal scapular nerve (C4-5) innervates the levator scapulae and rhomboids (major and minor).

      The levator scapulae elevates the scapula (as you might expect).

      The rhomboids adduct and lift the medial border of the scapula.

 Rhomboids have **4** sides, and the rhomboid muscles are innervated by C**4**, 5.

The Long Thoracic Nerve

The long thoracic nerve (C5-7) innervates the serratus anterior, which attaches the scapula to the chest wall.

Scapular winging occurs with weakness of the serratus anterior. (Scapular winging can also be seen with weakness of the trapezius. With scapular winging due to weakness of the serratus anterior, the scapula is displaced medially. With scapular weakness due to weakness of the trapezius, the scapula is displaced laterally.)

How do you recognize and remember medial versus lateral winging of the scapula?

Order a *SALTy wings meal*!

The **S**erratus **A**nterior muscle, innervated by the **L**ong **T**horacic nerve, causes **medial winging** (wings meal).

- and -

Don't get caught in a *late, 11th hour, accessory trap*!

(injury to the **trap**ezius muscle, innervated by the **accessory** nerve – CN **11** – causes **late**ral scapular winging)

Due to its superficial, supraclavicular position, the long thoracic nerve may be **injured by carrying heavy objects** on one's shoulder. It also can be **injured during mastectomy**.

Upper Extremity- Brachial Plexus

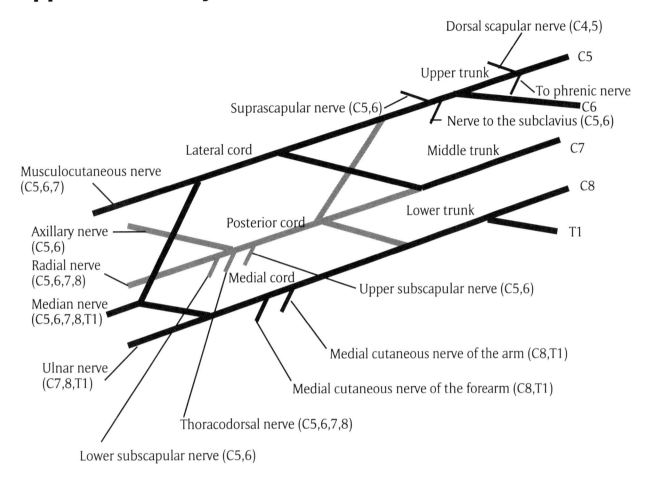

Dorsal scapular nerve (C4,5)

C5

Upper trunk

To phrenic nerve

Suprascapular nerve (C5,6)

C6

Nerve to the subclavius (C5,6)

Lateral cord

Middle trunk

C7

C8

Musculocutaneous nerve (C5,6,7)

Posterior cord

Lower trunk

T1

Axillary nerve (C5,6)

Medial cord

Radial nerve (C5,6,7,8)

Upper subscapular nerve (C5,6)

Median nerve (C5,6,7,8,T1)

Medial cutaneous nerve of the arm (C8,T1)

Ulnar nerve (C7,8,T1)

Medial cutaneous nerve of the forearm (C8,T1)

Thoracodorsal nerve (C5,6,7,8)

Lower subscapular nerve (C5,6)

MNEMONIC
Everyone remembers the brachial plexus mnemonic from med school: Republicans Think Democrats Can't Negotiate, which stands for Roots, Trunks, Divisions, Cords, Nerves.

Roots

The anterior primary rami of C5, C6, C7, C8, and T1 form the brachial plexus.

Trunks

There are 3 trunks:

> Upper trunk (C5-6)
> Middle trunk (C7)
> Lower trunk (C8-T1)

There are some branches off the upper trunk. See the Branches section below.

Divisions

There are anterior and posterior divisions.

- · The **anterior division** consists of fibers travelling to the **ventral arm**
- · The **posterior division** consists of fibers travelling to the **dorsal arm**.

Cords

There are lateral, medial, and posterior cords.

Lateral Cord

The lateral cord is formed by the anterior divisions of the upper trunk (C5,C6) and middle trunk (C7). So it consists of the anterior divisions of C5-C7.

To remember the location of the lateral cord, position your arm so that it is in the anatomical position. Now the lateral cord is lateral, and the medial cord is medial.

The L formed by the thumb and index finger tells you that that's the side where the lateral cord is.

Medial Cord

The medial cord is formed from the anterior divisions of the lower trunk, so it consists of the anterior divisions of C8-T1.

Posterior Cord

The posterior cord consists of the posterior divisions of all 3 trunks, so it consists of the posterior divisions of C5-T1.

Branches

Branches of the Trunks

 Branches of the trunks are the suprascapular nerve and nerve to the subclavius muscle. Both come off the upper trunk.

The Suprascapular Nerve

The suprascapular nerve innervates the **supraspinatus** and **infraspinatus muscles**.

The **suprascapular notch** (or scapular notch) is in the superior border of the scapula, medial to the coracoid process. A mass in the suprascapular notch can result in atrophy of the supraspinatus and infraspinatus muscles.

The **supra**scapular nerve innervates the **supra**spinatus and infraspinatus muscles.

- The supraspinatus muscle is responsible for the first 15 degrees of arm abduction.
- The infraspinatus muscle is responsible for external rotation of the arm.

The Nerve to the Subclavius

The nerve to the subclavius conveniently innervates the subclavius muscle.

Branches of the Lateral Cord

Branches of the lateral cord are:
- Lateral cutaneous nerve of the forearm
- Lateral pectoral nerve
- Musculocutaneous nerve
- Median nerve*

*Note that the medial cord also contributes to the median nerve.

A lesion of the lateral cord causes sensory loss over the lateral forearm and weakness of elbow and wrist flexion.

The Lateral Pectoral Nerve

The lateral pectoral nerve (C5-7) supplies the clavicular head of the pectoralis major muscle. It pulls the shoulder forward.

The Musculocutaneous Nerve

The **musculocutaneous nerve** is responsible for **supination of the forearm, elbow flexion**, and the **biceps reflex.**

The musculocutaneous nerve (C5-7) supplies the biceps, brachialis, and coracobrachialis muscles.

> The biceps (C5-6) is an elbow flexor and forearm supinator.
>
> The brachialis (C5-6) is an elbow flexor.
>
> The coracobrachialis (C6-7) elevates the arm forward.

The Median Nerve

Both the lateral and medial cords contribute to the median nerve, which is innervated by C5-T1.

As mentioned above, the lateral cord consists of the anterior divisions of C5-C7.

Sensation to the **thumb, middle**, and **index fingers** is supplied by **median nerve** sensory fibers from **the lateral cord.**

Sensation to the **lateral ring finger** is innervated by **sensory fibers from both the medial and lateral cord**.

The muscles that are supplied primarily from the part of the median nerve derived from the lateral cord are the pronator teres and flexor carpi radialis. (The lateral cord also contributes to other median-innervated muscles.)

> The pronator teres (C6-7) pronates the forearm.
>
> The flexor carpi radialis (C6-7) flexes and abducts the hand at the wrist.

Branches of the Medial Cord

Branches of the medial cord:

> · Medial cutaneous nerve of the arm (C8-T1)
>
> · Medial cutaneous nerve of the forearm (C8-T1)
>
> · Median nerve (C8, T1)*
>
> · Ulnar nerve (C7-T1)
>
> · Medial pectoral nerve (C8-T1)

*Note that the lateral cord also contributes to the median nerve.

A **lesion of the medial cord** causes **sensory loss over the medial forearm**, some **weakness of the long finger flexors**, and **weakness of the intrinsic hand muscles**.

Medial Pectoral Nerve (C8,T1)

The medial pectoral nerve innervates the pectoralis minor and part of the sternal head of the pectoralis major.

- The sternal head of the pectoralis major adducts the arm and rotates it medially.
- The pectoralis minor lowers the scapula and pulls the shoulder forward.

Median Nerve

The median nerve is responsible for flexion of the thumb, index and middle fingers, and wrist; opposition of the thumb; pronation of the forearm; and abduction of the hand.

As mentioned above, both the lateral and medial cords contribute to the median nerve, which is innervated by C5-T1. Recall that the lateral cord consists of the anterior divisions of C5-C7, and the medial cord consists of the anterior divisions of C8-T1.

The muscles that are supplied primarily from the part of the median nerve derived from the lateral cord are the pronator teres and flexor carpi radialis. (The lateral cord also contributes to other median-innervated muscles. Note the nerve roots.)

The **part of the median nerve that is a branch of the medial cord supplies**:

- Abductor pollicis brevis (C8-T1)
- Flexor digitorum profundus I and II (C7-8)
- Flexor digitorum superficialis (C7-T1)
- Flexor pollicis brevis (superficial head)[1] (C8-T1)
- Flexor pollicis longus (C7-8)
- Lumbricals I and II (C8-T1)
- Opponens pollicis (C8-T1)
- Palmaris longus (C7-T1)
- Pronator quadratus (C7-8)

The abductor pollicis brevis (APB) abducts the thumb perpendicular to the hand.

The flexor digitorum profundus I and II (FDP I and II) allows flexion of the terminal phalanges of the second and third digits.

---

[1] Recall that the **ulnar nerve supplies the <u>deep</u> head of the flexor pollicis brevis.**

The flexor digitorum superficialis flexes the middle phalanges of the second, third, fourth, and fifth fingers.

The superficial head of the flexor pollicis brevis (FPB) flexes the proximal phalanx of the thumb.

The flexor pollicis longus (FPL) is responsible for flexion of the terminal phalanx of the thumb.

Lumbricals I and II flex the metacarpophalangeal joint and extend the proximal and distal interphalangeal joints of the second and third digits.

The opponens pollicis allows opposition of the thumb.

The palmaris longus flexes the wrist.

The pronator quadratus (PQ) pronates the forearm.

Sensory branches of the median nerve supply the thenar eminence, the proximal palm (radial aspect of the hand), and the palmar aspect first 3 digits and half of the fourth digit.

Sensation to the thumb, middle, and index fingers is supplied by median nerve sensory fibers from the lateral cord. Sensation to the lateral ring finger is innervated by sensory fibers from both the medial and lateral cord.

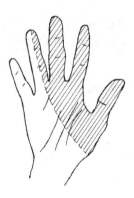 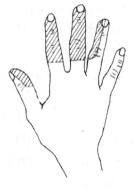

The Anterior Interosseous Nerve

The anterior interosseus nerve is the largest branch of the median nerve. It is purely motor.
It innervates:

- Flexor pollicis longus (C5-7)
- Flexor digitorum profundus I and II (C5-7)
- Pronator quadratus (C7-8)

flexion of distal phalanges thumb, index, middle

The median nerve proper and the anterior interosseous nerve, which is one of its branches, innervate similar sounding muscles.

Median nerve	Anterior interosseous nerve
Flexor Pollicis Brevis superficial head	Flexor Pollicis Longus
Flexor Digitorum Superficialis	Flexor Digitorum Profundus I and II
Pronator Teres	Pronator Quadratus

MNEMONIC To remember that the median nerve innervates the flexor pollicis brevis superficial head and flexor digitorum superficialis, remember that the **me**dian nerve is superficial and says, "It's all about me".

HOT TIP The pronator quadratus (PQ) is most accurately tested when the elbow is flexed, which prevents contribution from the pronator teres.

Injury to the anterior interosseous nerve results in the anterior interosseus nerve syndrome.

The **anterior interosseus nerve syndrome** is characterized by:

- Pain in the arm or forearm.
- Weakness of forearm pronation (due to weakness of PQ).
- Weakness of flexion of the terminal phalanx of the thumb (due to FPL weakness) and the terminal phalanges of the second and third digits (due to weakness of the FDP I and II).
- Normal sensation. (This is a pure motor nerve.)

A patient with the anterior interosseous syndrome is unable to make a circle using the thumb and index finger ₿ (as if saying OK) due to weakness of the FPL and FDP. (The circle looks squashed in anterior interosseous syndrome. It is called "the teardrop sign.")

MNEMONIC A patient with **a**nterior **i**nterosseous **n**europathy **ain't OK (they are tearful and crying)** because they can't make the OK sign.

Carpal Tunnel Syndrome (CTS)

Carpal Tunnel Syndrome (CTS) is a nerve entrapment syndrome due to compression of the median nerve as it passes through the carpal tunnel. **It is the most common nerve entrapment.**

Carpal tunnel is often bilateral; if it is unilateral, it tends to occur in the dominant hand (but not always).

Pain may be primarily at the wrist or radiate to the forearm, arm, or shoulder. It does not involve the neck.

Paresthesias occur in the median distribution, particularly at night. They may cause the patient to awaken at night and shake out the hand.

Wrist flexion or extension provokes symptoms.

The physical exam may be normal. There may be weakness of the abductor pollicis brevis, which abducts the thumb perpendicular to the hand.

There may be decreased sensation in the median distribution. However, **there is sparing of sensation over the thenar area because the palmar cutaneous sensory branch arises proximal to the carpal tunnel.**

Phalen's sign or Tinel's sign may be present.

- **Phalen's sign** is elicited when wrist flexion produces paresthesias in the median nerve distribution.

- **Tinel's sign** is present when tapping over the median nerve at the wrist elicits paresthesias in the median nerve distribution.

Remember that **Ph**alen's sign is when wrist flexion (**Ph**lexion) produces paresthesias in the median nerve distribution, and **T**inel's sign is when **T**apping produces them.

Carpal tunnel syndrome is typically due to demyelination, but there may be secondary axonal loss.

On nerve conduction studies (NCS), the distal latency is prolonged on the median sensory study before motor NCS are abnormal. However, **routine nerve conduction studies may be normal**.

Specific testing looking for focal slowing or conduction block of median nerve fibers across the carpal tunnel may be performed. For instance, the median nerve can be compared to the ulnar nerve, such as with the **palmar mixed study**, or **inching** may be performed (segmental stimulation of the median nerve across the carpal tunnel).

Ulnar Nerve

The ulnar nerve allows ulnar flexion at the wrist, flexion of the fourth and fifth digits, opposition and abduction of the 5th digit, thumb adduction, and finger abduction and adduction.

Weakness causes a **claw hand deformity** characterized by hyperextension of the last 3 digits at the metacarpophalangeal joints and flexion at the interphalangeal joints. The fourth and fifth digits are more affected than the third.

The ulnar nerve supplies sensation to the fifth digit and half of the fourth digit (medial aspect).

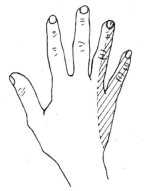 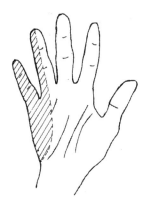

The ulnar nerve supplies:
- Abductor digiti minimi (C8-T1)
- Adductor pollicis (C8-T1)
- Flexor carpi ulnaris (C7-T1)
- Flexor digiti minimi (C8-T1)
- Flexor digitorum profundus III and IV (C7-8)
- Flexor pollicis brevis (deep head) (C8-T1)
- Interossei (C8-T1)
- Lumbricals III/IV (C8-T1)
- Opponens digiti minimi (C8-T1)
- Palmaris brevis (C8-T1)

The abductor digiti minimi (ADM) abducts the fifth digit.

The adductor pollicis adducts the metacarpal of the thumb.

The flexor carpi ulnaris (FCU) flexes the wrist and adducts the hand.

The flexor digiti minimi flexes the fifth digit.

The flexor digitorum profundus III and IV flexes the terminal phalanges of the fourth and fifth digits.

The deep head of the flexor pollicis brevis flexes and adducts the thumb.

Like the lumbricals, interossei flex the metacarpophalangeal joint and extend the proximal and distal interphalangeal joints.

Palmar interossei adduct the fingers.

Dorsal interossei abduct the fingers.

Lumbricals III/IV flex the metacarpophalangeal joint and extend the proximal and distal interphalangeal joints of the third and fourth digits.

The opponens digiti minimi allows opposition of the fifth digit.

Since the deep head of the flexor pollicis brevis can adduct the thumb, it may be used as an adductor if the adductor pollicis isn't working.

To **differentiate an ulnar nerve lesion from a T1 radiculopathy,** the abductor pollicis brevis (APB), which is innervated by the median nerve, can be tested.

The ulnar nerve tries to outdo the median nerve. The ulnar nerve may be trying to get revenge on the median nerve because of Martin-Gruber anastomosis. (See below.)

The ulnar nerve does for digiti minimi what the median nerve does for the thumb.

It works against the median nerve by adducting the thumb (adductor pollicis).

It also encroaches on the median nerve's territory by supplying the deep head of the flexor pollicis brevis.

The **u**lnar nerve supplies the deep head of the FPB, which is **u**nderneath. Remember the <u>median</u> nerve is superficial and only cares about <u>me, me, me</u>.

To remember the distal (hand) muscles supplied by both/either the Median or Ulnar nerves, think of holding a **LOAFF** of bread in your **hands**:

Median nerve	Ulnar nerve
L Lumbricals I and II	**L** Lumbricals III and IV
O Opponens pollicis	**O** Opponens digit minimi
A Abductor pollicis brevis	**A** Abductor digiti minimi
F Flexor pollicis brevis (superficial head)	**F** Flexor digiti minimi
F Flexor digitorum I and II	**F** Flexor digitorum III and IV

Martin-Gruber Anastomosis

A **Martin-Gruber anastomosis** is a communication from the median to the ulnar nerve. As a result, the median nerve innervates muscles usually innervated by the ulnar nerve: the **first dorsal interosseous (FDI), adductor pollicis,** and **abductor digiti minimi**. (Some books also list the deep head of the flexor pollicis brevis.)

 This is a communication from me to u: The FBI adds to police forces to catch the abductor of digiti minimi, Martin-Gruber. This is a communication from me to u (median to ulnar): The FBI (FDI) adds to police (adductor pollicis) forces to catch the abductor of digiti minimi, Martin-Gruber.

Cubital Tunnel Syndrome

Cubital tunnel syndrome is a nerve entrapment syndrome due to compression of the ulnar nerve in the cubital tunnel at the elbow.

Patients complain of **decreased grip and problems with finger dexterity.**

There may be **numbness and paresthesias in the ulnar distribution**.

A **claw-hand** may be seen.

The fifth digit may be abducted.

Froment's sign may be present. When trying to pinch a piece of paper between the thumb and finger, the patient uses the flexor pollicis longus and flexor digitorum profundus (which are innervated by the median nerve) because the adductor pollicis is weak.

Branches of the Posterior Cord

Branches of the posterior cord:
- Radial nerve (C5-8)
- Axillary nerve (C5-6)
- Thoracodorsal nerve (C5-8)
- Subscapular nerve (C5-7)

No one gives a RAT'S posterior about the posterior cord: Radial, Axillary, Thoracodorsal, Subscapular nerves.

A lesion of the posterior cord results in sensory loss over the posterior arm and hand, weak shoulder abduction, and weak extension of the fingers, wrist, and elbow.

Radial Nerve (C5-8)

The radial nerve is responsible for supination of the forearm, the brachioradialis reflex, and extension of the fingers, thumb, wrist, and elbow.

The radial nerve supplies:

- Abductor pollicis longus (C7-8)
- Anconeus (C6-8)
- Brachialis* (C5-6)
- Brachioradialis (C5-6)
- Extensor carpi radialis brevis (C5-7)
- Extensor carpi radialis longus (C5-6)
- Extensor carpi ulnaris (C7-8)
- Extensor digitorum (C7-8)
- Extensor digiti minimi (C7-8)
- Extensor indicis (C7-8)
- Extensor pollicis brevis (C7-8)
- Extensor pollicis longus (C7-8)
- Supinator (C6-7)
- Triceps (C6-8)

*The brachialis is also innervated by the musculocutaneous nerve.

The abductor pollicis longus abducts the metacarpal of the thumb.

The anconeus extends the elbow.

The brachialis flexes the elbow. It is also innervated by the musculocutaneous nerve.

The brachioradialis flexes the forearm.

The extensor carpi radialis brevis (ECRB) is a radial extensor of the hand.

The extensor carpi radialis longus (ECRL) extends and abducts the hand at the wrist.

The extensor carpi ulnaris extends and adducts the hand at the wrist.

The extensor digitorum extends the metacarpophalangeal joints of the 2nd –5th fingers.

The extensor digiti minimi (EDM) extends the metacarpophalangeal joint of the fifth finger.

The extensor indicis allows extension of the index finger while flexing the other fingers.

The extensor pollicis brevis extends the thumb; it is tested by asking the patient to extend the thumb at the metacarpophalangeal joint against resistance.

The extensor pollicis longus extends the thumb. It is tested by extending the thumb at the interphalangeal joint in a plane perpendicular to the palm.

The supinator supinates the forearm.

The triceps extends the forearm at the elbow.

 The brachioradialis is best tested midway between pronation and supination.

Radial nerve

- Triceps
- Anconeus

- Brachialis
- Brachioradialis
- Extensor carpi radialis longus

- Extensor carpi radialis brevis
- Supinator

- Extensor digitorum
- Extensor digiti minimi
- Extensor carpi ulnaris — Posterior interosseous nerve
- Abductor pollicis longus
- Extensor pollicis longus
- Extensor pollicis brevis
- Extensor indicis

Path of the Radial Nerve

Above the spiral groove of the humerus, the radial nerve gives off branches to the triceps and anconeus.

Below the spiral groove (but above the elbow), the radial nerve gives off branches to the brachialis, brachioradialis, and extensor carpi radialis longus. The posterior cutaneous nerves of the arm and forearm are also given off.

At or below the elbow, it divides into a superficial and a deep branch. The superficial branch provides sensation to the hand (dorsal digital nerve). The deep branch is the posterior interosseous nerve.

The posterior interosseous nerve passes through a slit in the supinator muscle (arcade of Frohse).

Above the arcade of Frohse, it gives branches to the extensor carpi radialis brevis and the supinator.

Below the arcade of Frohse, it gives off branches to the extensor digitorum, extensor digiti minimi, extensor carpi ulnaris, abductor pollicis longus, extensor pollicis longus, extensor pollicis brevis, extensor pollicis brevis, and extensor indicis.

Note that the extensor carpi ulnaris is innervated by a branch of the radial nerve, not the ulnar nerve. Remember that like the other extensors, the extensor carpi ulnaris is innervated by the radial nerve.

The posterior cutaneous nerve of the arm and the forearm are branches of the radial nerve.

The radial nerve supplies the lateral dorsum of the hand, part of the thumb, and the dorsal proximal phalanges of the index, middle, and ring fingers.

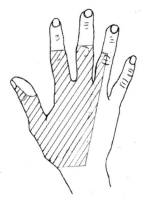
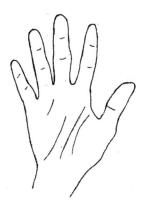

Posterior Interosseous Nerve

The posterior interosseous nerve supplies the extensor carpi radialis brevis, supinator, extensor digitorum, extensor digiti minimi, extensor carpi ulnaris, abductor pollicis longus, extensor pollicis longus, extensor pollicis brevis, and extensor indicis.

Lesions of the Radial Nerve

Radial Neuropathy at the Spiral Groove

The spiral groove is the most common site of radial neuropathy.

A humerus fracture can cause this.

Saturday night palsy is due to a radial neuropathy at the spiral groove.

MNEMONIC

If you stay up late on Saturday grooving to the radio, you may get a Saturday night palsy. If you stay up late on Saturday night grooving (spiral groove) to the radio (radial), you may get a Saturday night palsy.

Or

If your Saturday night <u>spirals</u> out of control, you may end up with a Saturday night palsy.

Radial neuropathy at the spiral groove causes wrist and fingerdrop and weakness of supination. Elbow flexion is mildly weak due to brachioradialis weakness. There is sensory loss over the lateral dorsal hand. The triceps and anconeus are spared because branches to these muscles are given off before the spiral groove. As a result, **elbow extension is spared**.

Radial Neuropathy in the Axilla

A radial neuropathy in the axilla is similar to radial neuropathy in the spiral groove, except the triceps and anconeus are weak, and there is sensory loss over the posterior forearm and arm.

Posterior Interosseous Neuropathy

BUZZ WORDS

Posterior interosseous neuropathy causes finger drop and weakness of wrist extension. When the wrist is extended, it deviates radially due to weakness of the extensor carpi ulnaris (which is innervated by the posterior interosseous nerve) and sparing of the extensor carpi radialis longus (which is innervated by the main trunk). **Thumb abduction and extension of the interphalangeal joint of the thumb are also weak.** There is no sensory loss.

Axillary Nerve (C5-6)

The axillary nerve supplies the deltoid (C5-6) and teres minor (C5-6) muscles.
- The deltoid muscle can be tested with shoulder abduction (15-90°).
- The teres minor is an external rotator of the shoulder.

The axillary nerve travels through the **quadrilateral space**, which is created by the teres major, triceps, humerus, and the teres minor.

It winds around the surgical head of the humerus.

It sends a sensory branch to the skin of the upper lateral arm over the deltoid.

The axillary nerve tends to be injured with **humerus fractures** and **shoulder dislocation**.

Thoracodorsal (C5-8)

The thoracodorsal nerve supplies the latissimus dorsi muscle.

The latissimus dorsi adducts and internally rotates the arm. It is innervated by C6-8.

 To remember that the latissimus dorsi is innervated by C6-8, think of latissimus dorsi as latsiximus dorsi.

Subscapular Nerve (C5-7)

The subscapular nerve supplies the teres major and subscapularis.

The teres major allows adduction of the elevated arm.

Injury to the subscapular nerve results in **difficulty scratching the lower back**.

Lower Extremity

Peripheral Nerves

Iliohypogastric Nerve (T12-L1)

The iliohypogastric nerve supplies the internal oblique and transversus abdominis muscles. It also supplies sensation to the hip/ outer buttocks and the anterior abdominal wall above the pubis.

Ilioinguinal Nerve (T12-L1)

The ilioinguinal nerve supplies the internal oblique and transversus abdominis, similar to the iliohypogastric nerve. It also provides sensation to the medial thigh, pubis, and external genitalia.

Genitofemoral Nerve (L1-L2)

The genitofemoral nerve provides sensation to the upper thigh (specifically the skin over the femoral triangle) and to the external genitalia.

The genitofemoral nerve (specifically the genital branch) is responsible for the **cremasteric reflex**.

This is the ***ultimate mnemonic*** for remembering the **nerves, compartments, and muscles** of the legs:

Frequently **A**sked **Q**uestions, **O**bviously **M**erit **G**raceful **A**nswers, **T**o **P**lease **S**ome **F**ine **F**olks.

(Note: the underlined letter of the each segment's first word represents the nerve, in each segment's second word represents the compartment, and in each segment's third, fourth, and fifth words represent the individual muscles innervated by the nerve in that compartment.)

FAQ: **F**emoral nerve, **A**nterior compartment, **Q**uadricep muscles

OMGA: **O**bturator nerve, **M**edial compartment, **G**racilis/**A**dductor muscles

TPSFF: **T**ibial nerve, **P**osterior compartment, **S**oleus/**F**oot **F**lexor muscles

Lateral Femoral Cutaneous Nerve of the Thigh (L2-3)

The lateral femoral cutaneous nerve provides sensation to the anterior thigh to the knee and to the upper part of the lateral thigh.

Meralgia Paresthetica

Compression of the lateral femoral cutaneous nerve of the thigh causes **meralgia paresthetica**.

This is characterized by paresthesias in the lateral thigh. It may be due to tight clothing, pregnancy, obesity, or heavy weights carried at the waist.

Femoral Nerve (L2-4)

The femoral nerve allows hip flexion and knee extension. It provides sensation to the anterior and medial thigh (medial cutaneous nerve of the thigh) and the medial calf (saphenous nerve).

The femoral nerve innervates:
- Iliacus (L2-4)
- Pectineus (L2-3)*
- Psoas (L2-4)
- Quadriceps femoris (L2-4)
- Sartorius (L2-4)

*The pectineus muscle is also innervated by the obturator nerve.

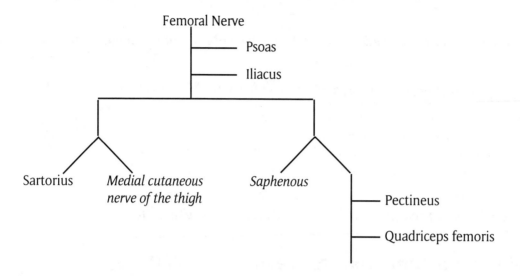

The iliacus and psoas muscles flex the thigh.

The sartorius flexes and everts the thigh.

The pectineus muscle adducts, everts, and flexes the thigh.

The quadriceps femoris (which consists of the rectus femoris, vastus lateralis, vastus intermedius, and vastus medialis muscles) extends the leg.

The tendon of the quadriceps is used to elicit the patellar reflex.

Obturator Nerve (L2-4)

The obturator nerve supplies:
- Adductor brevis (L2-4)
- Adductor longus (L2-4)
- Adductor magnus° (L2-4)
- Gracilis (L2-4)
- Obturator externus (L2-4)
- Pectineus* (L2-4)

°The adductor magnus is also innervated by the sciatic nerve.

*The pectineus is also innervated by the femoral nerve.

The obturator nerve supplies the AAA GOP: Adductor brevis, Adductor longus, Adductor magnus, Gracilis, Obturator externus, and Pectineus.

The adductor brevis, adductor longus, adductor magnus, obturator externus, and pectineus adduct the thigh.

The gracilis internally rotates the thigh and flexes the knee.

The obturator provides sensation to the medial thigh.

The obturator is quite an operator. Somehow it convinced the femoral nerve to help innervate the pectineus and the sciatic nerve to help innervate the adductor magnus. Maybe it's because it provides sensation to the medial thigh.

The obturator nerve can be injured in childbirth.

Gluteal Nerves (L4-S2)

Superior Gluteal Nerve

The superior gluteal nerve supplies the gluteus medius (L4-S1), gluteus minimus (L4-S1), and the tensor fasciae latae (L4-S1).

These muscles abduct and internally rotate the thigh.

Inferior Gluteal Nerve

The inferior gluteal nerve (L5-S2) supplies the gluteus maximus, which extends the hip.

Note it is the inferior gluteal nerve that supplies the gluteus maximus. The superior gluteal nerve supplies the gluteus medius and minimus. Innervation of the gluteal muscles is bass-ackward.

Posterior Femoral Cutaneous Nerve (S1-3)

The posterior femoral cutaneous nerve innervates the skin of the posterior thigh and popliteal fossa.

Pudendal Nerve (S1-4)

The pudendal nerve innervates perineal muscles such as the external urethral sphincter and external anal sphincter. It also provides sensation to the perineum, external genitalia, and anus.

Sciatic Nerve (L4-S3)

The sciatic nerve is the largest nerve in the body.

A complete sciatic neuropathy causes paralysis of knee flexion and loss of ankle and toe movement. Sensation loss occurs over the lateral knee, lateral and posterior calf, lateral foot, and the dorsum and sole of the foot. Also, **the ankle reflex is depressed.**

The sciatic nerve innervates:

- Hamstrings
  - ○ Semitendinosus (L4-S2)
  - ○ Semimembranosus (L4-S2)
  - ○ Biceps femoris (L4-S2)
- Adductor magnus (L2-L4)*

*Recall that the adductor magnus also receives innervation from the obturator muscle.

To remember the branches of the Sciatic Nerve and the muscles innervated by the Sciatic Nerve, think of this:

Science Awards HAMS To Common People

> **S**ciatic nerve
>
> **A**dductor muscles
>
> **HAMS**tring muscles
>
> **T**ibial nerve
>
> **C**ommon **P**eroneal nerve

To remember the hamstrings themselves, think of this:

HAMS SomeTimes SMell BeeFy

> **HAMS**trings
>
> **S**emi**M**embranosus
>
> **S**emi**T**endinosus
>
> **B**iceps **F**emoris

The hamstrings flex the knee.

The adductor magnus adducts the thigh.

The sciatic nerve branches into the tibial nerve and the common peroneal nerve.

Peroneal fibers in the sciatic nerve innervate the short head of the biceps femoris. **The short head of the biceps femoris is the only muscle innervated by the peroneal nerve that is above the fibular neck.**

The sciatic nerve can be injured by hip surgery, hip dislocation, hip fracture, and intramuscular injection in the buttocks.

The **piriformis syndrome** is caused by compression of the sciatic nerve by the piriformis muscle as it passes through the sciatic notch. It results in buttock pain and symptoms of sciatica.

Tibial Nerve (L4-S3)

The tibial nerve is responsible for plantar flexion and foot inversion. It is **the efferent limb of the Achilles tendon reflex.**

The tibial nerve innervates:
- Flexor digitorum longus (L5-S2)
- Flexor hallucis longus (S1-S2)
- Gastrocnemius (S1-S2)
- Soleus (S1-S2)
- Tibialis posterior (L4-L5)

The flexor digitorum longus plantar flexes the foot and all the toes except the great toe.

The flexor hallucis longus plantar flexes the foot and terminal phalanx of the great toe.

The gastrocnemius and soleus plantar flex the foot.

The tibialis posterior plantar flexes and inverts the foot.

 Inversion of the foot by the tibialis posterior should be tested while the foot is plantar flexed, to eliminate the action of the tibialis anterior.

The _ti_bial nerve allows you to _ti_ptoe. It innervates plantar flexors.

A branch of the tibial nerve joins the lateral sural cutaneous nerve to form the sural nerve. The sural nerve supplies the lateral aspect of the heel, foot, and small toe.

	Plantar flexion	Dorsi flexion
Inversion	Tibialis posterior	Tibialis anterior
Eversion	Peroneus brevis and longus	Peroneus tertius

The tibial nerve branches into the medial plantar, lateral plantar, and medial calcaneal nerves.

Medial Plantar Nerve (S1-S2)

The medial plantar nerve innervates:
- Abductor hallucis
- Flexor digitorum brevis
- Flexor hallucis brevis
- Lumbricals I and II
- Skin of the sole of the foot (medial 2/3)

Lateral Plantar Nerve (S1-S2)

The lateral plantar nerve innervates:
- Abductor digiti minimi
- Flexor digiti minimi
- Adductor hallucis
- Interossei
- Lumbricals III and IV
- Skin of the sole of the foot (lateral 1/3)

Medial Calcaneal Nerve

The medial calcaneal nerve supplies the sensation to the medial heel.

The **tarsal tunnel syndrome** is a focal neuropathy due to injury to the tibial nerve or its branches in the tarsal tunnel. It causes burning pain in the ankle and/or foot. Most often, patients have perimalleolar pain. The pain often is exacerbated by weight bearing and worsens at night. Patients also have paresthesias in the sole.

Common Peroneal Nerve (L4-S2)

Branches of the common peroneal nerve:
- Deep peroneal nerve
- Superficial peroneal nerve
  - ○ Lateral sural cutaneous nerve (forms sural nerve with branch from tibial nerve)
  - ○ Lateral cutaneous nerve of the calf

The common peroneal nerve is often injured at the fibular head due to its superficial location. For instance, crossing one's legs can result injure the nerve.

The deep peroneal branch is usually more affected in common peroneal neuropathies.

If both the superficial and deep branches are affected, there is weakness of toe and foot dorsiflexion and foot eversion. Sensory loss occurs over the dorsum of the foot and lateral distal lower extremity.

Deep Peroneal Nerve

The deep peroneal nerve innervates the ankle and toe dorsiflexors.

The **d**eep peroneal nerve **d**orsiflexes the foot.

The deep peroneal nerve innervates:
- Extensor digitorum brevis (L5-S1)*
- Extensor digitorum longus (L5-S1)
- Extensor hallucis longus (L5-S1)
- Peroneus tertius (L5-S1)
- Tibialis anterior (L4-5)

*In some people, a branch of the superficial peroneal nerve, the **accessory deep peroneal nerve**, may innervate part of the extensor digitorum brevis.

The extensor digitorum brevis extends the great toe and three medial toes.

The extensor digitorum longus dorsiflexes the foot and extends the four lateral toes.

The extensor hallucis longus dorsiflexes the foot and extends the great toe.

The peroneus tertius dorsiflexes and pronates the foot.

The tibialis anterior dorsiflexes and inverts the foot.

The deep peroneal nerve also innervates the skin between the first and second toes.

To remember that the deep peroneal nerve innervates the webspace between the big and 2nd toes, just think of a **"Deep Web of lies"**. *Don't fret – this mnemonic continues below ...*

The tibialis anterior (TA) is innervated by the deep peroneal nerve. The tibialis posterior (TP) is innervated by the tibial nerve.

To remember that the tibialis anterior (TA) is responsible for dorsiflexion: some people say TA-TA as they go out the door.

Alternatively, remember that the tibialis anterior is on the anterior aspect of the leg, with other muscles that allow dorsiflexion. The tibialis posterior is on the posterior aspect of the leg, with other muscles that allow plantar flexion. Both the tibialis anterior and tibialis posterior are innervated by L4-5.

Tibialis anterior (TA) and tibialis posterior (TP) are innervated by L4-5, and the L4-5 interspace is used for spinal TAPs.

Superficial Peroneal Nerve

The superficial peroneal nerve is responsible for foot eversion.

The superficial peroneal nerve innervates:
- Peroneus longus (L5-S1)
- Peroneus brevis (L5-S1)

The superficial peroneal nerve supplies sensation to the mid- and lower lateral calf.

The peroneus brevis and longus plantar flex and evert the foot.

Peroneus brevis and peroneus longus are supplied by the superficial peroneal. Peroneus tertius is supplied by the deep peroneal.

To remember that peroneus **ter**tius is supplied by the deep peroneal, which also innervates the webspace between the big and 2nd toes, just think of a "Deep, **Ter**rible Web of lies."

To remember the **superficial** peroneal nerve innervates the **peron**eus **B**revis and **L**ongus, and **e**version think of the Argentinean heroine, **Eva Peron** – who was a **superficial BL**onde!

Muscle Anatomy

Muscles are composed of muscle fibers.

Endomysium surrounds each muscle fiber.

A group of muscle fibers is surrounded by perimysium, forming a muscle fascicle.

Groups of fascicles are surrounded by epimysium.

Muscle fibers are composed of myofibrils, which allow contraction.

Myofibril Structure

Myofibrils are composed of sarcomeres.

Sarcomeres are separated by Z-discs.

Thin filaments, containing actin, are attached to the Z-discs.

Between the thin filaments are thick filaments, containing myosin.

These filaments create light and dark bands under the microscope.

- Light bands, referred to as **I-bands**, only contain actin. In this region, thick and thin filaments do not overlap.
- Dark bands, called **A-bands**, are where actin and myosin overlap.
- The **H band** contains only myosin.

Name of band	Type of filament in band
A band	Actin and Myosin
H band	Myosin
I band	Actin

MNEMONIC

To remember the band types, just link the A in **A** band to **A**ctin **A**nd myosin. The **H** band contains only my**H**osin, and the **I** band contains only act**I**n!

To remember that sarcomeres have a **Z**-disc at each end, think of our country: "From **Z** to shining **Z**!"

T-tubules (transverse tubules) are found near the junction of the A and I bands. These are structures that extend from the sarcoplasmic membrane. They allow an action potential to spread through the muscle fiber. Depolarization of the T-tubule leads to calcium release from the sarcoplasmic reticulum. Calcium binds to troponin, which sets into motion a chain of events that leads to muscle contraction.

Types of Muscle Fibers

There are three types of muscle fibers:

- Type I/ type S (slow)
- Type IIa/ type FR (fast, resistant)
- Type IIb/ type FF (fast, fatigable)

[handwritten: white]

*[handwritten:
type I atrophy
myotonic musc. dystrophy
centronuclear myopathy

type II atrophy
disuse
neurodegeneration
hyperthyroid
steroid]*

Type I or Type S (Slow) *[handwritten: red]*

[handwritten: dark – ATPase pH 4.2]

S stands for slow twitch. These contain **oxidative enzymes** and use **aerobic metabolism** to produce ATP. These produce the smallest force and contract the slowest. They produce **steady force** and are **fatigue-resistant**. Truncal postural muscles contain more type I fibers; muscles in the extremities have more type II fibers.

Type IIb or Type FF (Fast, Fatigable)

[handwritten: light – ATPase pH 4.2]

Type IIb fibers **produce the greatest force** but are **easily fatigable**. They contain **glycolytic enzymes** and use **anaerobic metabolism**. These fibers have the highest innervation ratio (number of muscle fibers innervated by one motor neuron) and largest cross-sectional area.

Type IIa or Type FR (Fast, Resistant)

These fibers have properties somewhere in between the other two types. They are fast twitch and resistant to fatigue. They contain both oxidative and glycolytic enzymes.

Muscle Receptors

There are 2 types of muscle receptors: muscle spindles and Golgi tendon organs.

Muscle Spindles

Muscle spindles **detect changes in muscle length**.

Muscle spindles consist of encapsulated muscle fibers. The muscle fibers in muscle spindles are referred to as **intrafusal** muscle fibers.

Muscle spindles are involved in the stretch reflex.

Information from the muscle spindles regarding the amount of activity a muscle is performing is carried to the central nervous system by fast conducting type A fibers. (See the nerve section below).

 The muscle **s**pindles are involved in the **s**tretch reflex.

 If you can remember that the spindles are involved in the stretch reflex, this may remind you that they detect changes in muscle length (stretching).

The Stretch Reflex

Hitting the tendon with a reflex hammer causes a stretch to be applied to a muscle, which is detected by the muscle spindles. Due to stimulation of the muscle spindles, an excitatory impulse is sent through **Ia afferent fibers** to the alpha motor neuron in the spinal cord. The alpha motor neuron then fires and causes contraction of the muscle. **This is a monosynaptic pathway**.

Golgi Tendon Organs

Golgi tendon organs are receptors found near the junction of a muscle and its tendon. They detect changes in muscle tension.

 Think of G-force to remember that the Golgi tendon organ is sensitive to force.

They help to prevent excess tension in a muscle. Stimulation of the Golgi tendon organ ultimately causes inhibition of the muscle.

When the Golgi tendon organ is stimulated, afferent signals are sent through **Ib afferent nerve fibers** to inhibitory interneurons in the spinal cord. As a result of a polysynaptic process, the alpha motor neuron is inhibited, which prevents contraction of the muscle. Also, the motor neurons of the antagonist muscle are excited. In addition, **gamma efferent nerves** cause the intrafusal spindle fibers to contract, so that they are again sensitive to stretch.

 Ib afferents synapse on **I**nhi**b**itory interneurons.

Nerve Anatomy

Peripheral Nerve Structure

Endoneurium, which is loose connective tissue, surrounds individual nerve fibers.

Nerve fibers are grouped into bundles, which are called fascicles. These fascicles are surrounded by connective tissue, which is called perineurium.

Groups of fascicles are surrounded by epimysium, which is dense connective tissue.

Classification of Nerve Fibers

Nerve fibers are classified into A, B, and C type fibers.[2]

Type A Fibers

Type A fibers are the largest and fastest conducting fibers. They are myelinated. Type A fibers include muscle afferent, muscle efferent, and cutaneous afferent fibers.

Type A alpha fibers innervate skeletal muscle and are fast conducting.

Type A delta fibers, which are the smallest type A fibers, carry pain and temperature.

Type A gamma fibers, which project from gamma motor neurons, innervate intrafusal skeletal muscle (muscle fibers in the muscle spindles).

Type B Fibers

Type B fibers are efferent, myelinated fibers that are smaller than type A fibers. These fibers are preganglionic autonomic axons.

 Think of B fibers as Before the ganglion (preganglionic).

---

[2] There are alternative classifications.

Type C Fibers

Type C fibers are the smallest fibers. They are unmyelinated. They function as efferent postganglionic fibers or afferent somatosensory fibers that carry temperature and deep, diffuse pain.

 Signals Creep along the C fibers, which are the slowest.

C fibers cause people to Cuss; they transmit pain sensation.

Myelin

Pzero (P_0) is the most common protein in peripheral myelin.

 The overwhelming majority of myelin is Po. It's the most **Po**pular.

Neuromuscular Junction

A synaptic vesicle contains 1 **quanta** of ACh, which is 10,000 molecules of ACh.

At rest, single vesicles are spontaneously released from the presynaptic membrane. This produces a change (about 1 mV) in the end plate potential at the postsynaptic membrane, which is called a **miniature end plate potential**.

When a descending nerve fiber action potential triggers release of acetylcholine, 60 to 100 vesicles are released.

(The action potential depolarizes the nerve terminal, which causes voltage gate calcium channels to open, resulting in the influx of calcium. This calcium binds with calmodulin, triggering a cascade of events that leads to release of acetylcholine.)

Myopathy

Channelopathies

Type of channel	Disease name
Calcium	Hypokalemic periodic paralysis
Chloride	Myotonia congenita, Paramyotonia congenita
Potassium	Hypokalemic periodic paralysis
Sodium	Hypokalemic periodic paralysis, Hyperkalemic periodic paralysis, Paramyotonia congenita, Sodium channel myotonia (acetazolamide-responsive myotonia, myotonia fluctuans, myotonia permanens)

Hypokalemic Periodic Paralysis

Hypokalemic periodic paralysis is most often due to a mutation on 1q in the gene that encodes the alpha-1 subunit of L-type calcium channels. It is an autosomal dominant condition. It also has been associated with sodium channel mutations and hyperthyroidism (**Thyrotoxic periodic paralysis**).

Hypokalemic periodic paralysis usually presents in the second decade.

It is characterized by episodes of weakness that last for hours or days. **The weakness is triggered by a large carbohydrate load or exercise**. Often the patient wakes up with weakness, the day after the trigger.

Hyperkalemic Periodic Paralysis

Hyperkalemic periodic paralysis is also known as **potassium-sensitive periodic paralysis**. (The potassium is not always elevated during an attack, but potassium worsens the attack.)

Hyperkalemic periodic paralysis is an autosomal dominant condition due to a mutation on **17q** in the gene that encodes the **alpha subunit of a skeletal muscle voltage-gated sodium channel (SCN4A)**. Mutations in this gene also cause paramyotonia congenita, acetazolamide-responsive myotonia, myotonia fluctuans, myotonia permanens, and a form of hypokalemic periodic paralysis.

Hyperkalemic periodic paralysis presents less than 10 years of age with episodes of weakness.

Usually the attacks are characterized by symmetric proximal weakness lasting for minutes to hours.

The attacks are **triggered by rest after exercise or fasting**. They are **relieved by eating carbohydrates or performing light exercise**.

	Hypokalemic Periodic Paralysis	**Hyperkalemic Periodic Paralysis**
Chromosome	1q	17q
Gene product	L-type calcium channel alpha1 subunit	SCN4A (Sodium channel)
Age	10-20s	<10 years old
Exercise	Lowers potassium→makes it WORSE	Lowers potassium→makes it BETTER
Carbohydrate loading	Lowers potassium→makes it WORSE	Lowers potassium→makes it BETTER
Treatment	Rest/fasting	Eat carbs and exercise

vacuolar dilatation of sarcoplasmic reticulum

MNEMONIC

To remember features of **HyperK**alemic PP, think of a **Hyper K**id who is **less than 10 years old** but thinks he's **17 q**uickly, and is **S**uper **C**razy **N**uts **4 A**nother **carb load** after he **exercises**.

Myotonia Congenita

Myotonia congenita is due to mutations in the gene on 7q that encodes a muscle chloride channel (CLCN1).

There are autosomal recessive and autosomal dominant forms.

BUZZ WORDS

Myotonia congenita presents in childhood with myotonia. The myotonia causes muscle stiffness and decreased speed. Muscle hypertrophy may be seen. Patients with the autosomal recessive form may have mild weakness On exam, grip and percussion myotonia can be seen.

Paramyotonia Congenita

Paramyotonia congenita may be due to a mutation in CLCN1, similar to myotonia congenita, or SCN4A, similar to hyperkalemic periodic paralysis.

BUZZ WORDS

Paramyotonia congenita is characterized by myotonia that *worsens* with exercise. (In other forms of myotonia, myotonia often improves with repeated muscle activity.) Paramyotonia congenita is also **triggered by cold**.

Congenital Myopathy

Congenital myopathy may present in the neonatal period/early infancy with hypotonia, weakness, and decreased reflexes. Creatine kinase may be normal or slightly elevated. Clinically, congenital myopathies are difficult to differentiate. Muscle biopsy is diagnostic.

Central Core Disease

Central core disease causes neonatal hypotonia and weakness. Skeletal abnormalities such as hip dislocation and clubfoot are seen.

 This is an autosomal dominant disorder due to a gene defect in the ***ryanodine receptor-1 gene*** (RYR1) on chromosome 19q. The ryanodine receptor mediates the release of calcium after sarcolemma depolarization. Mutations in this gene result in **malignant hyperthermia** as well.

Patients with central core disease may be at risk for malignant hyperthermia.

Cores are seen in type 1 fibers on histology. These areas lack mitochondria and oxidative enzyme activity.

Centronuclear (Myotubular) Myopathy

There are X-linked, dominant, and recessive forms of centronuclear (myotubular) myopathy.

These patients have ptosis and extraocular muscle weakness in addition to hypotonia and skeletal muscle weakness.

Centronuclear (**C**entro**N**uclear) myopathy involves cranial nerve (**CN**) innervated muscles. Patients have ptosis and extraocular muscle weakness.

In centronuclear myopathy, muscle biopsy shows central nuclei. Also, type I fibers predominate and are small.

Congenital Fiber Type Size Disproportion

There are dominant, recessive, and X-linked forms.

Some patients have arthrogryposis.

Muscle biopsy shows small type I fibers.

Congenital Muscular Dystrophy

See the muscular dystrophy section.

Nemaline (Rod) Myopathy

Nemaline myopathy may be static or progressive.

The neonatal form is associated with respiratory failure, severe hypotonia, and early death.

 Children with nemaline myopathy have a high-arched palate and a long, narrow face.

Multiple gene can cause nemaline myopathy e.g. alpha-actin, nebulin, tropomyosin.

Muscle biopsy shows rods in the cytoplasm of muscle fibers (dark red-blue structures seen with Gomori trichrome stain).

Electron microscopy shows that the **rods originate from Z-disks**.

Inflammatory Myopathy

Dermatomyositis

 Dermatomyositis is an **inflammatory myopathy** that can occur at **any age**.

It is a microangiopathy that is humorally mediated.

Patients with dermatomyositis have weakness in a limb-girdle distribution.

Dermatomyositis is accompanied by a characteristic rash.

Patients develop a **HELIOTROPE RASH – a purple discoloration on the eyelids and periorbital edema**. A scaly, red rash can be seen on the knuckles, known as **Gottron's papules**.

Subcutaneous calcifications are seen in some children with dermatomyositis.

In some adults, dermatomyositis is associated with malignancy, particularly GI/stomach cancer in men and GU/ovarian in women.

EKG abnormalities can be seen in patients with dermatomyositis.

Interstitial lung disease occurs in some cases of adult dermatomyositis. Frequently, these patients have anti-Jo-1 antibodies, which are the most common type of **Anti-Synthetase Antibody**.

Dermatomyositis is associated with **perifascicular atrophy**.

 Patients with dermatomyositis have a **fac**ial rash and peri**fasc**icular atrophy.

 Steroids are the treatment of choice.

Polymyositis

Polymyositis presents over 20 years of age.

 Like dermatomyositis, polymyositis has a limb-girdle distribution and can be associated with interstitial lung disease and cardiac arrhythmias.

However, **dermatomyositis is humoral mediated**, and **polymyositis is T-cell mediated**.

The CK is elevated in polymyositis.

Muscle biopsy shows **endomysial inflammation**. Definitive diagnosis of polymyositis requires the presence of CD8+ T cells in major histocompatibility complex class I positive muscle fibers.

Steroids are the treatment of choice.

Inclusion Body Myositis (IBM)

Inclusion body myositis is the most common inflammatory muscle disease in patients over 50 years of age.

The age of onset is greater than 50 years.

IBM involves the **quadriceps and wrist and finger flexors**.

To remember this, think of an IBM computer. You need your finger flexors to hit the keys of the keyboard and your quads to kick the hard drive if the computer acts up.

IBM is <u>not</u> associated with malignancy or systemic abnormalities.

CK is normal or slightly elevated (less than 10 times normal).

Light microscopy shows:

· Endomysial inflammation

· Eosinophilic cytoplasmic inclusions

· **Rimmed vacuoles**

· Amyloid deposition

IBM usually does not respond to immunomodulatory medications.

> EMG findings in myositis:
> • Increased insertional activity
> • Low amplitude, short duration motor unit action potentials
> • Early recruitment of motor unit action potentials

Medication-induced Myopathy

Steroid Myopathy

Usually steroid myopathy causes a proximal myopathy. The hip girdle muscles are the most involved.

Steroid myopathy is NOT associated with increased insertional activity.

Prednisone is associated with type 2 fiber atrophy.

Statins

Statins cause myopathy by inhibiting synthesis of mevalonic acid, which is a precursor of Coenzyme Q10.

Zidovudine (AZT)

AZT can cause a mitochondrial myopathy.

Ragged red fibers are found on muscle biopsy.

Myopathies associated with Systemic Disease

Hypothyroid Myopathy

 Hypothyroid myopathy is associated with **muscle cramps** and **mild proximal weakness**.

Muscle contraction is slow, and **reflexes may be delayed**.

Myoedema is seen with muscle percussion.

Muscle enlargement can be seen.

Myokymia may be present.

The CK is very elevated.

Critical Illness Myopathy

This is seen in ICU patients who have been treated with **steroids** and **neuromuscular junction blockers**.

 These patients are **ventilator dependent**, have a **flaccid paralysis**, and are **areflexic**. Extraocular muscles and sensation are spared.

CK is elevated initially.

Muscle biopsy shows loss of myosin.

 ICU (I see you) lost **myo**sin from critical illness **myopathy**.

Muscular Dystrophies

Type of muscular dystrophy	Inheritance pattern
Becker muscular dystrophy	X-linked recessive
Congenital muscular dystrophy	Autosomal recessive
Duchenne muscular dystrophy	X-linked recessive
Facioscapulohumeral muscular dystrophy	Autosomal dominant
Emery-Dreifuss muscular dystrophy	X-linked recessive, autosomal dominant, or rarely autosomal recessive
Oculopharyngeal muscular dystrophy	Autosomal dominant
Limb-girdle muscular dystrophy	Autosomal dominant or autosomal recessive

Duchenne Muscular Dystrophy (DMD) and Becker Muscular Dystrophy (BMD)

Duchenne muscular dystrophy (DMD) is the most common muscular dystrophy.

Clinical Course

DMD

 DMD usually presents by age 5 years.

Patients have **difficulty running, a waddling gait, lumbar lordosis, and calf pseudohypertrophy**.

Weakness is symmetric and proximal, involving the lower extremities more than the upper.

Patients with DMD also have **neck flexor weakness**, and use their hands to help them stand up from a lying down position (**Gowers sign**).

CK is very high.

DMD patients may have cognitive impairment.

Patients are usually wheelchair-dependent by age 13 years.

Eventually, all patients develop a **cardiomyopathy**.

Intestinal pseudo-obstruction can be life-threatening, but most patients with DMD die around 20 years of age from respiratory or cardiac failure.

BMD

 Patients with Becker Muscular Dystrophy have a later age of onset, milder clinical course, and live longer than patients with DMD.

The mean age of onset is 12 years, patients walk into adult life, and live beyond 30 years.

BMD patients are less likely to have cognitive delay, cardiac disease, contractures, scoliosis, and gastrointestinal problems.

Like DMD patients, BMD patients have calf pseudohypertrophy and early thigh weakness.

CK levels in DMD and BMD patients are similar.

 Patients with Becker do better than patients with Duchenne MD.

Genetics

 Becker and Duchenne are both due to mutations in the **dystrophin gene on Xp**.

Becker patients have in-frame mutations, and Duchenne patients have out of frame mutations.

 Becker patients are in luck compared to Duchenne patients, and have in-frame mutations.

Pathology

Duchenne patients have no dystrophin when muscle biopsies are stained with antidystrophin antibodies. Staining shows reduced dystrophin in patients with BMD.

There is variability of muscle fiber size with degenerating and regenerating fibers. Fat and connective tissue replace muscle. Later endomysial and perimysial fibrosis are seen.

Treatment

 Prednisone can be used to improve strength in DMD.

Congenital Muscular Dystrophy

There are multiple types of congenital muscular dystrophy. These disorders are **autosomal recessive**.

 They present at birth or in infancy. They are characterized by **weakness, hypotonia, and often an elevated creatine kinase**.

Muscle biopsy is consistent with myopathy or a dystrophic process.

To remember congenital muscular dystrophy is autosomal recessive and appears in infancy: Infants with congenital muscular dystrophy attend recess.

Classic Congenital Muscular Dystrophy

Classic congenital muscular dystrophy is divided into merosin-positive and merosin-negative forms. Merosin is also known as **laminin α-2** because it is the heavy α-2 chain of laminin 2. It is found in the basement membrane of muscle fibers. **The gene for merosin is located on chromosome 6q.**

To remember that the gene for merosin is located on chromosome 6, think of merosin as merosix.

Merosin-negative Congenital Muscular Dystrophy

Merosin-negative congenital muscular dystrophy is the most common form of congenital muscular dystrophy.

It presents with hypotonia, weakness, and feeding difficulties. Patients have progressive contractures and usually do not attain ambulation.

MRI shows **cerebral white matter changes** (indicated by increased T2 signal).

Merosin-positive Congenital Muscular Dystrophy

Patients with merosin-positive congenital muscular dystrophy present at birth with hypotonia, diffuse weakness, facial weakness, and contractures.

Merosin-positive congenital muscular dystrophy is less severe than the merosin negative form. Patients with merosin-positive congenital muscular dystrophy are more likely to ambulate. Also, these patients lack cerebral white matter abnormalities.

Syndromic Congenital Muscular Dystrophy

Syndromic congenital muscular dystrophies are associated with cobblestone lissencephaly, eye abnormalities, and muscle weakness. In cobblestone lissencephaly, the cortex lacks recognizable layers. The neurons are present on the brain surface and in the meninges because they migrate too far.

There are **3 forms of syndromic congenital muscular dystrophy**:

1. Fukuyama congenital muscular dystrophy
2. Muscle-eye-brain disease
3. Walker-Warburg syndrome

Fukuyama congenital muscular dystrophy, which is found primarily in Japan, is associated with mutations in the gene on 9q that encodes **fukutin**.

Muscle-eye-brain disease, which is found common in Finland, is due to a defect in **POMGnT1** on 1p, which encodes *O*-mannoside β1,2-*N*-acetylglucosaminyl-transferase.

Walker-Warburg syndrome is due to a mutation in **POMT1** on 9q, which encodes *O*-mannosyltransferase 1.

All 3 forms are associated with **hypoglycosylated α-dystroglycan** in skeletal muscle.

Distal Muscular Dystrophies

Miyoshi Myopathy (Early Adult Onset Distal Myopathy Type II)

Miyoshi myopathy causes myopathy, which first affects the posterior compartment of the legs.

The gastrocnemius and soleus are involved. The **extensor digiti minimi is spared.**

Patients have a very high CK.

Since Miyoshi looks a bit like My sushi, remember the phrase, "My sushi is a gastronomical delight" to remember that Miyoshi myopathy is associated with gastrocnemius weakness.

Miyoshi myopathy is autosomal recessive or sporadic.

It is due to a mutation in the *dysferlin* gene on 2p; **it is allelic with LGMD type 2B**.

 In keeping with the previous mnemonic, and to remember the mutation associated with Miyoshi Myopathy, just think that the sushi is even better when it's given as a gift to your friend Lynn: dys-fer-lin!

Welander (Late Adult Type 1) Distal Myopathy

Like Miyoshi myopathy, this is due to a defect on 2p. However, it is <u>not</u> allelic to Miyoshi myopathy.

Welander myopathy is an autosomal dominant myopathy that starts in the hands, primarily affecting the fingers and wrist extensors.

 Remember the association with distal hand onset and Welander, think of We-**hand**-er Myopathy.

Emery-Dreifuss Muscular Dystrophy (EDMD)

EDMD can be X-linked recessive, autosomal dominant, or autosomal recessive (rare).

X-linked EDMD is due to a mutation in the gene *EMD* on Xq, which encodes **emerin**.

Autosomal EDMD is due to a mutation in the *LMNA* gene on 1q, which encodes **lamin A/C**.

EDMD is associated with **early joint contractures, weakness in a humeroperoneal distribution, and cardiac abnormalities**.

Joint contractures are seen in childhood, usually involving the elbows and ankles. Toe-walking may be a presentation of EDMD.

Later joint contractures involve the neck, causing reduced neck flexion. As the disease progresses, movement of the spine and lower limbs may be limited, which interfere with the ability to walk.

Weakness in EDMD is said to occur in a humeroperoneal distribution. The biceps and triceps are often affected first. Then the peroneal muscles in the distal leg are affected. Later, the scapular and pelvic girdle muscles are affected.

 Patients with EDMD can have cardiac conduction defects that can lead to sudden death.

When you see Emery-Dreifuss, think Emergency-Department because cardiac conduction defects can cause sudden death. Also for Emery, think of the 3 **E**'s: **E**mery **E**arly **El**bow contractures, and for Dreifus, think of **Drei-Bi-Tri** for **Bi**ceps and **Tri**ceps involvement.

Facioscapulohumeral Muscular Dystrophy (FSHD)

FSHD usually presents by age 20.

It is associated with <u>asymmetric</u> weakness involving the face, muscles that stabilize the scapula, proximal upper extremities, and dorsiflexors of the foot.

Facial weakness results in difficulty closing the eyes tightly, whistling, and using a straw. Patients with FSHD sleep with their eyes open.

FSHD is associated with a **Popeye effect**; patients have weak biceps and triceps but the deltoids spared.

Scapular winging is seen in FSHD.

Sensorineural hearing loss may occur.

FSHD may be associated with **Coats' disease**, which is characterized by an exudate telangiectasia of the retina and retinal detachment.

FSHD is **autosomal dominant**. It is due to a **deletion of D4Z4 repeats on chromosome 4q**.

Think of Four when you see F in FSHD to remind you that FSHD is due to a deletion of D4Z4 repeats on chromosome 4q.

Limb Girdle Muscular Dystrophy

Limb girdle muscular dystrophy (LGMD) includes a number of diseases that are characterized by proximal muscle weakness, affecting the shoulder and/or pelvic girdle. The facial and extraocular muscles tend to be spared. Some patients have cardiomyopathy.

Muscle biopsy shows dystrophic changes.

The autosomal dominant forms of LGMD are categorized as LGMD 1; the autosomal recessive forms are called LGMD 2.

The age of onset varies from childhood to adulthood, but usually they are not congenital. Most forms of LGMD are slowly progressive. LGMD 2 tends to present earlier and progress faster than LGMD 1. The CK tends to be higher in LGMD 2. One exception to this is LGMD1C, which does cause a high CK.

LGMD1

LGMD1A is due to defective myotilin.
LGMD1B is due to defective lamin A/C.
LGMD1C is due to defective caveolin-3.

The defective protein is unknown for the other types of LGMD1.

 Lamin A/C gene mutations are found in LGMD1B and autosomal dominant Emery-Dreifuss muscular dystrophy (EDMD). **Like EDMD, LGMD1B is associated with cardiac problems.** LGMD1B is associated with cardiomyopathy and cardiac conduction defects.

In LGMD1**C**, which is due to defective **c**aveolin-3, you see a high **C**K.

LGMD2

There are more than 10 types of LGMD2.

LGMD2A, which is due to calpain deficiency, is associated with early contractures.

LGMD2B, which is due to defective dysferlin, is allelic with Miyoshi myopathy and causes similar findings (early gastrocnemius and soleus weakness).

The **sarcoglycanopathies** (LGMD 2C, 2D, 2E, and 2F) and LGMD2I (due to defective fukutin-related protein) resemble DMD or BMD.

Myotonic Dystrophy Type 1 (DM1)

Myotonic dystrophy is the most common muscular dystrophy in adults.

DM1 is characterized by myotonia, facial and distal weakness, and involvement of multiple organ systems.

Myotonia (delayed muscle relaxation) is seen in DM1. This results in difficulty releasing one's grasp or opening one's eyes after tight closure. It can be elicited with percussion.

Weakness affects the facial muscles and distal limbs. The wrist extensors, finger extensors, grip, and ankle dorsiflexors are particularly affected.

Patients have neck weakness, temporal and masseter wasting, ptosis, and pharyngeal weakness resulting in dysphagia and dysarthria. Eye and mouth closure are weak.

Multiple organ systems are involved. The following may be found in DM1:
- Apathy
- Christmas tree cataracts
- Cardiomyopathy and conduction defects
- Dysphagia, megacolon, cholelithiasis
- Frontal balding (males)
- Hypersomnia
- Hypogonadism e.g. testicular atrophy, gynecomastia
- Hypoventilation
- Insulin resistance.

Death is often due to respiratory insufficiency, pneumonia, or cardiac arrhythmia.

There is a congenital form of DM1. See congenital myotonic dystrophy below.

EMG/NCS shows **myotonic discharges** and myopathic MUAPs.

Muscle biopsy shows type 1 fiber atrophy. There are **increased central nuclei**.

DM1 is autosomal dominant. It is due to an amplified **CTG repeat** in the *DMPK* **(dystrophia myotonica protein kinase) gene on chromosome 19q.**

Congenital Myotonic Dystrophy

Congenital myotonic dystrophy is the most common myopathic disorder to appear in the neonatal period.

Congenital myotonic dystrophy is associated with > 1,000 CTG repeats in the *DMPK* gene on 19q. This large number of repeats is due to anticipation. The mother is usually the affected parent. If you are suspicious of congenital myotonic dystrophy, check Mom's grip. If she doesn't let go, you may be right.

Patients with congenital myotonic dystrophy exhibit hypotonia, facial diplegia, feeding and respiratory difficulties, and decreased reflexes. "fish mouth"

They may have joint deformities ranging from clubfoot to arthrogryposis.

The hypotonia and feeding and respiratory problems improve.

Development is delayed. Cognition is impaired.

Myotonia develops around age 2 years.

 EMG does not demonstrate myotonia until the patient is older.

Myotonic Dystrophy Type 2 (DM2)

DM2 is also known as **Proximal Myotonic Myopathy (PROMM)**.

Similar to DM1, DM2 causes facial weakness, ptosis, myotonia, and progressive weakness. Unlike DM1, DM2 causes primarily proximal muscle weakness.

Calf pseudohypertrophy may be seen in DM2.

DM2 is associated with proximal weakness rather than distal, has less cardiac and pulmonary involvement than DM1, has no congenital form, is associated with less atrophy, and is due to a tetranucleotide repeat.

DM2 is due to a CCTG repeat expansion in the *ZNF9* (zinc finger protein 9) at 3q.

To remember this, think of a **C**rushing **C**losing of **T**hat **G**rip! The **grip was so tight**, that the DM2 patient squeezed the other person's hand into **3 q**uivering **Zinc Fingers**!

Oculopharyngeal Muscular Dystrophy (OPMD)

OPMD presents in middle age with <u>asymmetric</u> ptosis, due to asymmetric involvement of the levator palpebrae muscles. Ptosis is progressive and extraocular muscle weakness develops.

Unlike myasthenia gravis, OPMD is <u>not</u> associated with diplopia.

 Pharyngeal weakness results in dysphagia and dysarthria.

Mild neck and proximal limb weakness is seen.

OPMD is **autosomal dominant**. It is due to a **GCG repeat expansion in the gene encoding PAPB2 (poly-A binding protein-2) on 14q**.

 The GCG expansion in OPMD could stand for Gag, Choke, Gag because OPMD causes dysphagia.

 To remember the clinical features of OPMD and the gene product acronym, think of the **PAPB**2 gene standing for **P**rogressive **A**symmetric **P**tosis & **B**ulbar weakness.

Muscle biopsy shows **rimmed vacuoles** and fiber size variation.

Metabolic Myopathies

Carnitine Deficiency

 Carnitine is important for fatty acid oxidation; it's required for transport of fatty acids into mitochondria.

There are primary and secondary forms of carnitine deficiency. For instance, zidovudine and valproate can cause secondary carnitine deficiency.

Primary Myopathic Carnitine Deficiency

Primary myopathic carnitine deficiency causes progressive proximal muscle weakness and atrophy beginning in childhood or early adulthood.

Muscle biopsy shows **lipid storage**.

 Primary myopathic carnitine deficiency is treated with carnitine.

Primary Systemic Deficiency of Carnitine

 Primary systemic deficiency of carnitine presents in childhood.

It causes **episodes resembling Reye's syndrome** characterized by vomiting, encephalopathy, hepatomegaly, hyperammonemia, and hypoglycemia.

Patients also have **progressive weakness and cardiomyopathy**.

Muscle biopsy shows **lipid storage**.

 Some patients with primary systemic deficiency of carnitine respond to treatment with carnitine.

Carnitine Palmitoyl Transferase-II Deficiency (CPT-II Deficiency)

The adult myopathic form of CPT-II deficiency is the most common metabolic cause of recurrent myoglobinuria.

The defect is on chromosome 1. CPT-II has a role in fatty acid β-oxidation. It's involved in transport of fatty acids across the inner mitochondrial membrane; it mediates formation of fatty acid-CoA.

CPT-II deficiency usually presents in adolescence.

Patients with CPT-II deficiency have tenderness and swelling of muscles with sustained aerobic exercise (or other stressors such as infection). This is associated with an increased CK and myoglobinuria. Patients are normal between episodes.

 In patients with CPT-II (2) deficiency, you C (see) P (pee) T (tea) with 2 (too) much exercise.

Glycogen Storage Diseases

Type	Eponym	Enzyme Defect
II	Pompe	Acid maltase (1,4 glucosidase)
III	Cori-Forbes	Debranching
IV	Andersen	Transglucosidase
V	McArdle	Muscle phosphorylase
VII	Tarui	Muscle phosphofructokinase
VIII	—————	Phosphorylase kinase
IX	—————	Phosphoglycerate kinase
X	—————	Phosphoglycerate mutase
XI	—————	Lactic dehydrogenase

All of the glycogenoses are autosomal recessive except phosphoglycerate kinase deficiency, which is X-linked recessive.

Types I and VI do not involve muscle, but all the others cause myopathy.

Acid Maltase Deficiency

 Acid maltase deficiency is also known as **Pompe's disease** and Glycogen Storage Disease Type II. It is autosomal recessive.

Infantile-Type Acid Maltase Deficiency

The infantile form of acid maltase deficiency causes neonatal hypotonia.[3]

Adult Acid Maltase Deficiency

Adults with acid maltase deficiency present in their 20s or 30s.

In younger adults, it may present with fatigue. In older adults, it may present with leg and trunk weakness.

---

[3] Please see the Metabolic Diseases chapter.

Patients can present with **respiratory failure** or develop it later.

Adults with acid maltase deficiency have an increased CK and **myotonia** on EMG particularly in the **paraspinal** muscles (but have no clinical myotonia).

They may have **intracranial aneurysms** due to glycogen deposition.

A **vacuolar myopathy** is seen on muscle biopsy. Due to glycogen storage, **lysosomes stain with PAS**.

 Acid **M**altase deficiency in adults is associated with **A**neurysms and **M**yopathy (vacuolar), and **A**symptomatic **M**yotonia (in the paraspinal muscles on EMG). Folks with **AM** say, "I **AM** what I **AM**."

McArdle's Disease/ Muscle Phosphorylase Deficiency/ GSD V

This is an autosomal recessive metabolic myopathy that causes **fatigue and cramps**.

Fifty percent of patients have **myoglobinuria,** which may cause renal failure.

McArdle's disease is associated with a **second-wind phenomenon**.

The **forearm ischemic lactate test is abnormal** in McArdle's disease; these patients lack a rise in lactate.

Muscle biopsy shows **subsarcolemmal vacuoles**.

To remember that McArdle's disease is associated with a second wind phenomenon, think of this as McArnold disease. Arnold Schwarzenegger's career had a second wind. First he was a weight lifter, then an actor, then governor.

Tarui's Disease/ Phosphofructokinase deficiency/ GSD VII

This is an autosomal recessive metabolic myopathy that causes exercise intolerance (cramps and fatigue) and exercise-induced myoglobinuria.

Similar to McArdle disease, **the forearm ischemic lactate test is abnormal**; however, there is no second wind phenomenon in Tarui's disease.

Just think of Commander Sulu from Star Trek, played by actor George **Takei** (sounds like **Tarui's** Disease), who's career **didn't** have a second wind. This is in contrast to Arnold Schwarzenegger, (**McArnold** sounds like **McArdle** Disease) who's career **did** have a second wind.

Mitochondrial Myopathies

Mitochondrial diseases are discussed in the Metabolic Diseases chapter.

They can cause weakness or muscle fatigue.

Neuromuscular Junction Diseases

Botulism

Infantile Botulism

In infants, botulism is due to a **toxin produced by** **ingested** *Clostridium botulinum*.

Infants **living near construction sites are at risk**, but classically (on exams) infantile botulism has been associated with **ingestion of honey**.

First the infant develops **constipation**. Then **generalized weakness** including bulbar and skeletal muscles, **hypotonia, decreased reflexes, ptosis, and dilated pupils** are seen. Respiratory failure may occur.

Stool cultures and EMG/NCS help with the diagnosis. Specifically, **posttetanic facilitation** and **absence of posttetanic exhaustion** are seen.

Adult Botulism

In adults, botulism is due to **toxin produced by germinated *Clostridium botulinum* spores**. Spores can be found in improperly prepared canned foods, undercooked food, and anaerobic wounds.

There are 7 types of Botox subtoxins, each named alphabetically: **A,B,C,D,E,F and G**.

Subtypes **A**&**E** work by cleaving the protein **SNAP-25**.
Think of turning off the ***A&E*** network (channel **25**) in a **SNAP** because your show was cancelled.

Subtypes **B,D,F and G** work by cleaving **VAMP** (Vesicle Associated Membrane Protein).
Think of a **BaD FanGed VAMP**ire...

Subtype **C** is perhaps the most **C**lever toxin: it **C**leaves **SNAP-25** and **synaptotaxin**!
Subtype **C C**leaves a **C**ombo of proteins in a **SNAP**!

The toxin blocks release of acetylcholine.

Patients have **dry mouth, vomiting, ophthalmoplegia, loss of pupillary reflexes, and a symmetric DESCENDING weakness**, which can lead to respiratory failure.

If patients present at that point, they can look like Guillain-Barré patients. However, Guillain-Barré usually causes ascending weakness and does not usually cause loss of pupillary reflexes. EMG also differentiates the two diseases.

In botulism, EMG/NCS show low-amplitude muscle action potentials. **With repetitive stimulation at 20-50 Hz, there is potentiation of the response**. *Prolonged posttetanic facilitation and absence of posttetanic exhaustion* are seen in adult botulism as well as infantile botulism.

Congenital Myasthenia Gravis

Congenital myasthenia gravis causes weakness in infancy/childhood.

Some patients have ptosis or ophthalmoparesis.

Bulbar and respiratory weakness are also seen.

Some patients respond to Tensilon; an exception is endplate Acetylcholinesterase deficiency.

A number of neuromuscular transmission defects cause congenital myasthenia gravis: defects in acetylcholine synthesis or mobilization, a decreased number of acetylcholine receptors, defective breakdown of acetylcholine at the end plate, or prolonged open time of the acetylcholine receptor channel. Note that the defect may be presynaptic or postsynaptic.

 Congenital myasthenia gravis is <u>not</u> associated with acetylcholine receptor antibodies.

Lambert-Eaton Myasthenic Syndrome

Lambert-Eaton syndrome is a neuromuscular junction disorder due to **antibodies directed against P/Q-type voltage-gated calcium channels**.

 It may be due to an underlying malignancy such as small cell lung cancer.

Treatment

 3,4-DiAminoPyridine

Although not a cure, therapy with **3,4-DiAminoPyridine** may help LEMS patients function better.

3,4-DAP inhibits **potassium-channels** which in turn permit calcium entry into the cell, despite the LEMS-antibodies produced against the voltage-gated **calcium channels**.

To remember the features, antibodies and treatment of LEMS, think of this mnemonic:

A **small** (small cell lung cancer) **lamb** (LEMS) tries to escape a **Voltage Gate**, because he doesn't like getting **milked (calcium)**. He tries to jump the gate **3 or 4 times** (3,4-DAP) **repetitively** (rep stim), and his **muscle strength improves with this exercise**, so finally he **Kicks** (**K+**=potassium) the gate open to freedom.

Lambert-Eaton syndrome usually presents in adults. Patients have a **dry mouth; constipation; proximal muscle weakness**, especially **the thighs; and decreased reflexes**.

Strength may improve temporarily after exercise.

Patients with Lambert-Eaton syndrome have low amplitude CMAPs. Lambert-Eaton (and myasthenia gravis) patients have a **CMAP decrement (greater than 10% drop) with repetitive stimulation at 2-5 Hz.**

In Lambert-Eaton patients, the **CMAP increases significantly with repetitive stimulation at 20-50 Hz,** which can also be seen in severe myasthenia gravis.

Myasthenia Gravis (MG)

Autoimmune Myasthenia Gravis

Autoimmune myasthenia gravis is due to a decrease in the number of functioning acetylcholine receptors at the neuromuscular junction due to antibodies. Antibodies may bind to the receptor and cause complement-mediated destruction of the receptor. There are also blocking and modulating antibodies.

Patients with MG have **fluctuating weakness**. They **fatigue with exercise and improve with rest**.

Weakness occurs in the proximal more than distal extremities. Patients also have **neck weakness**.

Diplopia, dysphagia, and **ptosis** are common in patients with MG.

Symptoms **worsen when the patient is hot**.

The **Tensilon test** may be used for diagnosis.

EMG/NCS are also helpful in the diagnosis. Myasthenia gravis patients often have a **CMAP decrement** (greater than 10% drop) **with repetitive stimulation at 2-5 Hz.**

EMG may show motor unit potential amplitude variation.

Single fiber EMG (SFEMG) shows **blocking** (failure of transmission at the NMJ) and **increased jitter** of muscle fiber potentials.

Some patients have lymphoid hyperplasia, and some have thymoma. Thymectomy may eventually decrease symptoms.

Anticholinesterase medications such as **pyridostigmine (Mestinon®)** are used to treat the symptoms of MG.

Immunosuppressants are used such as *prednisone, azathioprine, cyclosporine*, and *mycophenolate mofetil.*

Myasthenic crises *may be treated with*:

· IVIG

· Methylprednisolone

· Plasma exchange.

Certain medications can <u>worsen</u> MG and should be avoided. Examples include aminoglycosides, beta-blockers, procainamide, quinine, quinidine, and magnesium.

Toxicity from cholinesterase inhibitors causes diarrhea, increased secretions, and sweating due to its muscarinic effects. Fasciculations and weakness result from the effect on nicotinic receptors.

Myasthenia Gravis with anti-MuSK Antibodies

There are patients who are diagnosed with MG based on clinical and electrodiagnostic criteria who do not have antibodies to the acetylcholine receptor.

Some of these patients have antibodies to **muscle specific kinase (MuSK)**.

These patients may not respond to anticholinesterase medications. Thymectomy is not as helpful.

Neonatal Myasthenia Gravis

Neonatal myasthenia gravis is the most common illness resulting in a neuromuscular transmission defect in newborns.

It is a **transient condition** due to transfer of maternal acetylcholine receptor antibodies across the placenta.

It presents within the **first 3 days of life** and **resolves by 6 weeks of age**.

It causes **weakness** and may **result in respiratory depression**.

Neonatal myasthenia gravis can be treated with anticholinesterase inhibitors.

Tick Paralysis

Tick paralysis is usually due to the ticks of the ***Dermacentor* species**.

It most commonly occurs in **small children in the spring**. The tick tends to attach to the scalp or neck.

It is thought that a neurotoxin produced by the tick causes **reduced release of acetylcholine**.

Tick paralysis causes an ascending flaccid paralysis with areflexia, which **resembles Guillain-Barré syndrome.**

Patients with tick paralysis often have **ophthalmoplegia**, which is also found in the Miller-Fisher variant of GBS.

However, **patients with tick paralysis have normal CSF.**

EMG/NCS show decreased CMAP amplitudes and a normal response to repetitive nerve stimulation.

Symptoms significantly improve after the tick is removed!!

Neuropathy

Polyneuropathy

Please also see the Neurotoxins chapter and the Infectious Diseases chapter (for HIV and Leprosy).

Critical Illness Neuropathy

This is an axonal neuropathy that occurs in ICU patients, often in the setting of multiorgan failure and sepsis.

Diabetes

Diabetes can cause almost any kind of neuropathy. The most common type is a distal symmetric chronic sensorimotor polyneuropathy (sensory > motor).

Diphtheritic Polyneuropathy

The exotoxin from *Corynebacterium diphtheriae* causes Diphtheria.

Diphtheria produces a demyelinating neuropathy that may resemble Guillain-Barré Syndrome.

 Initially, patients with diphtheria have **pharyngitis with a gray membrane in the throat**.

There may be a palatal neuropathy.

Later, paralysis of accommodation may occur. Some patients develop a diffuse motor and sensory polyneuropathy 2 –3 months after the infection. The CSF protein is elevated.

Familial Amyloid Polyneuropathy

There are 4 types **Familial Amyloid Polyneuropathy (FAP)**.

FAP type 1, which is due to a defect in **TransThyRetin**, causes a primarily **Small Fiber Neuropathy (SFN)**.

Patients initially have pain in the lower limbs. Pain and temperature sensation are lost.

Autonomic Nervous System (ANS) symptoms include orthostatic hypotension, impotence, and urinary difficulties.

FAP type 1 is also associated with **Carpal Tunnel Syndrome (CTS)**.

Congestive heart failure **(CHF)** may result in death.

To remember the features of Familial Amyloid Polyneuropathy, think of the **FACTS**:

F = **F**AP

A = **A**NS

C = **C**TS and **C**HF

T = **T**TR

S = **S**FN

Friedreich's Ataxia

Friedreich's ataxia causes a sensory polyneuropathy.[4]

GALOP

GALOP stands for:

Gait disorder

Autoantibody

Late age

Onset

Polyneuropathy

GALOP presents over age 50 years.

These patients have a symmetric polyneuropathy, distal sensory loss, and IgM against central myelin antigen.

 The name GALOP is a misnomer; **these patients have trouble walking, let alone galloping.**

Hereditary Motor and Sensory Neuropathies (HMSN) / Charcot-Marie-Tooth disease (CMT)

HMSN is also known as Charcot-Marie-Tooth disease (CMT).

There are multiple types.

---

[4] For more information about this disease, please see the Movement Disorders chapter.

Type of CMT	Inheritance (mostly)	% CMT patients affected	Type of neuropathy
CMT type 1	AD	30%	Demyelinating
CMT type 2	AD >AR	20-40%	Axonal
CMT type 3	AR	<5%	Demyelinating
CMT type 4	AR	<5%	Demyelinating
CMT type "X"	X-linked	10-20%	Demyelinating

Symptoms of CMT (usually foot drop or claw toe) can begin in childhood/teens up to the early 30s/40s. Muscle wasting in the lower legs can manifest as a "stork leg" or "inverted champagne bottle." Patients with CMT are extremely sensitive to vincristine.

Type 1A (95%) – PMP22 (peripheral myelin protein) duplication, chromosome 17
Type 1B (5%) – MPZ or P0 (myelin protein zero) mutation, chromosome 1

CMT1A shows up most often on tests.

CMT1A is associated with foot deformity (pes cavus and hammer toes), wasting of the hands, feet, and distal leg muscles, and mild distal sensory loss. They have enlarged nerves. **Nerve conduction studies show very slow conduction velocities**. Pathology shows demyelination and **onion bulbs**.

Type 1 primarily affects the ***myelin sheath***, whereas type 2 primarily affects ***axons***, so EMG/NCS will show markedly slowed velocities in ***demyelinating*** types of CMT (type 1)!

You can **SEND** for a glass of inverted champagne to get a CMT diagnosis any of 4 ways: **S**ymptoms, **E**lectromyography, **N**erve biopsy, or **D**NA/gene testing.

Hereditary neuropathy with liability to pressure palsies (HNPP) is allelic with CMT1A. It is characterized by multiple or recurrent compression neuropathies or a mild generalized demyelinating neuropathy. It is also known as **tomaculous neuropathy**, due to focal myelin thickening called **tomaculi**.

Sites for compression neuropathies: **"MR. UP"** -- the **M**edian nerve at the wrist, the **R**adial nerve at the spiral groove, the **U**lnar nerve at the elbow, and the **P**eroneal nerve at the knee.

Charcot-Marie-Tooth 1A versus Hereditary Neuropathy with Liability to Pressure Palsies (HNPP):

Both are due to a defect in PMP-22 (Peripheral myelin protein-22) on chromosome 17 (17p).

CMT 1A is due to a <u>duplication</u> or point mutation in PMP-22, but most exams expect you to know that it is due to a duplication.

<u>HNPP</u> is due to a <u>deletion</u> of PMP-22.

 You see 2 abnormal feet (pes cavus) in patients with CMT1A, which is due to duplication (2 copies) of PMP-22.

CMT2A is the most common axonal CMT. It is autosomal dominant and is due to mutations in Mitofusin 2, which is associated with mitochondrial transport and fusion. Restless leg syndrome is common in patients with the axonal form of CMT.

CMT3/Dejerine-Sottas disease is associated with a severe demyelinating neuropathy in infancy.

CMT X is due to a point mutation in the connexin-32 gene on the X chromosome.

 CMTX is due to ConneXin-32 gene mutations.

Multifocal Motor Neuropathy with Conduction Block

This is a chronic immune demyelinating polyneuropathy.

It usually presents around age 40 years and is more common in males.

It causes **asymmetric distal weakness and atrophy, usually in the upper extremities**.

It is associated with **anti-GM1 antibodies** and conduction blocks along motor fibers at sites where compression usually does not occur.

POEMS Syndrome

POEMS stands for:

> **P**olyneuropathy
>
> **O**rganomegaly
>
> **E**ndocrinopathy
>
> **M** protein – due to an underlying plasma-cell proliferative disorder (typically multiple myeloma)
>
> **S**kin changes

In many (up to 80%) but not all of POEMS patients, a serum paraprotein can be detected.

 This is usually IgG or IgA, with a lambda light chain type.

This is unlike most other paraproteinaemic neuropathies, in which the paraprotein is usually an IgM antibody.

The average age at onset of POEMS is 50.

POEMS affects up to twice as many men as women.

If untreated it is progressive and often fatal, with only 60% of POEMS patients alive at 5 years.

 To remember details of a typical POEMS patient, think of a man who just started writing POEMS at age 50, and writes them for 5 years until he dies at age 55 from liver failure with dark, jaundiced skin.

Tangier Disease

Tangier disease is due to **deficiency of alpha-lipoprotein**.

 It is associated with a mutation in the ATP-binding-cassette-1 gene (ABCA1) on 9q.

Patients with Tangier disease have a **sensory neuropathy affecting the distal upper extremities and atrophy of the intrinsic muscles of the hand**.

They also have **large orange tonsils**, lymphadenopathy, and splenomegaly.

Electrodiagnostic studies show both axonal and demyelinating features.

Laboratory findings in Tangier disease include: decreased cholesterol and LDL, very low HDL

Macrophages contain cholesterol esters. Vacuolization occurs in Schwann cells.

 Remember: You hold a tangerine in your hand, which is where the atrophy occurs.

Vasculitis

Vasculitis most often causes mononeuritis multiplex, but it can cause a distal sensorimotor polyneuropathy.

Plexopathies

Brachial Plexopathies

Erb-Duchenne Paralysis/Erb's Palsy

 Erb's palsy is a brachial plexus injury at birth involving the upper trunk or C5-C6 roots.

This is the most common brachial plexus injury in newborns.

It results in weakness of the deltoid, biceps, brachioradialis, and supinator muscles. Therefore, the arm is adducted, internally rotated, and extended, and the forearm is pronated. This is called the **waiter's tip position**.

To remember that Erb-Duchenne paralysis/ **Erb's** palsy is associated with a waiter's tip position, and that it results in weakness of the **D**eltoid, **BR**achioradialis, **B**iceps, and **S**upinator muscles, remember this request, "Waiter, **D**o **BR**ing **B**ack **S**ome h**ERB**s."

Klumpke's Paralysis

Klumpke's paralysis is a brachial plexus injury involving the lower trunk (C8-T1).

It is a rare plexus injury.

Patients with Klumpke's paralysis have weakness of the intrinsic hand muscles, forearm extensors, and wrist and finger flexors.

The hand has a **claw-like deformity**, the elbow is flexed, the forearm is supinated, and the wrist is extended.

Horner's syndrome may be seen because sympathetic fibers accompany T1.

The finger flexor reflex, which is mediated by C8-T1, is decreased.

 Klumpke's paralysis is associated with a Klaw (claw).

 Ulnar neuropathy causes a different claw-hand deformity.

Neoplastic Plexopathy

 Neoplastic plexopathy may be due to local tumor invasion (e.g. Pancoast's tumor of the lung) or metastases.

This is most commonly due to lung cancer, breast cancer, or lymphoma.

Pain is prominent in neoplastic plexopathy.

Patients with neoplastic plexopathy may have a **Horner's syndrome**.

Radiation Plexopathy

Radiation exposure may cause radiation plexopathy.

Sensory symptoms are more prominent in radiation plexopathy than brachial plexopathy due to recurrent tumor.

Also, **myokymia** is a characteristic finding in radiation plexopathy.

Neurogenic Thoracic Outlet Syndrome (TOS)

The thoracic outlet is the space between the first rib and clavicle where the brachial plexus passes into the arm from the shoulder and axilla.

Neurogenic TOS is usually due to a fibrous band between a cervical rib and the first thoracic rib that entraps the lower trunk of the plexus. This causes weakness and sensory loss in the C8-T1 distribution.

Parsonage-Turner Syndrome/Brachial Plexus Neuritis

Parsonage-Turner syndrome is also known as **neuralgic amyotrophy** and **idiopathic brachial plexopathy**.

It may be **preceded by a viral syndrome or immunization**.

It is characterized by **pain in the shoulder girdle followed by weakness**. Paresthesias may be present. **Muscle atrophy** follows the weakness.

The long thoracic, musculocutaneous, axillary, and anterior interosseous nerves are commonly affected.

Lumbosacral Plexopathy

Lumbosacral plexopathies have structural and nonstructural etiologies. Diabetes is a common nonstructural cause. **Diabetic amyotrophy** affects the lumbosacral plexus and nerve roots, so it is discussed in the polyradiculoneuropathy section.

Polyradiculoneuropathy

Acute Inflammatory Demyelinating Polyradiculoneuropathy / Guillain-Barré Syndrome (GBS)

Acute Inflammatory Demyelinating Polyradiculoneuropathy (AIDP) is also known as **Guillain-Barré Syndrome (GBS)**.

GBS causes a severe ascending, symmetric weakness with areflexia.

There may be a preceding illness. Of all the possible precursors, *C. jejuni* is the most commonly identified agent.

It begins with distal paresthesias, pain in the back and lower legs, and leg weakness.

The cranial nerves may be affected.

Respiratory failure may result.

Autonomic instability is found in some cases resulting in arrhythmia and blood pressure changes.

The disease may progress for up to a few weeks.

The CSF protein is increased, but the white blood cell count is usually normal. This is termed **"albumino-cytological dissociation"** because the **albumin (protein)** is so much **higher** than the **leukocytes (cytological)**, and is part of the AIDP diagnostic criteria.

On EMG/NCS, the first finding is loss of F-waves.

Steroids are <u>not</u> useful in the treatment of Guillain-Barré syndrome.

 Plasma exchange or IVIG are helpful for GBS.

Acute Motor Axonal Neuropathy (AMAN)

This is a form of Guillain-Barré syndrome that is characterized by early axonal involvement.

It has a poor prognosis.

It is associated with Campylobacter infections, anti-GD1a antibodies, and anti-GM1 antibodies.

Acute Motor and Sensory Axonal Neuropathy (AMSAN)

Clinically, this is similar to AMAN, **but there is sensory involvement**.

Miller-Fisher Syndrome

The Miller-Fisher variant of GBS is characterized by **ophthalmoparesis, ataxia,** and **areflexia**.

Accounting for only 5% of GBS cases, Miller Fisher variant manifests as a **descending weakness** -- in the reverse order of classic GBS, with eye muscles paralyzed first. The ataxia that occurs is typically truncal as limbs are less often involved. In about 90% of Miller Fisher cases, anti-GQ1b antibodies are present.

Chronic Inflammatory Demyelinating Polyradiculoneuropathy (CIDP)

CIDP is characterized by slowly progressive weakness, which is usually symmetric.

There is sensory loss to all modalities, which is worse in the legs.

 Patients with CIDP have generalized hyporeflexia.

Nerves may be enlarged.

The CSF protein is elevated. An increased number of cells may occur if the patient has HIV.

Nerve conduction studies show prolonged distal latencies, significantly slowed conduction velocities, conduction block, temporal dispersion, and abnormal F-waves (prolonged latencies).

CIDP is treated with steroids, plasmapheresis, IVIG, and immunosuppressants.

Diabetic Amyotrophy

Diabetic amyotrophy affects the upper lumbosacral plexus and nerve roots.

It causes **asymmetric proximal weakness**, particularly affecting the *quadriceps and psoas muscles.*

The patient also has **significant weight loss and pain**.

Guillain-Barré Syndrome

Please see Acute Inflammatory Demyelinating Polyradiculoneuropathy (AIDP) above.

Radiculopathy

A radiculopathy is due to damage to a nerve root.

Radiculopathies are characterized by sensory complaints in a dermatomal distribution and weakness in the muscles innervated by the root. If the nerve root subserves a reflex, the reflex may be decreased.

On nerve conduction studies, the sensory nerve action potentials (SNAPs) should be normal **because SNAPs are normal with lesions proximal to the dorsal root ganglion**.

The needle exam is the most sensitive test for diagnosing a radiculopathy.

Fibrillations in the paraspinal muscles are helpful in diagnosis of an acute radiculopathy, but they usually present until the symptoms have been present for 2 weeks.

In chronic radiculopathy, the motor unit morphology in affected muscles is consistent with chronic neurogenic changes such as increased duration, increased amplitude, and polyphasia.

Disc herniation is the most common cause of radiculopathy.

Motor Neuron Disease

Amyotrophic Lateral Sclerosis (ALS)

ALS is also known as Lou Gehrig disease.

 It is a **neurodegenerative disease of the upper and lower motor neurons**.

Clinical Features of ALS

ALS tends to begin in the 6th decade.

There is a slight male predominance.

Patients with ALS have upper and lower motor neuron signs; these may be present in the same myotome.

- **Upper motor neuron signs include**: hyperreflexia, spasticity, stiffness, Hoffman's sign, Babinski sign, and a brisk jaw jerk.
- **Lower motor neuron signs** include fasciculations, atrophy, weakness, and muscle cramps. Tongue fasciculations are associated with ALS but can be found in other diseases. Bulbar dysfunction is seen including dysarthria, dysphagia, and a hyperactive gag reflex. Patients with ALS may have pseudobulbar affect.

The **extraocular muscles** and **sensation are usually spared**.

Late in the course, spasticity may result in urinary frequency or urgency. Prior to that bowel and bladder function are usually spared.

Patients often present with **asymmetric distal weakness**. Usually weakness starts in one region, spreads to adjacent regions, and then spreads to the contralateral limb.

A recent study showed that about half of patients with ALS have cognitive impairment. Most often, executive dysfunction is seen. For example, ALS patients had problems with concentration. When more severe impairment occurred, patients had features seen in frontotemporal dementia (FTD).[5]

Patients often die from respiratory insufficiency or aspiration pneumonia.

Mean survival is less than 5 years after the disease onset.

Malnutrition is associated with a worse prognosis.

---

[5] Ringholz GM, Appel SH, Bradshaw M, et al. Prevalence and patterns of cognitive impairment in sporadic ALS. Neurology 2005;65:586-590.

Laboratory Findings of ALS

CK may be normal or mildly elevated.

EMG shows denervation in several body regions characterized by fibrillations and positive sharp waves. Fasciculations are characteristic of ALS. As the disease progresses, **motor units increase in duration and amplitude due to collateral sprouting. The motor units vary in configuration and demonstrate polyphasia**.

Diagnosis of ALS

The World Federation of Neurology created criteria for the diagnosis of ALS in 1990 in El Escorial, Spain. These criteria were revised in 1998. The revised criteria are available at: www.wfnals.org/guidelines/1998elescorial/elescorial1998.htm.

Superoxide dismutase mutation

Pathology of ALS

Grossly, atrophy of the motor strip, spinal cord, and the anterior roots of the spinal cord are seen.

Microscopically, there is a **loss of motor neurons** in the cord and brainstem with sparing of the extraocular nuclei.

In the precentral cortex, Betz cells are lost.

Involved muscles show atrophy with **fiber-type grouping**.

Bunina bodies (intracytoplasmic eosinophilic inclusions) and **axonal spheroids** are found in the **anterior horn cells**.

Treatment of ALS

Percutaneous endoscopic gastrostomy (PEG) is recommended early when patients have dysphagia.[6] It is safest if this is done when the patient's vital capacity is greater than 50% of predicted.

It is also recommended that noninvasive mechanical ventilation be initiated while the patient's vital capacity is > 50% predicted.

---

[6] These treatment recommendations were taken from AAN Pocket Guidelines, 2003 edition.

Multiple treatment options are available for sialorrhea, such as glycopyrrolate, benztropine, and trihexyphenidyl. Amitriptyline treats sialorrhea and pseudobulbar affect.

Riluzole (Rilutek®) may prolong survival. It may cause gastrointestinal side effects, and ALT should be monitored.

Riluzole, which **inhibits the release of glutamate**, is used because **ALS patients were found to have elevated CSF glutamate**.

Familial ALS

There are multiple familial forms of ALS.

One cause of familial ALS is a defect in the **SOD1 (superoxide dismutase) gene**, which is on chromosome 21q.

Hyaline conglomerate inclusions (HCI) can be found in motor neurons in patients with familial ALS due to a mutation in SOD but are not found in sporadic ALS.

A locus was found on 9p that is linked to ALS and frontotemporal dementia.[7]

Fazio-Londe Syndrome

Fazio-Londe syndrome is also known as **juvenile progressive bulbar palsy**.

It presents in late childhood and is characterized by **facial weakness and dysarthria**.

Patients also have **dysphagia** and **lingual fasciculations**.

Think of face when you seen Fazio, to remember that the patients have facial weakness.

When you see Londe, think of Lingual for Lingual fasciculations, dysarthria and dysphagia. Alternatively, Londe may you remind you of London, where British speakers may be difficult to understand, like patients with Fazio-Londe who have dysarthria.

---

[7] Morita M, Al-Chalabi A, Andersen PM, et al. A locus on chromosome 9p confers susceptibility to ALS and frontotemporal dementia. Neurology 2006;66:839-844.

Spinobulbar Muscular Atrophy (Kennedy's Disease)

Spinobulbar muscular atrophy is an **X-linked recessive motor neuron disease** found in males.

This is the **most common form of adult onset spinal muscular atrophy**.

It is due to **CAG expansion in the androgen-receptor (*AR*) gene**.

 In adolescence, the patient may have muscle cramps.

Later, proximal limb and facial weakness are seen. Facial fasciculations may be present.

Tongue fasciculations and atrophy are also seen. There may be a **midline furrow in the tongue**.

Patients have **dysarthria** and **swallowing difficulties**.

 You can imagine that a fasciculating tongue can cause problems with swallowing and talking.

Reflexes are reduced.

Patients have **decreased vibration**, particularly in the legs.

Kennedy's disease is associated with **gynecomastia, impotence,** and **testicular atrophy**. Patients have **abnormal sex hormone levels**.

Some patients have **diabetes mellitus**.

Spinal Muscular Atrophy (SMA)

The types of spinal muscular atrophy described below are autosomal recessive disorders. They are due to deletions or mutations in exons 7 and 8 of the ***SMN1* (survival motor neuron) gene on 5q**. This gene is the telomeric copy of the SMN gene. *SMN2* is the centromeric copy of the *SMN* gene. It is a disease-modifying gene.

SMA Type I (Werdnig-Hoffman Syndrome)

This is the most severe form of SMA.

 SMA type 1 **presents before 6 months of age with hypotonia, weakness, and areflexia**.

The patients are alert but move very little. They have some movement of the hands and feet.

arthrogryposis - hand/feet/joint deformities at birth

Most patients are unable to sit.

Weakness of the intercostal muscles causes paradoxical breathing.

Tongue fasciculations are seen.

Death due to respiratory failure often occurs by age 2 years of life.

EMG shows signs of denervation.

In these patients, *SMN1* is deleted on both chromosomes. The patient still has 2 copies of the *SMN2* gene.

SMA Type II

The **onset of SMA type II is less than 18 months**.

Patients have symmetric proximal weakness.

 These patients can sit but **don't walk**.

They have problems with scoliosis.

These patients usually have a deletion of *SMN1* from one chromosome and the other *SMN1* gene has been converted to a *SMN2* gene. As a result, the patient has 3 copies of the *SMN2* gene.

SMA Type III

SMA type III **begins after 18 months**.

 Patients have symmetric proximal weakness.

Patients with SMA Type III are able to **walk eventually, but often lose the ability**.

Scoliosis is also a concern for these patients.

In this situation there are more than 3 copies of the *SMN2* gene.

The Most

Duchenne muscular dystrophy (DMD) is the most **common muscular dystrophy in children**.

Merosin-negative congenital muscular dystrophy is the most common **form of <u>congenital</u> muscular dystrophy**.

Myotonic dystrophy is the most common **muscular dystrophy in adults**.

Congenital myotonic dystrophy is the most common **myopathic disorder to appear in the neonatal period**.

CMT 1 is the most common **form of hereditary motor and sensory neuropathy**.

Carnitine palmitoyltransferase II deficiency is the most common **metabolic cause of recurrent myoglobinuria**.

Spinobulbar muscular atrophy (Kennedy's disease) is the most common **form of adult onset spinal muscular atrophy**.

Neonatal myasthenia gravis is the most common **illness resulting in a neuromuscular transmission defect in newborns**.

Tips from the Authors

Alan Pestronk's Neuromuscular Website at www.neuro.wustl.edu/neuromuscular/index.html is a wonderful resource.

Neuromuscular Diseases Quiz

(Answers on page 747)

1. Which nerve innervates the supinator?

    A. The anterior interosseous nerve

    B. The median nerve

    C. The radial nerve

    D. The ulnar nerve

2. Which of the following muscles is spared in a radial neuropathy at the spiral groove?

    A. Anconeus

    B. Extensor carpi radialis brevis

    C. Extensor carpi ulnaris

    D. Abductor pollicis longus

3. Which nerve innervates the pectineus muscle (in addition to the obturator nerve)?

    A. Femoral nerve

    B. Sciatic nerve

    C. Superior gluteal nerve

    D. Inferior gluteal nerve

4. Which nerve innervates the adductor magnus (in addition to the obturator nerve)?

    A. Femoral nerve

    B. Sciatic nerve

    C. Superior gluteal nerve

    D. Inferior gluteal nerve

5. Match the nerve with the muscles it innervates.

    1) Inferior gluteal nerve   A. Hip extensors

    2) Obturator nerve   B. Thigh abductors

    3) Superior gluteal nerve   C. Thigh adductors

6. When present, which muscle does the accessory peroneal nerve usually innervate?

    A. Extensor digitorum brevis

    B. Extensor digitorum longus

    C. Extensor hallucis longus

    D. Peroneus tertius

7. Which finding may be present in radiation-induced plexopathy?

    A. Complex repetitive discharges

    B. Myokymia

    C. Myotonia

    D. Neuromyotonia

8. Which muscular dystrophy is associated with a triplet repeat?

    A. Becker muscular dystrophy

    B. Duchenne muscular dystrophy

    C. Emery-Dreifuss muscular dystrophy

    D. Fascioscapulohumeral muscular dystrophy

    E. Oculopharyngeal muscular dystrophy

9. Which muscular dystrophy is associated with rimmed vacuoles on muscle biopsy?

    A. Becker muscular dystrophy

    B. Duchenne muscular dystrophy

    C. Emery-Dreifuss muscular dystrophy

    D. Fascioscapulohumeral muscular dystrophy

    E. Oculopharyngeal muscular dystrophy

10. Tomaculous neuropathy is another name for which disease?

    A. CMT1A

    B. Fabry's disease

    C. Fazio-Londe syndrome

    D. Hereditary neuropathy with liability to pressure palsies

11. Anti-GM1 antibodies are found in which disease?
   A. Multifocal motor neuropathy with conduction block
   B. Parsonage-Turner syndrome
   C. Riley-Day syndrome
   D. Tarui's disease

12. Match the disease and the histologic finding.
   1) Bunina bodies and axonal spheroids   A. Amyotrophic lateral sclerosis (ALS)
   2) Increased central nuclei   B. Charcot-Marie-Tooth (CMT) 1A
   3) Onion bulbs   C. Inclusion body myositis
   4) Ragged red fibers   D. Myotonic dystrophy
   5) Rimmed vacuoles   E. Zidovudine (AZT) myopathy

Chapter 10

Neuro-Oncology

Primary Brain Tumors

Microcellular features of CNS tumors (and hence their malignancy potential) – makes you want to say "AMEN" that you don't have them!: Anaplasia, Mitoses, Endothelial proliferation, Necrosis.

Astrocytic Tumor Grading[1,2]

WHO Grade	Description	Tumors
I	Circumscribed.	Juvenile Pilocytic Astrocytoma (JPA), Subependymal Giant-cell Astrocytoma (SEGA)
II	Cytological atypia.	Diffuse astrocytoma, Pleomorphic Xanthoastrocytoma (PXA), Pilomyxoid astrocytoma
III	Anaplasia and increased mitotic activity. (MIB-1 staining helps to differentiate grade II from grade III.)	Anaplastic Astrocytoma
IV	Endothelial proliferation or glomeruloid microvascular proliferation, necrosis of any kind (in addition to a high mitotic rate and anaplasia).	Glioblastoma Multiforme

Astrocytoma

Although there are lots of ways to classify tumors, the **World Health Organization (WHO) classification** is the most widely used classification.

---

1 Louis DN, Ohgaki H, et al. The 2007 WHO Classification of Tumours of the Central Nervous System. Acta Neuropathol 2007;114:97-109.

2 Louis DN, Ohgaki H, Wiestler OD, Cavenee WK. (eds). WHO Classification of Tumours of the Central Nervous System, 4th edition. Lyon: International Agency for Research on Cancer, 2007.

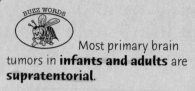 Most primary brain tumors in **infants and adults** are **supratentorial**.

Most primary brain tumors in **children** are **infratentorial**.

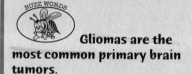 **Gliomas are the most common primary brain tumors.**

Gliomas arise from glial cells, which include astrocytes, oligodendrocytes, and ependymal cells.

WHO Grade Tumor

Juvenile Pilocytic Astrocytomas (JPA) and SubEpendymal Giant-cell Astrocytomas (SEGA)

Grade I/Astrocytoma

Juvenile **P**ilocytic **A**strocytomas **(JPA)** and **S**ub**E**pendymal **G**iant cell **A**strocytomas **(SEGA)** are grade I astrocytomas.

Juvenile Pilocytic Astrocytoma (JPA)

Rosenthal fibers and **intracellular eosinophilic granular bodies (EGBs)** are found in juvenile pilocytic astrocytomas[3].

(handwritten) round ubiquitin of GFAP ⊕

 Rosenthal fibers are elongated eosinophilic inclusions that contain glial fibrillary acidic (GFAP protein).

They look a bit like red worms.

Since **ro**ses are **red**, **Rose**nthal fibers are **red**/eosinophilic.

 Rosenthal fibers are also found in Alexander's disease. Please see the Metabolic Diseases chapter for more details.

Additional microscopic findings in JPA include:

1. A biphasic appearance
2. Neovascularization
3. Immunopositivity for glial fibrillary acidic protein (GFAP)
4. Microcystic change

JPAs are said to be *biphasic* because in some areas bundles of elongated cells are seen while other areas are hypocellular. The resemblance of these bundles of elongated cells to hair led to the name *pilocytic*. The hypocellular regions are characterized by stellate cells and microcysts.

---

3 Some neuropathologists simply refer to this tumor as pilocytic astrocytoma because it also appears in adults.

The neovascularization does not mean anaplastic transformation has occurred. This neovascularization leads to contrast enhancement on MRI.

When you see the word **pilocytic** in Juvenile Pilocytic Astrocytoma, think of **red hair** because there's *lots of red with this tumor: eosinophilic granular bodies (EGBs), Rosenthal fibers*, and *neovascularization.*

PXA | epend.
JPA | gang.
HB | cell

If you are presented with a **child** who has a cerebellar cyst associated with a mural nodule think of **juvenile pilocytic astrocytoma.**

If it's an **adult**, think of a **hemangioblastoma** and **Von Hippel-Lindau disease.**

SubEpendymal Giant Cell Astrocytoma (SEGA)

Subependymal giant cell astrocytomas are usually associated with tuberous sclerosis (TS).

This tumor is in the differential for an intraventricular tumor.

TS is characterized by Vogt's triad and spells out SAM:

    1) **S**eizures/Epilepsy
    2) **A**denoma Sebaceum
    3) **M**ental retardation

SEGA
subependymomas
colloid cysts
central neurocytomas

Sub**E**pendymal **G**iant cell **A**strocytoma—SEGA—**now SAM is playing SEGA in your Tub!**

The FDA approved everolimus (Afinitor), which is a mTOR inhibitor, to treat SEGA in TS patients. **Vigabatrin** is the drug of choice to treat infantile spasms in patients with TS.

Grade II/Astrocytoma

Low-grade astrocytoma- more cells than normal and occasional nuclear atypia. Examples include pilomyxoid astrocytoma, diffuse astrocytoma, and pleomorphic xanthoastrocytoma.

Pleomorphic Xanthoastrocytoma (PXA)

Pleomorphic xanthoastrocytoma is classified as WHO grade II. It tends to present in the second decade of life with **seizures**.

Like JPAs, PXAs can present as a **cyst with an enhancing mural nodule** on MRI. However, PXAs tend to occur in the **temporal lobe**.

Like JPAs, PXAs have **eosinophilic granular bodies (EGBs)**. However, PXAs do <u>not</u> have a biphasic appearance or Rosenthal fibers, as seen in JPAs.

Since these tumors are very pleomorphic, they can be mistaken for glioblastoma multiforme (GBM). The absence of necrosis or microvascular proliferation and the presence of eosinophilic granular bodies help to differentiate PXA from GBM.

Grade III/ Astrocytoma

Anaplastic astrocytoma- more cells than normal, mitoses, moderate nuclear atypia, and pleomorphism.

Grade IV/ Astrocytoma

Glioblastoma multiforme- microvascular proliferation and/or necrosis are present.

You can see **pseudopalisading** around areas of necrosis in GBM.

The glial cells have a **blast** in glioblastoma; they have a **parade/ palisade** around areas of necrosis.

A butterfly glioblastoma is a glioblastoma that spreads across the corpus callosum.

Beware of the Butterfly. A tumor that spreads across the corpus callosum may be a glioblastoma or CNS lymphoma.

> ## IDH Mutations
>
> Isocitrate dehydrogenase 1 and 2 (IDH 1 and 2) genes are mutated in many tumors:
>
> - Grade II and III astrocytomas
> - Oligodendrogliomas
> - Oligoastrocytomas
> - Seconday (NOT primary) GBMs
>
> Tumors with these mutations have TP53 mutations or loss of 1p/19p. Patients with IDH mutations have a better prognosis.

HMB45 - ⊕ melanoma
        ⊖ GBM

Oligodendroglioma

Oligodendrogliomas are gliomas that originate from oligodendrocytes. They usually are located in the cerebral hemispheres and present with seizures. Most oligodendrogliomas are grade II; however, anaplastic oligodendrogliomas, like anaplastic astrocytomas, are grade III.

Patients with oligodendroglioma who have loss of heterozygosity (LOH) for chromosomes 1p and 19q respond better to chemotherapy.

Microscopic features: **calcifications, perinuclear halos,** and **delicate vessels**.

Perineuronal satellitosis and perivascular satellitosis are also seen.

Delicate branching capillaries, which look like chicken wire, and cells with a **fried egg appearance (perinuclear halos)**, are characteristic of oligodendroglioma.

Pronounce this **Ol-egg-odendroglioma** *to remember that this is the tumor where you see the chicken (wire) and the egg.*

To remember its microscopic features, think of the SHOCK of cracking an egg:

- **S** - **S**eizures and **S**atellitosis (perineuronal and perivascular),
- **H** - **H**alos (perinuclear) and **H**emispheric involvement,
- **O** - **O**=loss of heterozygosity (1p, 19q)
- **C** - **C**alcifications: **Wash down that egg with some milk.** *Calcifications are common in oligodendrogliomas.*
- **K** - **K**illed with Khemotherapy (1p, 19q)

If you remember the delicate blood vessels, which resemble chicken wire, it will help you remember that **this is the most common primary brain tumor to bleed**.

ODG - Oh Dear God He's Bleeding!

Wash down that egg with some milk. *Calcifications are common in oligodendrogliomas.*

Patients with oligodendroglioma who have loss of heterozygosity (LOH) for chromosomes 1p and 19q respond better to chemotherapy.

Ependymoma

Ependymomas are gliomas that originate from ependymal cells. They can be supratentorial or infratentorial.

Infratentorial ependymomas may be intraventricular and can fill the fourth ventricle.

Ependymomas are the most common spinal cord glioma.

One variant, myxopapillary ependymoma, arises in the filum terminale.

 Ependymomas are characterized by **perivascular pseudorosettes** on microscopy.

 Ependymal cells form rings around vessels, with their fibrillary processes adjacent to the vessel. These structures are called perivascular pseudorosettes.

Ependymomas may also have true rosettes. See War of the Roses below.

multifocal in SC ∝ NF2

Meningioma

Meningiomas arise from arachnoid cells.

Characteristic Features

 MRI shows a **dural tail sign** and homogenous enhancement.

Microscopy shows **whorls, psammoma bodies**, and **positive staining for EMA** (epithelial membrane antigen).

Desmosomes are seen on electron microscopy.

 Psammoma bodies are found in meningioma.

You check a PSA in men, so **PSA**mmoma bodies are in **men**ingiomas.

progesterone receptors

How to remember all the *microscopic features* of meningiomas?

Man/**Men**, I'm **WHiPPED** from trying to remember the microscopic features of meningiomas.

Meningioma:

W-*whorls*,

H-*homogeneous enhancement*,

P-*psammoma bodies*,

P-*positive staining for...*

E-*epithelial membrane antigen*, and

D-*desmosomes*.

Meningiomas are associated with monosomy 22, leading to loss of the tumor suppressor gene (merlin).

Merlin is mutated in NF2, which is associated with multiple meningiomas.

Higher Grade Meningiomas

These meningiomas are more aggressive and/or more likely to recur:

· Atypical meningioma (WHO grade II)

· Clear cell meningioma (WHO grade II)

· Choroid meningioma (WHO grade II)

· Papillary meningioma (WHO grade III)

· Rhabdoid meningioma (WHO grade III)

· Anaplastic (malignant) meningioma (WHO grade III)

Atypical meningiomas have an increased mitotic rate defined as more than 4 but less than 20 per 10 high power fields

Or

Demonstrate *three or more of the following*:

1. Sheeting

2. Increased cellularity

3. Necrosis

4. Prominent nucleoli

5. Small cells with a high nucleus to cytoplasm ratio

Aggressive meningiomas:

· Choroid (WHO grade II)

· Clear cell (WHO grade II)

· Rhabdoid (WHO grade III)

· Papillary (WHO grade III)

Aggressive meningiomas include **c**horoid, **c**lear cell, **r**habdoid, and **p**apillary, (C.C.R.P.).

Question: Which meningomas are the more aggressive/malignant types?
Answer: the ones that are a **Clear-Cut Real Problem** – C.C.R.P.:

Clear cell (stage II), **Choroid** (stage II), **Rhabdoid** (stage III) & **Papillary** (stage III).
Note the II's and III's are lumped together for easy recall of type and stage!

Anaplastic Meningiomas (WHO grade III) have a mitotic rate of greater than or equal to 20 per 10 high power fields and have features similar to sarcoma, carcinoma, or melanoma. These meningiomas are usually fatal (median survival less than 2 years).

Craniopharyngioma

Craniopharyngioma is *the most common supratentorial tumor in childhood.*

It is a WHO grade I tumor found in the suprasellar region and/or the third ventricle.

Craniopharyngiomas are thought to **arise from remnants of Rathke's pouch**.

Craniopharyngiomas typically present with **hypopituitarism, visual changes (diplopia), and hydrocephalus**.

Adamantinomatous Craniopharyngioma

The adamantinomatous type is the most common type of craniopharyngioma.

Craniopharyngiomas contain *solid areas* and *cystic areas* containing dark fluid, which resembles motor oil/ "crank-case oil" due to cholesterol crystals. **Calcification** frequently occurs and nodules of **wet keratin** are seen.

Pituitary Tumors

Pituitary tumors can cause bitemporal hemianopsia due to compression of the optic chiasm.

Visual field defect:

Pituitary adenomas are the most common pituitary tumor.

Prolactinomas are the most common type of pituitary adenoma.

Sometimes prolactinomas may be treated with bromocriptine.

 To be classified as pituitary **carcinoma**, there has to be **metastasis**.

Atypical Teratoid/Rhabdoid Tumor (ATRT)

ATRTs in the central nervous system are found in the posterior fossa, usually in infants and young children.

Most are associated with loss of heterozygosity (LOH) or partial deletion of chromosome 22, which results in the loss of the tumor suppressor gene INI1.

 ATRT has **Two T's** so it is associated with LOH or partial deletion of **Twenty-Two** (22).

(Ependymoma, meningioma, and schwannoma also are associated with LOH of chromosome 22.) ATRTs are WHO grade IV. (2+2=4).

CNS PNETs (Primitive Neuroectodermal Tumors)

PNETs are also known as **small round blue cell tumors**.

Lots of –blastomas, such as medulloblastoma, pineoblastoma, and retinoblastoma, are classified as PNETs.

One of the histologic features of PNETs is **Homer Wright rosettes**.

To remember that Homer Wright rosettes are associated with PNETs, remember that Homer Simpson likes peanuts (PNETs). Homer Simpson is a very primitive cartoon, like the PNETs are primitive neuroectodermal tumors, and Homer is always having a blast in every episode, just like the PNETs include many blastomas.

Medulloblastoma

Medulloblastomas are the most common intracranial PNET. *most common malignant tumor in children*

They arise in the **cerebellum** and can spread through CSF pathways resulting in spinal **drop metastases**. They are WHO grade IV.

cause hydrocephalus   *⊕T-K℗ → favorable outcome*

Retinoblastoma

Retinoblastoma is an intraocular PNET found in young children due to deletion of the Rb suppressor gene on chromosome 13.

In addition to Homer Wright rosettes, **Flexner-Wintersteiner rosettes (true rosettes)** are seen. See below.

Some patients have trilateral tumors. Talk about the number 13 being unlucky! These kids deserve real rosettes.

Trilateral tumor- when patients have bilateral retinoblastomas and a pineoblastoma.

Neuroblastoma

These PNETs most frequently arise from the sympathetic chain or adrenal gland.

 Neuroblastoma is classically associated with **opsoclonus-myoclonus,** which is also known as **Dancing eyes-dancing feet syndrome**. Children with neuroblastoma also have ataxia.

Urine catecholamines (homovanillic acid or vanillylmandelic acid) may be elevated.

Patients with amplification of the N-myc oncogene on chromosome 2 have a worse prognosis.

Think of the **2** houses you have on **N**orth **B**each -- **NB** is associated with all the **2**'s:

2 cats in the yard (**2** catecholamines: HVA and VMA),

2 houses in North Beach (sympathetic chain/Aorta and adrenal medulla),

2 age groups (adults anti-Ri; children Dancing eyes/feet)

2 markers (Neuro-N and synaptophysin), and

chromosome **2**!

Neuroblastoma has a blast causing neurological symptoms. It causes Dancing eyes-dancing feet syndrome (opsoclonus-myoclonus).

War of the Roses

Type of rosette	Histology	Tumors classically associated with the rosette
Flexner-Wintersteiner (True rosette)	There is a central lumen.	Retinoblastoma
Homer Wright	Cytoplasmic processes are in the center.	Neuroblastoma, medulloblastoma
Perivascular Pseudorosette	A vessel is at the center.	Ependymoma[4] (glioma)

4 Remember that **ependymoma is a glioma**, not a PNET.

Flexner-Wintersteiner (True Rosette)

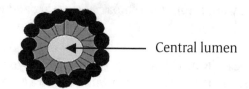

Central lumen

 Real rosettes are found in retinoblastoma.

Homer Wright Rosette

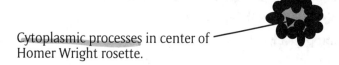

Cytoplasmic processes in center of
Homer Wright rosette.

 Homer Wright rosettes are seen in **neuroblastoma** and **medulloblastoma**.

Perivascular Pseudorosette

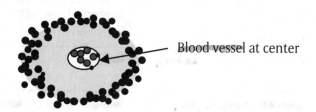

Blood vessel at center

 Perivascular pseudorosettes are seen in **ependymomas**.

 To remember that pseudorosettes occur in ependymomas, notice that **ependymoma sounds like pretendymoma.** You can imagine that *pseudorosettes could be seen in pretendymomas.*

Cancer Syndromes with Primary Brain Tumors

Syndrome	Tumor
Cowden's disease	Lhermitte Duclos (dysplastic gangliocytoma of the cerebellum)
Gorlin's syndrome	Medulloblastoma
Li-Fraumeni syndrome	Diffuse astrocytomas
Von Hippel-Lindau disease[5]	Hemangioblastoma
Tuberous Sclerosis	Subependymal Giant Cell Astrocytoma (SEGA)
Turcot's syndrome	Glioblastoma or medulloblastoma

Gorlin's syndrome

Also known as Nevoid Basal Cell Carcinoma Syndrome

 To remember that medulloblastomas are associated with Gorlin's syndrome, remember that medicine can be gory.

Gorlin's syndrome has been associated with defects in the PTCH gene.

Li-Fraumeni Syndrome

This is an autosomal dominant condition associated with a mutation in the tumor suppressor gene p53.

As a result, patients are at risk for sarcomas, breast cancer, and brain tumors such as diffuse astrocytomas.

Lhermitte Duclos

Lhermitte Duclos is a dysplastic gangliocytoma found in the cerebellum.

Lhermitte Duclos is associated with Cowden syndrome.

---

[5] Please see the Neurocutaneous Disorders chapter for more information about Von Hippel-Lindau disease, Tuberous Sclerosis, and Neurofibromatosis.

Cowden syndrome is associated with multiple hamartomas. Patients have breast cancer, thyroid neoplasms, and colon polyps.

Remember that Lhermitte Duclos is associated with Cowden syndrome by thinking of Lhermitte Duclos as **Lhermitte DuCOW**.

For the sports fans out there....

Think of coach **Cower** (Cowden) and the Pittsburgh Steelers winning their **5**th Super Bowl championship – Cowden's Little Ducks (Lhermitte Duclos) are a **dy**namic **gang** that **C**an **B**eat **T**eams **H**ard: Cerebellar **dy**splastic **gang**liocytoma, **C**olon polyps, **B**reast cancer, **T**hyroid neoplasms, and **H**armartomas. *Their **5** Super Bowl rings represent the 5 neoplasms you need to know for this disorder!*

Metastases

Brain metastases are the most common intracranial tumor in adults.

Often multiple metastases are found.

Brain metastases are most commonly found at the gray-white junction.

Tumors that tend to metastasize to the brain are:

· Gastrointestinal
· Renal
· Melanoma
· Breast —→ *most epidural SC compression*
· Lung.

Tumors that metastasize to the brain GRuMBLe: Gastrointestinal, Renal, Melanoma, Breast, and Lung.

Which metastatic tumors are hemorrhagic in the brain?

My Cranium Really Bleeds Terribly!

My	**M**-melanoma
Cranium	**C**-choriocarcinoma
Really	**R**-renal cell carcinoma
Bleeds	**B**-bronchogenic
Terribly	**T**-thyroid

Tumors of the Filum Terminale

Myxopapillary ependymoma and paraganglioglioma of the filum terminale are two tumors of the filum terminale.

Myxopapillary ependymoma is associated with mucin. When you see myxo in myxopapillary ependymoma, think of myxoid / mucin.

Paraneoplastic Syndromes

Paraneoplastic syndromes are syndromes that are associated with a cancer but the effects are far away from where the tumor is located.

If you have to guess a cancer with which a paraneoplastic autoantibody is associated, choose small cell lung carcinoma.

Paraneoplastic Syndromes

Autoantibody	Presentation	Cancer
Amphiphysin	Stiff person syndrome, (GAD if φ para neo) encephalomyelitis	Small cell lung carcinoma, breast
CV-2 (CRMP-5)	Limbic encephalitis, cerebellar degeneration, encephalomyelitis, chorea, peripheral neuropathy, Chronic gastrointestinal pseudo-obstruction	Small cell lung carcinoma, thymoma
Hu	Encephalomyelitis, sensory neuronopathy, cerebellar degeneration, limbic encephalitis	Small cell lung carcinoma neuroblastoma prostate CA
Ma2	Limbic, diencephalic, and brainstem encephalitis	Testicular, lung
Ri **(ANNA-2)**	Ataxia, opsoclonus-myoclonus, brainstem encephalitis	Breast, gynecological, small cell lung carcinoma
Ta	Limbic encephalitis, brainstem dysfunction	Testicular
Tr and **mGluR1**	Cerebellar degeneration	Hodgkin's disease
Yo	Cerebellar degeneration	Ovary, breast
Zic4	Cerebellar degeneration	Small cell lung carcinoma

Hugh Hefner gets around and *Hu gets around the CNS.* Hugh Hefner wears a *smoking jacket,* and *smokers get small cell lung carcinoma. Or, to remember all the various malignancies/disorders linked to Hu antibodies, think of this mnemonic:* **Hu kNeu that Pretty women Crush** *men with a* **Small Limbic system?** *(anti-***Hu**, **Neu***roblastoma,* **Pr***ostate cancer,* **C***erebellar degeneration,* **Small** *cell lung cancer,* **Limbic** *Encephalitis)*

If a man has anti-*Ta* autoantibody, he may have to say *Ta-Ta* to his testicles.

Syndrome	Pathological involvement
Limbic encephalitis	Hippocampus, Amygdala
Brainstem encephalitis (mostly bulbar)	Medulla oblongata
Cerebellar degeneration	Purkinje cells
Myelitis (anterior horn)	Motor neurons
Sensory neuronopathy	Dorsal Root Ganglia
Chronic gastrointestinal pseudo-obstruction	Myenteric plexus

J Neurol Neurosurg Psychiatry 2004;75:1135–1140.

Like a *yo-yo*, patients with *Yo autoantibody* lurch around due to cerebellar degeneration.

Some people use the eloquent phrase "yo momma". This phrase may help you remember that Yo is associated with female cancers such as ovarian and breast cancer.

Other paraneoplastic syndromes include dermatomyositis, cancer-associated retinopathy, and Lambert-Eaton syndrome. More information on Lambert-Eaton syndrome is in the Neuromuscular Diseases chapter.

Chemotherapy

Asparaginase can cause stroke/central venous thrombosis. Maybe patients on **Asp**araginase should take **Asp**irin to prevent stroke. (**This is just a mnemonic, not a clinical recommendation**.)

Cyclophosphamide can make you psycho due to SIADH.

Cytarabine (**Ara-C**) causes **Ara**chnoiditis and **C**erebellar dysfunction. It also can cause seizures. You can also think of Ara-C as *Aura-C-zure* (Aura-seizure).

Iphosphamide can cause encephalopathy.

Methotrexate causes a reversible posterior leukoencephalopathy. *PRES*

Methotrexate and cytarabine are the most commonly used agents for intrathecal therapy.

Suramin probably will knock out your *sural nerve* due to *peripheral neuropathy.*

 Etoposide, vincristine, cisplatin, and taxol EViCT cancer but leave you numb due to peripheral neuropathy.

Taxol causes a dose-dependent **peripheral neuropathy** with **painful dysesthesias**.

 Taxes are painful.

Vincristine causes **s**ensory and **m**otor neuropathy.

 Sorry, no S & M mnemonics allowed; we have a reputation to protect. One day we will be **vin**dicated!

Most Common Roll Call

The most common **category of primary brain tumors** is **gliomas**.

Ependymomas are the most common **spinal cord glioma**.

Prolactinoma is the most common **pituitary adenoma**.

Oligodendroglioma is the most common **primary brain tumor to bleed**.

Medulloblastoma is the most common intracranial **primitive neuroectodermal tumor**. *AND most common malignant tumor - children*

Acoustic schwannoma is the most common **cerebellopontine angle** tumor.

biphasic architecture-
① clear cytoplasm in nests
② small reactive T cells

Germinoma is the most common **tumor of the pineal gland**.

Craniopharyngioma is the most common **supratentorial tumor in childhood**.

Epidural metastases are the most common **spinal tumor in the elderly**.

Glioblastoma multiforme is the most common **primary brain tumor in adults**.

Chordoma is the most common **neural crest-derived tumor of the sacrum**.

Brain metastases are the most common **intracranial tumor in adults**.

Lung cancer is the most common **primary tumor to metastasize to the spinal cord**.

Neuro-Oncology Quiz

(Answers on page 749)

1. Which agent can cause peripheral neuropathy?
>   A. Vincristine
>
>   B. Taxol
>
>   C. Cisplatin
>
>   D. Etoposide
>
>   E. All of the above.

2. Which autoantibody is least likely to be found in a patient with lung cancer?
>   A. Tr
>
>   B. Hu
>
>   C. Ri
>
>   D. Amphiphysin
>
>   E. Ma2

3. Which of these is a grade I meningioma?
>   A. Metaplastic
>
>   B. Rhabdoid
>
>   C. Choroid
>
>   D. Clear Cell
>
>   E. Papillary

4. Match the tumor with the description

1) Oligodendroglioma	A. The most common supratentorial tumor in childhood.
2) Schwannoma	B. The most common tumor found in the cerebello-pontine angle.
3) Germinoma	C. Stains positive for epithelial membrane antigen.
4) Meningioma	D. The most common tumor of the pineal gland.
5) Craniopharyngioma	E. The primary brain tumor that is most likely to bleed.

Chapter 11

Neuro-Ophthalmology

Eye on Anatomy

The Eye

The Lens

The lens of the eye causes images to be **upside-down and reversed** on the retina.

The **ciliary muscle** changes the shape of the lens, allowing **accommodation**.

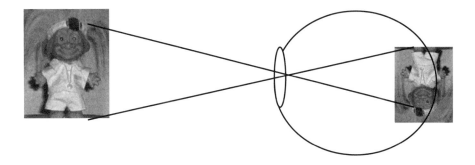

The Retina by Parts

 The **macula** is in the middle of the retina and is responsible for central vision.

 The **fovea**, which is the *center of the macula*, is the region of the retina with the highest visual acuity; it represents the central one to two degrees of visual space.

As mentioned above, the lens of the eye causes images to be upside-down and reversed on the retina.
· The **temporal field** of vision is represented on the *nasal aspect* of the retina.
· The **nasal field** is represented on the *temporal aspect* of the retina.

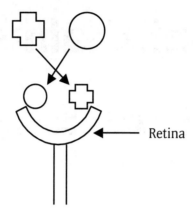

Retina

Vascular supply to the retina is by the *central retinal artery*, which is a *branch of the ophthalmic artery*.

Emboli to the Eye

Hollenhorst Plaques versus **Calcific Emboli** versus **Platelet-Fibrin Emboli**.

Recall that the ophthalmic artery is the first major branch of the internal carotid artery.

The **retina has 3 cell layers**:

      1) Outer nuclear layer containing photoreceptors

      2) Bipolar cell layer

      3) Ganglion cell layer (innermost layer)

 The retina has *Photos of Bipolar Gangs* (Photoreceptors, Bipolar cell layer, and Ganglion cell layer).

The retina has **two types of photoreceptors: rods** and **cones**.

    · **Rods** are more numerous and are useful for **night vision**. They are found at the **periphery of the retina**.

    · **Cones** detect **color** and are concentrated at the **fovea**.

 Think of **orange cones** to remember that cones detect **color**.

Alternatively **c**one begins with C and **c**olor begins with C.

 Rods are relegated to the rim of the retina. The **c**ones are at the **c**enter and detect **c**olor.

The **optic disc**, which leads to the optic nerve, **has no photoreceptors** and produces a blind spot, which is about 15 degrees lateral to the central fixation point.

The photoreceptors synapse on the ——————————→ bipolar cells.
The bipolar cells synapse onto ——————————→ ganglion cells.
Axons of the ganglion cells form the ——————————→ optic nerve.

To remember that the **optic disc has no photoreceptors** and produces a blind spot, think of the last time you used a floppy disc to store pictures – it didn't work: This disc has no photos!

The Optic Nerve (Cranial Nerve Two)

An optic nerve lesion causes an ipsilateral visual field defect.

A right optic nerve lesion could cause this visual field defect:

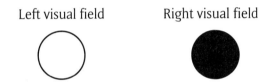

Left visual field   Right visual field

The optic nerves unite at the optic chiasm, where their fibers partially cross.

The Optic Chiasm

At the chiasm:
        Fibers from the nasal aspect of the retina cross.
        Temporal fibers don't cross.

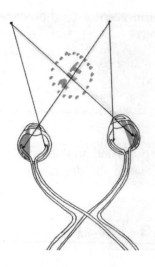

Nasal fibers cross;
temporal fibers don't cross.

The optic chiasm usually is above the pituitary fossa.

Pituitary tumors can cause bitemporal hemianopia due to compression of the optic chiasm. Recall that pituitary adenomas are the most common pituitary tumor, and prolactinomas are the most common type of pituitary adenoma.

Bitemporal hemianopia can be seen with a **pituitary tumor** causing compression of the optic chiasm:

Binasal hemianopia can occur with **bilateral lateral compression** of the optic chiasm, as seen with **calcified internal carotid arteries.**

Eyelid

Eye Opening

The levator palpebrae superior (skeletal muscle supplied by CN III) and Müller's smooth muscle (supplied by sympathetics) perform eye opening.

Eye Closure

The orbicularis oculi muscle (innervated by the facial nerve) closes the eye.

Corneal Reflex

 When the cornea is touched, the corneal reflex causes the eyelids to close.

- **Afferent limb**: ophthalmic division of the trigeminal nerve.
- **Efferent limb**: facial nerve.

Eye Muscles

 There are 6 eye muscles:

1. Inferior oblique
2. Inferior rectus
3. Lateral rectus
4. Medial rectus
5. Superior oblique
6. Superior rectus

These 6 muscles are supplied by the cranial nerves outlined below.

Muscle	Cranial nerve by which it is innervated
Inferior oblique	III (Oculomotor)
Inferior rectus	III (Oculomotor)
Lateral rectus	VI (Abducens)
Medial rectus	III (Oculomotor)
Superior oblique	IV (Trochlear)
Superior rectus	III (Oculomotor)

The purposes of these 6 muscles are as follows:

Muscle	Function
Inferior oblique (IO)	Elevation and extorsion
Inferior rectus (IR)	Depression and extorsion
Lateral rectus (LR)	Abduction
Medial rectus (MR)	Adduction
Superior oblique (SO)	Depression and intorsion
Superior rectus (SR)	Elevation and intorsion

When the eye is abducted (rotated outward) 23 degrees, the superior rectus acts as a pure elevator and the inferior rectus acts as a pure depressor.

When the eye is adducted 51 degrees (pulled inward), the superior oblique acts as a pure depressor and the inferior oblique acts as a pure elevator.

The inferiors extort.

· Inferior rectus (IR) depresses and extorts.
· Inferior oblique (IO) elevates and extorts.

To remember that the inferior oblique and inferior rectus extort, **remember that inferiors extort money.**

The **IRS** (Internal Revenue Service) makes us **SO depressed**, and the **IRs** (inferior rectus muscles) and **SO** (**S**uperior **O**blique muscles)) **depress.**

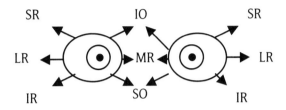

The superior rectus (SR) is above the inferior rectus (IR), so S**R** and I**R** are **rightly** placed.

However, inferior oblique (IO) is above the superior oblique (SO), so I**O** and S**O** are **O**ut-of-place.

To remember the location of IO, MR and SO, and to remember that a 51-degree adducted eye lets the SO act as a pure depressor and the IO act as a pure elevator, remember the phrase: "I owe Mr. So **$51** when the bill is **added**."

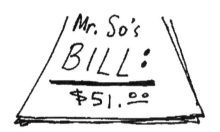

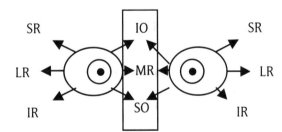

Cranial Nerves

Cranial nerve	Name of cranial nerve	Foramina through which CN exits skull
II	Optic nerve	Optic canal
III	Oculomotor nerve	Superior orbital fissure
IV	Trochlear nerve	Superior orbital fissure
VI	Abducens	Superior orbital fissure

Cranial nerve	Muscles Innervated
III (Oculomotor)	Inferior oblique, inferior rectus, medial rectus, superior rectus
IV (Trochlear)	Superior oblique
VI (Abducens)	Lateral rectus

Cranial Nerve II (Optic Nerve)

 The optic nerve provides input to the visual pathway:

Optic nerve ➔ optic chiasm ➔ optic tract ➔ lateral geniculate nucleus ➔ optic radiations ➔ visual cortex.

The optic nerve is also important in the pupillary light reflex:

Optic nerve ➔ optic chiasm ➔ optic tract ➔ pretectal nuclei ➔ Edinger-Westphal nuclei ➔ ciliary ganglion ➔ short ciliary nerves.

The pupillary light reflex pathway does **not** include the lateral geniculate nucleus, optic radiations, or visual cortex.

The optic nerve also provides input to the **suprachiasmatic nucleus** of the hypothalamus, which is responsible for *circadian rhythms*, and to the **superior colliculus**, which is important in *generating saccades*.

Cranial Nerve III (Oculomotor Nerve)

 The oculomotor nerve supplies these muscles:

- Inferior oblique
- Inferior rectus
- Medial rectus
- Superior rectus

- Levator palpebrae
- Pupillary sphincter.

The oculomotor nerve supplies parasympathetic innervation to the eye allowing **pupil constriction** and **accommodation**.

A **complete oculomotor palsy** causes the **eye to look down and out**. It also causes **ptosis** and a **dilated nonreactive pupil**.

Patients have less diplopia when looking far than near due to impaired convergence.

Internal Ophthalmoplegia is defined as loss of parasympathetic innervation to the sphincter pupillae (iris) and ciliary muscle.

External Ophthalmoplegia is defined as paralysis of the external ocular muscles.

Total Ophthalmoplegia is defined as paralysis of all the eye muscles, both intraocular and extraocular.

CN III palsy may be due to compression.

One cause is a **P**osterior **COM**municating artery aneurysm. A PCOM aneurysm can compress the CN III in the SAS (anterior to the cerebral peduncle and prior to the entry of CN III into the cavernous sinus).

Also, recall that CN III passes between the posterior cerebral and superior cerebellar arteries. Aneurysms at the junction of these arteries and the basilar artery may also compress CN III.

Transtentorial herniation can also result in compression of CN III.

The parasympathetic fibers are near the surface of the nerve, so **compressive lesions tend to first cause a dilated pupil** prior to extraocular muscle weakness.

Parasympathetic **p**upilloconstrictor fibers are along the **p**eriphery of CN III.

The pupil is usually spared in ischemic lesions of the nerve.

Diabetes is a cause of a CN III palsy sparing the pupil. It tends to affect the central fibers and not the pupilloconstrictor fibers.

Myasthenia gravis is another cause of a CN III palsy sparing the pupil.

Mnemonic for causes of a CN III palsy sparing the pupil: Inside the **I**, it is **DiM** (**D**iabetes and **M**yasthenia), and Ischemic lesions are usually **I**ncomplete there.

In the orbit, CN III divides into superior and inferior divisions.

· The **superior division** innervates the **superior rectus** and **levator**.

· The **inferior division** innervates the **inferior oblique**, **inferior rectus**, **medial rectus**, and **pupillary sphincter.**

The **oculomotor nerve** has **2 nuclei**:

· **Main oculomotor nucleus**

· **Edinger-Westphal nucleus** (also known as the *accessory parasympathetic nucleus*).

See the Brainstem section below.

Cranial Nerve IV (Trochlear nerve)

The trochlear nerve is the longest and most slender cranial nerve. It is the only cranial nerve that exits from the **D**orsal aspect of the brainstem. It is also the only cranial nerve that **D**ecussates (at the medullary velum).

A patient with trochlear **nerve palsy** experiences **D**ouble vision that is worst when looking **D**own and away from the lesion.

The patient will have a **head tilt;** the **involved eye is elevated in primary gaze.**

Elevation is greatest when head is tilted toward side of involved eye. It ~~improves when the head is tilted away from the side of the involved eye~~. Patients tend to ~~tuck down their heads~~ and tilt them away from the involved eye.

 The *FOUR* **D**'s of Cranial Nerve *FOUR*:

> **D**ouble vision **Deteriorates** when looking **D**own and away from the lesion,
>
> **D**orsal brainstem exit point, and
>
> **D**ecussates in medulla.

 A ~~trochlear palsy makes one tuck and turn one's head~~ (away from the involved eye).

 Troch in trochlear sounds like truck.

When a patient with a **tr**ochlear nerve palsy tilts his/her head **t**oward the lesion, **you can drive a truck beneath the involved eye because it's elevated so high**.

Elevation is **a**ttenuated when head is tilted **a**way from the side of the lesion.

Cranial Nerve VI (Abducens Nerve)

The abducens nerve, CN VI, supplies the **lateral rectus**.

 Recall that **increased intracranial pressure** is a cause of CN VI palsy.

Patients with a CN VI palsy experience the **worst diplopia when looking laterally <u>toward</u> the side of the lesion**.

Lesions Involving Multiple Cranial Nerves

Site of lesion/Name of syndrome	Cranial nerves involved
Orbital Apex Lesion	**2**, 3, 4, 6, V1
Superior Orbital Fissure Abnormality (SOFA)	3, 4, 6, V1***
Tolosa-Hunt and other causes of cavernous sinus syndrome	3, 4, 6, V1, **V2**

Orbital apex lesions, the cavernous sinus syndrome, and superior orbital fissure lesions all involve cranial nerves 3,4,6, and V1.

Orbital Apex Lesion

In an **O**rbital apex lesion you have CN II (**O**ptic nerve) involvement and may have a bulging eye.

Superior Orbital Fissure Abnormality (SOFA)***

A mnemonic for structures that pass through the SOFA: LOST IN FAO's Superior SOFA. *Lacrimal nerve, Ophthalmic veins, Sympathetic nerves, Trochlear nerve, Inferior branch of oculomotor nerve, Nasociliary nerve, Frontal nerve, Abducens nerve, Oculomotor nerve's **Superior** branch **SOFA**.*

Tolosa-Hunt Syndrome

Tolosa-Hunt syndrome is a granulomatous inflammation in the cavernous sinus that results in painful ophthalmoplegia. It is treated with prednisone.

In Tolosa-Hunt and other cavernous sinus syndromes you can have V2 (maxillary branch of the trigeminal nerve) involvement.

Brainstem

Oculomotor Nucleus

The oculomotor nucleus is a wacky thing. It has **multiple subnuclei**.

 The superior rectus muscle is innervated by the **contralateral subnucleus**. I kid thee not!

One subnucleus located at the midline innervates both levators.

The inferior oblique, inferior rectus, and medial rectus are innervated by ipsilateral subnuclei.

Edinger-Westphal Nucleus

The Edinger-Westphal nucleus contains preganglionic parasympathetic neurons, which synapse in the ciliary ganglion.

The Edinger-Westphal nucleus innervates both pupillary sphincters and ciliary bodies.

It is important in **pupil constriction** and **accommodation**.

To remember that preganglionic parasympathetic fibers travel from the Edinger-Westphal nucleus (EW) to the ciliary ganglion, remember it as the "**Eeewww! Cilia!**" nucleus.

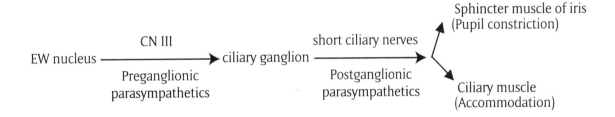

 The **long ciliary nerve** carries sympathetic fibers to the **dilator of the pupil**.
The **short ciliary nerves** carry parasympathetic fibers to the **pupil constrictor** and **ciliary muscles**.

The **l**ong ciliary nerve makes the pupil **l**arge and the **s**hort ciliary nerves make it **s**mall.

Abducens Nucleus

 The abducens nucleus is important in **lateral gaze**.

The medial longitudinal fasciculus (MLF) travels from the abducens nucleus to the contralateral oculomotor nucleus.

As a result, a left abducens nucleus lesion causes left gaze palsy, due to inability of the left eye to abduct and the right eye to adduct.

Medial Longitudinal Fasciculus (MLF)

As mentioned above, the MLF connects the abducens nucleus and contralateral oculomotor nucleus.

(It also connects the vestibular nucleus and trochlear nucleus with these nuclei.)

Internuclear Ophthalmoplegia (INO)

 A **lesion of the MLF** interrupts the connection between the abducens and contralateral oculomotor nucleus. This causes **difficulty adducting the ipsilateral eye**. This is called **internuclear ophthalmoplegia (INO)**.

A lesion of the left MLF prevents adduction of the left eye when looking to the right. The right eye can abduct and exhibits nystagmus.

INO can be seen in **Multiple Sclerosis** (MS) or Stroke. In fact, bilateral INO can be seen in MS.

 INO versus CN III Palsy

If a patient has an INO, the eye can adduct during convergence; this is not possible with an oculomotor palsy.

 I kNOw how to add even when you get close to my face (during convergence).

Paramedian Pontine Reticular Formation (PPRF)

 The PPRF also has a role in horizontal gaze.

The PPRF projects to the ipsilateral CN VI nucleus and contralateral oculomotor nucleus through the MLF.

It receives information from the frontal eye fields.

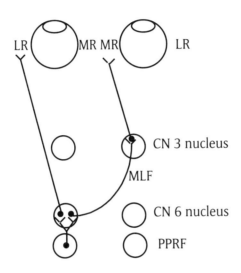

One-and-a-half Syndrome

ipsi Ⅵ, contra Ⅲ

 One and a half syndrome is due to a pontine lesion involving the PPRF <u>or</u> the abducens nucleus <u>and</u> the MLF. ipsi Ⅲ via MLF

The ipsilateral eye can't move. **The only movement seen is abduction and nystagmus of contralateral eye.**

Visual Cortex

Area of cortex	Brodmann's area
Frontal eye fields	8
Primary visual cortex	17
Visual association cortex	39,19,18

The primary visual cortex surrounds the calcarine fissure in the occipital lobe.

The primary visual cortex is also called striate cortex, due to the stria of Gennari (layer 4B of the cortex), which has a pale appearance.

Most information arrives at cortical layer 4 of the visual cortex.

Visual association cortex is nearby at Brodmann's areas 18, 19, and 39. (Brodmann's area 39 is the angular gyrus.)

The upper bank of calcarine cortex is called the cuneus, and the lower bank is lingual gyrus.

 The **L**ower bank is **L**ingual gyrus. The **U**pper bank is the c**U**ne**U**s.

Information from the **right lower visual field** is projected to the **left cuneus** (upper bank of calcarine cortex); Information from the **right upper visual field** is projected to the **left lingual gyrus**.

 The fovea has a large area of representation in the cortex because it is responsible for central vision.

The macula, including the fovea, is represented by posterior calcarine cortex. The peripheral retina has more anterior representation.

 To remember that the macula is represented posteriorly, remember that the **mac is in the back**.

Cortical Blindness

 Patients with cortical blindness do not blink to threat and have no optokinetic responses.

 To differentiate cortical blindness from pregeniculate lesions: patients with cortical blindness have pupillary responses to light.

Optokinetic Nystagmus (OKN)

OKN is generated by asking the patient to watch a tape with vertical stripes of alternating colors.

 The eyes follow slowly in the direction of movement and then jerk in the opposite direction.

> · The **slow phase** is the smooth pursuit phase. It tests parieto-occipital pathways ipsilaterally.
>
> · The **fast phase** is the saccadic phase. It tests pathways that originate in the contralateral frontal lobe.

Slow is P-O (**P**arietal-**O**ccipital). **F**ast is **f**rontal.

Visual Field Defects

General Principles

 General principles of visual field defects:

A unilateral prechiasmal lesion can cause a **visual field defect in** one eye, **the ipsilateral eye.**
Chiasmal lesions can cause **nonhomonymous visual field defects** in **both eyes.**
Retrochiasmal lesions cause **homonymous** visual field defects.

> · Lesions of the **cortex** tend to cause **congruous visual field defects** and the **macula may be spared.**
>
> · More anterior but still retrochiasmal lesions tend to cause incongruent visual field defects.

Specific Lesions

Optic Nerve Lesion

As mentioned above, a right optic nerve lesion could cause this visual field defect:

Left visual field   Right visual field

Junctional Scotoma/Anterior Chiasm Syndrome

A junctional scotoma is due to a lesion of the optic nerve at the optic chiasm that involves the nasal fibers from the contralateral optic nerve as they cross. It results in **ipsilateral blindness** and a **contralateral defect of the upper temporal quadrant.**

Superior Homonymous Quadrantanopia

Superior homonymous quadrantanopia, also known as **pie-in-the-sky lesions,** are due to lesions of the lower optic radiations traveling through the temporal lobe. Specifically, temporal lobe lesions may cause a contralateral superior homonymous quadrantanopia. This may occur with **temporal lobectomy**.

A right temporal lobe lesion could cause this visual field defect.

Inferior Homonymous Quadrantanopia

Parietal lesions cause a contralateral inferior homonymous quadrantanopia, otherwise known as **pie-on-the-floor**.

A left parietal lesion could cause this defect:

 Poor me. My **pi**e is on the floor and I have a **p**arietal lobe lesion.

Homonymous Hemianopia

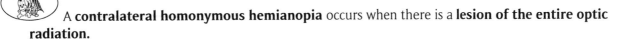 A **contralateral homonymous hemianopia** occurs when there is a **lesion of the entire optic radiation.**

A lesion of the left optic radiations causes a right homonymous hemianopia.

Anterior Choroidal Artery Lesion

A stroke in the **anterior choroidal artery distribution**, which causes a lateral geniculate body lesion, can cause a quadruple sectoranopia. The upper and lower quadrants have a homonymous defect with sparing of a horizontal sector.

The visual field defect with a stroke in the **anterior choroidal artery distribution**, which causes a lateral geniculate body lesion, looks a bit like an arch on its side.

Occipital Lobe Lesions

Lesions of the occipital cortex tend to cause homonymous hemianopia **with macular sparing** (due to dual blood supply). An exception is a lesion of the anterior calcarine cortex, which is described below.

A lesion of the left occipital cortex could cause this lesion:

 The occipital **c**ortex causes lesions that look like a **c**.

Anterior Calcarine Cortex Lesion

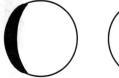 **Monocular visual field defects** can be seen with lesions of the **anterior calcarine cortex**. *This is the only way a cortical lesion can cause a monocular defect.*

This visual field defect is consistent with an anterior calcarine cortex lesion on the right:

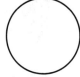

Eye Movements

Saccades

Saccades are fast conjugate eye movements used to bring a target into view. There is some voluntary control.

 The frontal lobe (Brodmann's area 8) generates contralateral saccades through connections with the PPRF.

Smooth Pursuit

Smooth pursuit is not under voluntary control. It allows one to view a moving object.

The parieto-occipital cortex generates ipsilateral smooth pursuit movements.

Vertical Eye Movements

The **posterior commissure** is important in **upgaze**.

The **rostral interstitial nucleus of the MLF** is important in **downgaze**.

Remember **UPC** and **DRINK** to remember vertical eye movements. **U**pgaze-**P**osterior **C**ommissure. **D**owngaze-**R**ostral **I**nterstitial **N**uc**K**leus-.

Disorders of the Eye

Anterior Ischemic Optic Neuropathy (AION)

AION causes **painless vision loss of sudden onset**.

It is due to infarction of the optic disc.

HOT TIP

This is the most common cause of persistent monocular vision loss in patients over 50 years old. It may occur in **giant cell arteritis**.

How can you distinguish Acute Ischemic Optic Neuropathy (AION) from Optic Neuritis (ON)?

· Disc swelling is bland and present in only 30% of ON patients. **In AION, the disc is swollen with splinter hemorrhages.**

· Pain in ON is common and worse with eye movements. **Only 10% of AION** patients note eye pain, which does not change with eye motion.

· Recurrent ON is common but **Recurrent AION is rare**.

· Although both conditions might show a reduced amplitude in the visual evoked response, ON is more likely to show a prolonged or delayed response.

Horner's Syndrome

TAKE HOME MESSAGE

Horner's syndrome includes **Miosis** due to loss of sympathetic innervation to the dilator of the pupil. It can also be associated with **Ptosis** (due to loss of innervation to Müller's smooth muscle) and **Anhydrosis**.

The *miotic pupil will react to light*. Anisocoria is more prominent in the dark.

HOT TIP

10% cocaine (norepinephrine reuptake inhibitor) will dilate a normal pupil but not the pupil of a patient with Horner's syndrome.

Horner's syndrome may be due to a central, preganglionic, or postganglionic lesion in the oculosympathetic pathway:

1) Hypothalamus to ciliospinal center of Budge.

2) Ciliospinal center of Budge to superior cervical ganglion.

3) Superior cervical ganglion to iris dilator muscle.

Honing in on Horner's

HOT TIP Eye drops help to localize the lesion.

1% hydroxyamphetamine (**HO**) hydrobromide (which releases **NE** into cleft) dilates the pupil in Horner's syndrome if the lesion is **PRE**-ganglionic.

1% phenylephrine hydrochloride (**Neo**-synephrine), which is a direct **A**lpha-**A**gonist, dilates the pupil if Horner's is due to a **POST**-ganglionic lesion. Post-ganglionic Horner's syndrome is not associated with anhidrosis.

All you need to remember is:

1% HO→NE→dilates if PRE-G lesion,

1% NEO→AA→dilates if POST-G!

(H in HO comes before N in Neo, and Pre precedes Post.)

Hornblower PAM will **not use cocaine**. Her **hypothesis** (hypothalamus 1st) is that she absolutely won't **Budge** (ciliospinal center of Budge 2nd) even if her **superior gang** (superior cervical ganglion 3rd) of friends tries to use peer pressure and persuade her with a beautiful **iris** (iris dilator muscle).

BUZZ WORDS

Carotid dissection can cause a **painful Horner's syndrome**.

MNEMONIC

Horner's Syndrome from a **COMMON** Carotid Artery (CCA) dissection involves all 3 **PAM** signs and **PAM Horner** is a **COMMON** name.

MNEMONIC

For **EXTERNAL** Carotid Artery (ECA) dissections, only **A**nhydrosis is seen **A**lone, sparing oculosympathetics. Pam's mother **An**n **Horner** (**An**hydrosis) is **A**lone **outside** (**EXTERNAL** Carotid Artery), where nobody can see her (sparing oculosympathetics).

MNEMONIC

Conversely, for **INTERNAL** Carotid Artery (ICA) dissections, only **P**tosis-**M**iosis is seen, sparing facial sweat glands. Pam's grampa, ol' **P.M. Horner** (**P**tosis-**M**iosis) is secretly **P**retty **M**ad to be stuck **inside** (**INTERNAL** Carotid Artery) but tells everyone it's "No sweat!" (sparing facial sweat glands).

Optic Neuritis

Optic neuritis (ON) is due to demyelination of the optic nerve.

Patients with ON complain of **eye pain, which increases with movement**. Usually the patient has a **central scotoma**.

In the Optic Neuritis Treatment Trial (ONTT), mild-to-severe eye pain was present in 92% of patients. ONTT also showed that oral steroids demonstrated an *increased* incidence of recurrent optic neuritis, while IV steroids increased the rate of *recovery* of optic neuritis and decreased the incidence of the development of MS over a 2-year period.

Patients have **decreased visual acuity**, **red desaturation** (objects look less red with the affected eye), and an **afferent pupillary defect**.

There may be swelling of the optic disc or it may look normal.

Visual field defect with optic neuritis affecting the right optic nerve:

ON is often the first sign of Multiple Sclerosis (MS). MRI looking for white matter lesions helps to predict risk for MS.

 Methylprednisolone increases the rate of recovery of ON.

Reflexes

Accommodation Reflex

 There are 3 components of the accommodation reflex:

1. Ocular convergence (contraction of medial rectus muscles)

2. Pupillary constriction

3. Change in the lens shape.

A pathway from the cortex to the oculomotor nuclei via the superior colliculus allows ocular convergence.

Pupillary constriction and change in lens shape are parasympathetic responses. Please see the Edinger-Westphal section above.

Pupillary Light Reflex

Afferent limb: CN II
Efferent limb: CN III

See the section about the optic nerve above.

Eye Phenomena

Adie's Pupil

 Adie's pupil is also known as Adie's tonic pupil or **myotonic pupillary reaction**.

This pupil, which is enlarged compared to the normal pupil, reacts very slowly to light but reacts to accommodation. Once it has constricted, it stays constricted for awhile.

Adie's pupil is due to defect in parasympathetic innervation of the iris sphincter e.g. degeneration of the ciliary ganglion or postganglionic parasympathetic neurons.

Asymmetric pupils, **A**ccommodation produces some constriction
Dilated slightly, **D**egeneration of ciliary ganglion or postganglionic parasympathetic fibers
Increased sensitivity to pilocarpine, **I**mpaired reaction to light
Eye bigger **E**specially in light

 Holmes-Adie syndrome- Adie's tonic pupil with absence of knee or ankle jerks.

Afferent Pupillary Defect

A pupil that demonstrates an afferent pupillary defect responds poorly to direct light but responds consensually. It usually is due to optic nerve damage anterior to the chiasm.

Amaurosis Fugax

Amaurosis fugax is a **temporary monocular loss of vision**. Amaurosis means darkening or black and fugax means fugitive or fleeting, in Latin.

It is due to emboli causing temporary occlusion of the retinal artery, which is a branch of the ophthalmic artery.

It is often described as a **shade coming down.**

A noninvasive carotid duplex ultrasound is typically ordered after a patient complains of Amaurosis fugax. If carotid atherosclerosis is identified, aspirin is indicated, as is a surgical consult for a carotid endarterectomy based on the location and grade of stenosis, to prevent a future stroke.

Emboli to the Eye

XOL emboli - yellow/orange, refractile

A Hollenhorst Plaque is a small, shiny, cholesterol embolus lodged in a retinal arteriole. It typically originates from an atheromatous plaque in a proximal artery, usually a severely atherosclerotic internal carotid. When identified, it signifies prior ischemic damage to the eye; treating the upstream vessel may prevent further embolization and injury.

Calcific Emboli originate from diseased heart valves and are more likely to **C**ompletely o**CC**lude retina vessels than Hollenhorst plaques. Calcific Emboli are gray and globular.

/white, non-refractile

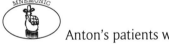

Platelet-Fibrin Emboli are ~~gray~~ *white* and long. They are endogenous and friable, often breaking up into smaller pieces that can occlude distal retinal branches. *lodge @ bifurcations*

from ulcerative atheromas

Anton's Syndrome

Anton's syndrome is the denial of cortical blindness.

It is due to bilateral occipital lobe damage. It can occur with **bilateral PCA infarcts**.

Anton's patients will say, "I ain't blind".

Argyll-Robertson Pupil

An Argyll-Robertson pupil is an irregular, small pupil that reacts poorly to light but reacts to accommodation.

Argyll-Robertson pupil is associated with **CNS syphilis**.

Bálint's Syndrome

Bálint's syndrome is a disconnection syndrome, which is associated with a triad:

    1) Simultagnosia

    2) Oculomotor-apraxia

    3) Optic-ataxia

 Simultagnosia is the inability to attend to multiple objects in one's view.

Optic-ataxia is difficulty reaching for objects using visual information, as if there is a disturbance of hand and eye coordination.

Oculomotor-apraxia is difficulty with visual scanning despite normal extraocular movements.

Patients with Balint's syndrome have difficulty voluntarily looking at particular points in space.

Balint's syndrome is due to **bilateral parietal-occipital damage.**

When you see **BAL** in **Bál**int's syndrome, think of base**Bál**l and the Boston Red **S.O.X.** who have difficulty getting 3 outs sometimes because of 3 visual deficits:

- **S**imultagnosia (they cannot perceive simultaneous objects -- only focusing on their huge salary and not the baseball),

- **O**culomotor-apra**X**ia (they cannot change to a new location of visual fixation -- the fielder cannot look over to see the baserunner), and

- **O**ptic-ata**X**ia (they cannot guide their hand toward an object using visual information -- the fielder is unable to tag the runner out!)

When you see **Bál** in **Bál**int's syndrome, think of eye**bál**l off **bál**ance. Patients have oculomotor-apraxia, optic-ataxia, problems with depth perception, and simultanagnosia.

Balint's Syndrome

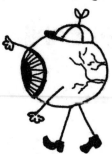

Ciliospinal Reflex

Pinching the neck causes pupil dilation. Afferents are C2 and C3. Efferent pathway: sympathetic fibers.

 If there's a Horner syndrome, the pupil will not dilate.

Duane Syndrome

Duane syndrome is a congenital disorder due to hypoplasia of the abducens nucleus and nerve with aberrant innervation of the lateral rectus by branches of CN III. During adduction, narrowing of the palpebral fissure and globe retraction are seen.

Foster Kennedy Syndrome

Foster Kennedy syndrome is characterized by a triad:

       1) Ipsilateral anosmia

       2) Ipsilateral optic atrophy

       3) Contralateral papilledema

Foster Kennedy syndrome is classically associated with a mass, such as a meningioma, involving the olfactory groove or sphenoid ridge. The mass compresses one optic nerve, causing optic atrophy, and increases intracranial pressure, resulting in papilledema of the contralateral eye.

To remember <u>Foster</u> Kennedy syndrome, picture some **groov**y *men* (olfactory **groove** *men*ingioma) wearing <u>Foster</u> Grant™ sunglasses.

The glasses cover the eyes and sit on the nose. One eye has optic atrophy and one has papilledema. The nose doesn't work (anosmia) if the sunglasses are too tight on the nose.

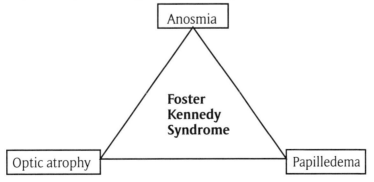

Marcus Gunn Jaw-winking

Marcus Gunn jaw – winking is characterized by unilateral ptosis and synkinesis of cranial nerves V and III, which causes the eyelid to move when the jaw moves.

Marcus Gunn Pupil

 Marcus Gunn pupil is also known as relative afferent pupillary defect.

During the swinging flashlight test, the abnormal pupil appears to dilate when the light is pointed at it, rather than constricting. It does react consensually when the normal pupil is illuminated.

An optic nerve lesion is one possible cause.

If someone pointed a gun at your pupil, your eye would dilate wide open in horror and you'd ask the police to put out an **APB**.

Likewise, if someone has a Marcus Gunn pupil, the eye dilates when it's pointed at and there's an **APD** (**A**fferent **P**upillary **D**efect).

Möbius Syndrome

Möbius Syndrome is also known as congenital **facial diplegia syndrome**.

It is characterized by **congenital bilateral facial** weakness palsy that is often associated with **Bilateral abducens palsy**. With a palsy of both cranial nerves VI and VII, abducens and facial nerve diplegia cause a **"stone" face** appearance.

Patients can have other cranial nerve findings and neuromuscular abnormalities.

 How can you remember the **Möb**ius syndrome?

Even after they've killed their **6th and 7th** victim, the **Möb** must show no expression on the job, so they have **stone faces**!

Oculogyric Crisis

An oculogyric crisis is an attack of conjugate eye deviation. It is seen with neuroleptic use and in **postencephalitic Parkinsonism**.

Parinaud's Syndrome

Parinaud's syndrome is due to a lesion of the dorsal midbrain affecting the superior colliculi and pretectum.

 A **CRUEL** constellation of eye findings are seen in Parinaud's syndrome:

1. **C**onvergence-**R**etraction nystagmus on attempted up-gaze.
2. Paralysis of **U**pgaze and accommodation
3. **E**yelid retraction (Collier sign)
4. **L**ight-near dissociation

Patients with Parinaud's syndrome and paranoia should be pitied, because they can't look to see if someone is dropping something on them.

 To remember that Parinaud's syndrome is associated with the **pretectal area**, remember that *when one is paranoid, one **protects** oneself.* **When one is paranoid (Parinaud's), one protects (pretectal) oneself from CRUEL people.**

Pinpoint Pupils

 Pinpoint, reactive pupils can be seen with "**point-ine**" lesions.

Riddoch Phenomenon

Riddoch phenomenon is when a person can see the examiner's fingers if they are moving but not if they are still.

 The examiner **looks ridiculous wiggling his fingers but Riddoch phenomenon can then be demonstrated**.

Spasmus Nutans

Spasmus nutans is a condition seen in early childhood characterized by a triad:

       1) Titubation / nodding of head

       2) Nystagmus

       3) Torticollis / neck in weird position

 To remember that spasmus nutans is associated with **T**itubation, **N**ystagmus, and **T**orticollis, remember the phrase: **I would spaz if I saw T.N.T. in my grandma's cellar!** (supracellar glioma = grandma's super cellar)

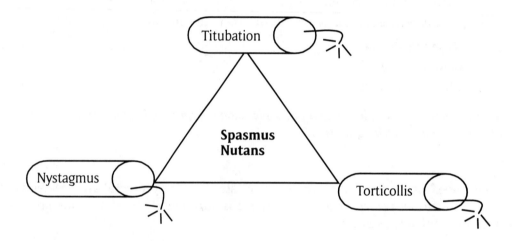

Uhthoff's Phenomenon

Uhthoff's phenomenon is **decreased visual acuity associated with increased temperature**.

It is seen in optic nerve disease.

Under
Heat
The
Optic nerve
Fatigues
Fast

Von Graefe Sign

Von Graefe sign is observed when **during downward gaze there is a lag of the upper lid.**

 Von Graefe sign is seen in **thyrotoxicosis**.

Weber's Syndrome

Patients with Weber's syndrome have an ipsilateral CN III palsy and contralateral weakness due to a lesion in the ventral midbrain involving CN III and the cerebral peduncle.

Diseases with Eye Findings

The following are various systemic disorders and the eye findings that are associated with them. [1]

Systemic disease	Eye findings
Aicardi syndrome	Optic nerve coloboma, chorioretinal lacunae
Ataxia-telangiectasia	Telangiectasias
Behçet disease	Uveitis
Cytomegalovirus (CMV)	Chorioretinitis, cataracts, keratitis, optic atrophy, microphthalmia
Down syndrome	Brushfield spots
Homocystinuria	Downward subluxation of the lens
Lowe syndrome	Cataracts, glaucoma
Marfan syndrome	Upward subluxation of the lens
Myotonic dystrophy	Cataracts
Neurofibromatosis I	Lisch nodules
Sturge-Weber	Choroidal hemangioma, glaucoma
Susac's syndrome	Branch retinal artery occlusions
Tuberous sclerosis	Retinal nodular hamartomas
Von Hippel-Lindau	Retinal angiomas
Whipple's disease	Oculomasticatory myokymia
Wilson's disease	Kayser-Fleischer ring

[1] See also: Tran T, Kaufman L. The child's eye in systemic diseases. Pediatr Clin N Am 2003;50:241-258.

Aicardi Syndrome

Aicardi syndrome is a condition that is characterized by a triad:

 1) **Ag**enesis of the corpus callosum

 2) **I**nfantile spasms

 3) **C**horioretinal lacunae

 AICardi syndrome is a rare disorder that is **X-linked dominant**.

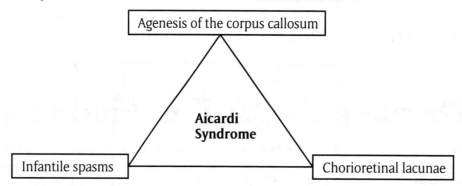

Behçet Disease

Behçet Disease is a type of vasculitis that can be associated with recurrent meningoencephalitis.

It is characterized by a triad:

 1. Oral ulcers

 2. Genital ulcers

 3. Uveitis

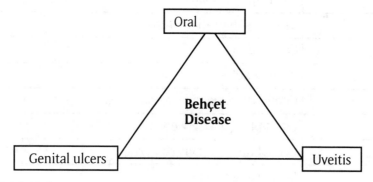

When you see Behçet, think **Betcha It hurts**. These poor patients have **oral and genital ulcers** as well as **uveitis**.

Cancer Associated Retinopathy Syndrome

Cancer associated retinopathy syndrome is a paraneoplastic syndrome that causes visual loss.

It may be seen in patients with small cell lung cancer (SCLC).

Patients with cancer associated retinopathy syndrome may have antibodies to **recoverin**.

Chronic Progressive External Ophthalmoplegia (CPEO)

CPEO is a mitochondrial disease that begins after age 20. It is characterized by progressive bilateral ptosis and loss of eye movements.

External ophthalmoplegia is defined as paralysis of the extraocular muscles.

Devic's Disease/NeuroMyelitis Optica (NMO)

NMO/Devic's disease is a demyelinating disease which causes **transverse myelitis and optic neuritis**.

On spinal MRI, cord lesions typically extend 3 or more segments during acute attacks.

CSF pleocytosis and the absence of oligoclonal bands help to distinguish this from MS. Unlike MS, NMO is associated with other autoimmune disorders. Also, patients with Devic's disease have seropositivity for NMO-IgG. This autoantibody targets aquaporin-4, and is not found in MS patients.[2]

The female to male ratio is >4:1.

Onset of NMO varies, with two peaks, one in childhood and the other in adults in their 40s.

Treatment with Rituxan (rituximab, a monoclonal antibody against CD20 on B-cells) may reduce frequency of NMO attacks, and stabilize or improve disability.

---

[2] Please see the Neurodegenerative Diseases chapter for more information.

Homocystinuria

 To remember that Marfan syndrome is associated with upward lens deviation and homocystinuria is associated with downward deviation: Marfan's patients are really, really **tall,** so their lens dislocation is **upwards**. As for the homocysteinemic patient, the goal of vitamin treatment is to bring down their homocysteine level, so their lens dislocation is downwards![3]

Kearns-Sayre Syndrome (KSS)

Kearns-Sayre Syndrome (KSS) is a mitochondrial disorder that can cause **Progressive External Ophthalmoplegia** and **pigmentary retinopathy**.

Patients with Kearns-Sayre syndrome may also have:

- Cerebellar syndrome
- Elevated CSF protein
- Endocrine abnormalities.
- Heart block
- Mitochondrial myopathy

How can you remember <u>Kearne Sayer Syndrome</u> is associated with **Pig**mentary retinopathy, **endo**crine abnormalities, and **heart** arrhythmias? Easy – just remember to **KiSS** the **Pig** in the rear **end or** else you'll break his **heart**.

Leber's Hereditary Optic Neuropathy

Leber's Hereditary Optic Neuropathy is a bilateral optic neuropathy due to a mitochondrial DNA point mutation. It presents as a *painless* **loss of central vision** usually beginning in **adolescence or early adulthood.**

Locked-in Syndrome

Locked-in syndrome is due to bilateral ventral pontine lesions.

Is the **V**ice-**P**resident (**V**entral **P**ons) **locked-in** a bunker somewhere??

---

[3] For more information, please see the Metabolic Diseases chapter.

It can occur with central pontine myelinolysis, which may be due to rapid correction of hyponatremia.

Patients with locked-in syndrome are quadriparetic due to corticospinal tract involvement and can't speak due to corticobulbar involvement. **Horizontal eye movements are also impaired**, but **patients can blink and move their eyes vertically.**

Oculopharyngeal Muscular Dystrophy

Oculopharyngeal muscular dystrophy is an autosomal dominant disorder that causes **ptosis** and **impairment of movement of extraocular muscles without diplopia** in the fifth decade of life. Patients also have **swallowing difficulties**.

Oculopharyngeal muscular dystrophy is due to **GCG repeat expansion in the gene encoding PABP2 on chromosome 14**. Pathology shows **rimmed vacuoles**.

NARP (Neuropathy, Ataxia, Retinitis Pigmentosa)

NARP is a mitochondrial disease associated with retinitis pigmentosa. It is due to an ATPase point mutation.

The most common presentation of NARP is <u>night blindness</u>.

Patients with NARP do **not** have ragged-red fibers and may not have lactic acidosis.

Niemann-Pick Disease

Niemann-Pick Disease Type A is associated with a cherry-red spot.

Type C is associated with vertical supranuclear gaze palsy.

For more information, please see the Metabolic Diseases chapter.

A cherry-red spot mnemonic: Farber Salivates Getting **cherry-picked**, half-off Sales at Sacks Fifth Ave & Nieman Marcus! **(Farber's disease, Sialidosis, GM1-Gangliosidosis, Sandhoff's, Tay-Sachs, and Niemann-Pick type A)**.

> ### Cherry Picking
> Other diseases that cause a cherry-red spot:
> - Farber's lipogranulomatosis
> - GM1 gangliosidosis
> - Sandhoff disease
> - Sialidosis
> - Tay Sachs disease

Opsoclonus-Myoclonus

Opsoclonus- **my**oclonus is associated with **child**hood **N**euro**B**lastoma, which may be diagnosed with **Ur**ine **Cat**echolamines and imaging of the brain, chest, and abdomen.

"**O, my**! **N**o**B**ody loves **Ur Cats**!" said the **child**.

Opsoclonus- **my**oclonus may be seen in adults with **Anti-Ri** antibody, which is associated with **B**reast, **G**ynecologic, and **L**ung cancers.

"**O, my**! An **Anti-Ri**publican **BLoG**!" said the **adult**.

Progressive Supranuclear Palsy (PSP)

PSP is one of the atypical parkinsonian disorders/Parkinsonism-plus syndromes.

Slow vertical saccades and **square-wave jerks** of the eyes are early eye findings.

Septo-optic Dysplasia (DeMorsier Syndrome)

Septo-optic dysplasia is characterized by optic nerve hypoplasia, absence of the septum pellucidum, and hypopituitarism. The gene locus is 3p.

Susac's Syndrome

Susac's Syndrome is a microangiopathy involving the brain, retina, and cochlea that usual presents in young women.

Susac's syndrome is associated with a triad:

    1) Branch retinal artery occlusions (BRAO)

    2) Encephalopathy

    3) Sensorineural hearing loss

Brain MRI findings in Susac's syndrome may resemble Multiple Sclerosis. There are multiple areas of high T2 signal on brain MRI involving white and gray matter. The corpus callosum is often involved.

To remember the features of Susac's syndrome, think of this as Sumac's syndrome. *Sumac* has *branches*, just as **Susac's syndrome** is associated with **branch retinal artery occlusions**.

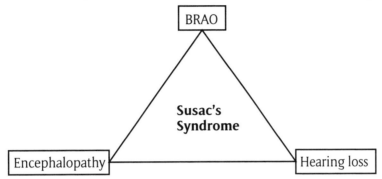

Temporal Arteritis (Giant-Cell Arteritis)

Temporal arteritis, which is due to inflammation of the temporal artery, usually presents after age 50 years. The artery itself can become pulseless and thickened upon palpation.

Patients with temporal arteritis have **headache, an elevated ESR, jaw and tongue claudication**, and **scalp tenderness**. **Systemic signs** such as fever and weight loss may be present. The patient may also carry a diagnosis of PolyMyalgia Rheumatica (PMR).

Temporal artery biopsy shows **multinucleated giant cells** in the media.

Temporal arteritis requires prompt treatment with steroids to prevent vision loss.

The treating physician can follow the ESR as a guide as it falls with steroids.

Prednisone can be given 1-2mg/kg/day and may be tapered over 1-2 years in some cases.

To remember the features of **Giant** Cell Arteritis, think of a **Giant CHEST of multinucleated cells**:

<ul style="list-style:none">
<li><u>C</u> – <u>C</u>laudication (of jaw and tongue)</li>
<li><u>H</u> – <u>H</u>eadache</li>
<li><u>E</u> – <u>E</u>SR Elevation</li>
<li><u>S</u> – <u>S</u>calp tenderness</li>
<li><u>T</u> – <u>T</u>emperature (fever)</li>
</ul>

It's important to remember both large-vessel vasculidities: Temporal Arteritis and Takayasu's Arteritis

The **T**wo Arteritises both start with **T**: **T**emporal and **T**akayasu's

Wernicke Encephalopathy/Wernicke Disease

Wernicke encephalopathy is due to **thiamine deficiency**.
It is most often observed in **alcoholics**.[4]

Wernicke encephalopathy is characterized by a triad:

> 1) Oculomotor palsies
>
> 2) Ataxia of gait
>
> 3) Confusion

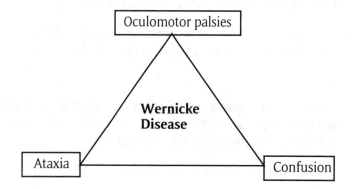

Whipple's Disease

Whipple's disease is due to a gram-positive bacillus (*Tropheryma whippelii*), which is PAS positive.

Diagnostic triad for Whipple's disease:

> 1) Dementia
>
> 2) Supranuclear gaze palsy
>
> 3) Myoclonus

Oculomasticatory and skeletal myorhythmias are pathognomonic for Whipple's disease.
Patients with Whipple's disease also may have **convergence-divergence nystagmus.**

---

4 For more information, see Behavioral Neurology chapter.

Symptoms of Whipple's Disease *(triad first: My Super Duodenum)*

My Super Duodenum Smells Like We Can't Digest Nothing!

Myoclonus-**Supra**nuclear palsy-**D**ementia, **S**teatorrhea, **L**ymphadenopathy, **W**eight loss, **C**onvergence/**D**ivergence-**N**ystagmus!

 In Whipple's disease, **pendular convergent-divergent oscillations of the eyes** are seen. The **jaw moves simultaneously**.

Bursts of myoclonus may be seen in the *eyes, jaw, and face.*

Pathognomonic for Whipple's disease: oculomasticatory and skeletal myorhythmias.

> ### Whipple Eyes
>
> Eye findings in Whipple's disease may include:
>
> • Papilledema or postpapilledema optic atrophy
> • Supranuclear gaze palsy
> • Pendular eye movements

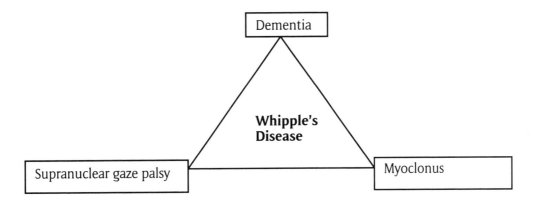

Wilson's Disease (Hepatolenticular Degeneration)

Wilson's disease is an autosomal recessive condition resulting in defective copper metabolism.

Copper is deposited in Descemet's membrane in the lens. This is called a **Kayser-Fleischer ring**.

Also **"sunflower" cataracts** are seen.

Wilson's disease is treated with **Chelation**. D-penicillamine, ammonium tetrathiomolybdate, zinc, and triethylene tetramine dihydrochloride have been used.

To remember how to treat Wilson's, **TRI DAZ Chelation**:

TRIethylene tetramine dihydrochloride,

D-penicillamine,

Ammonium tetrathiomolybdate,

Zinc.

Chelation

Wolfram Syndrome

Wolfram syndrome is also known as DIDMOAD, which stands for **D**iabetes Insipidus, **D**iabetes **M**ellitus, **O**ptic **A**trophy, **D**eafness.

Drugs and Toxins

Cocaine

Cocaine causes opsoclonus, stroke (both ischemic and hemorrhagic), vasospasm, and even rarely vasculitis.

Cocaine makes the eyes (and the blood vessels in the brain) dance around crazy, similar to a person on cocaine.

Ethylene Glycol

Ethylene glycol is found in antifreeze. It causes nonreactive pupils and loss of corneal reflexes.[5]

---

[5] Please see the Neurotoxins chapter for more information.

Ethambutol

Ethambutol, which is used to treat tuberculosis, can cause optic neuropathy.

Vigabatrin

Vigabatrin, which is an anti-epileptic drug, causes bilateral concentric visual field defects with relative temporal sparing.

It is an irreversible inhibitor of GABA transaminase, which breaks down GABA.

 Vigabatrin causes **vi**sual field defects.

Thioridazine (Mellaril)

Thioridazine can cause a severe retinopathy.

Visual Hallucinations

Charles Bonnet's Syndrome

In Charles Bonnet's syndrome patients with vision loss may see things in the space where vision is lost.

Charles Bonnet's Syndrome is abbreviated **CBS**, which is a TV network that advertises an "Eye on America" – quite appropriate for this disorder! To remember the lilliput images associated with Charles Bonnet Syndrome, think of **CBS** airing the TV movie "Gulliver's Travels" which featured the miniature people known as Lilliputians from the island of **Lilliput**!

Dementia with Lewy Bodies

Dementia with Lewy bodies is a degenerative dementia associated with **fluctuating levels of alertness**, **visual hallucinations**, **parkinsonian features**, and **sensitivity to neuroleptics**.[6]

---

6 Please see the Neurodegenerative Diseases chapter for more details.

Epilepsy

Patients with epilepsy can have visual auras.

      · **Formed visual auras** arise from the temporal-occipital region.

      · **Simple, unformed visual auras** such as flashes arise from the occipital lobe.

The letter "**T**" is a formed aura and arises from the **T**emporal lobe.
The letter "**O**" is a circular, primitive, unformed aura and arises from the **O**ccipital lobe.

Migraine

Visual auras associated with **M**igraine usually develop over several **M**inutes and last less than one hour.

MMMMM, so MMMMMarvelous, I'm getting a **M**igraine!

In addition to flashes and fortification spectra, patients with migraine can have **M**icropsia (objects look small), **M**acropsia (objects look large), or **M**etamorphopsia (objects are distorted).

Narcolepsy

Narcolepsy can be associated with **hypnopompic** (while awakening) or **hypnagogic** (while falling asleep) **hallucinations**.

To remember **hypnopompic** means **awakening** (pompic) **from sleep** (hypno), think of the volcano **awakening** the city of **Pompeii** (remember that from history class or were you sleeping?); to remember **hypnagogic** means **while falling asleep**, think of how **groggy** (gogic) you get when it's your bedtime!

Peduncular Hallucinosis

Peduncular hallucinations are **vivid images seen following midbrain injury**.

The Most

The most **common genetic cause of visual impairment**: <u>Leber congenital amaurosis</u>.

The **fovea** is the <u>area of the retina with the highest visual acuity</u>.

Neuro-ophthalmology Quiz

(Answers on page 751)

1. Match the condition to its eye findings.

    1. Down syndrome   A. Brushfield spots

    2. Neurofibromatosis I   B. Cataracts

    3. Lowe syndrome   C. Kayser-Fleischer ring

    4. Wilson's disease   D. Lisch nodules

2. Match the eye findings to the condition

    1. Chorioretinal lacunae   A. Aicardi syndrome

    2. Chorioretinitis   B. Cytomegalovirus

    3. Oculomasticatory myokymia   C. Homocystinuria

    4. Downward lens subluxation   D. Marfan syndrome

    5. Upward lens subluxation   E. Whipple disease

3. Which nerve does not exit the skull through the superior orbital fissure?

    A. Optic nerve

    B. Oculomotor nerve

    C. Trochlear nerve

    D. Abducens nerve

4. Match the disease with its eye findings.

    1. Olfactory groove meningioma   A. Branch retinal artery occlusion

    2. Neuroblastoma   B. Cherry red spot

    3. Niemann-Pick Disease Type A   C. Foster Kennedy syndrome

    4. Susac's syndrome   D. Opsoclonus-myoclonus

5. Match the visual field defect with the anatomic lesion.
      A. Right temporal lesion
      B. Optic chiasm compression
      C. Left parietal lesion
      D. Anterior choroidal artery lesion
      E. Occipital lobe lesion

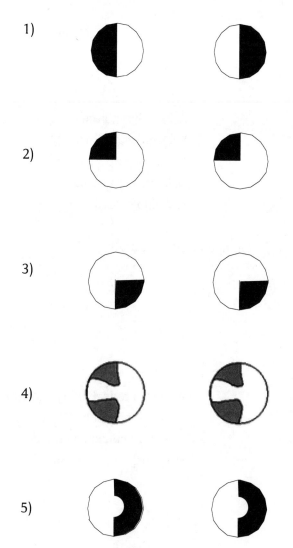

1)

2)

3)

4)

5)

Chapter 12

Neuropathology

Alzheimer Type I and Alzheimer Type II Astrocytes

Alzheimer type I astrocytes and Alzheimer type II astrocytes are both found in hyperammonemia, but type II astrocytes are more common.

Alzheimer type I astrocytes are more often found in Wilson's disease than type II.

 Alzheimer type II astrocytes are particularly common when there's too (two) much ammonia.

 Alzheimer cells are **not found** in Alzheimer's disease.

Pathologic features of Alzheimer's disease[1]:
· Neuritic plaques
· Neurofibrillary tangles
· Hirano bodies
· Granulovacuolar degeneration
· Amyloid deposition

Ballooned Neurons

 Ballooned neurons are swollen neurons found in **corticobasal ganglionic degeneration (CBGD)** and **Pick's disease**.

In **Pick's disease** the cytoplasm is eosinophilic and the nucleus is not in the center.

 The *nucleus picks one side* of the cell in ballooned neurons in Pick's disease.

---

1 Please see the Neurodegenerative Diseases chapter for more information on Alzheimer's disease.

Bizarre Astrocytes

Bizarre as it may seem, this is an actual pathology term.

 Bizarre astrocytes are enlarged and have hyperchromatic, pleomorphic nuclei.

They are found in **progressive multifocal leukoencephalopathy (PML)**, a subacute CNS demyelinating disease due to infection of oligodendrocytes with JC virus.

The pathology of PML:

Oligodendrocytes have intranuclear inclusions.

Bizarre astrocytes.

Multifocal demyelination that begins in the occipital lobes.

PML is seen in AIDS and other immuncompromised patients.

 Remember that PML is associated with AIDS, the disease and acronym.

Astrocytes are bizarre.

Inclusions in oligodendrocytes.

Demyelination that begins in the occipital region.

Subcortical white matter.

For more information on PML, please see the Infectious Diseases chapter.

Creutzfeldt Astrocyte

The Crux of Creutfeldt- Jakob Disease[2]

Spongiform change/ vacuolation of neuropil

Loss of neurons

Proliferation of astrocytes

Loss of synapses on electron microscopy

Deposition of prion protein

 Creutzfeldt astrocytes are associated with demyelination.

 Creutzfeldt astrocytes are **not** characteristic of Creutzfeldt-Jakob disease (CJD).

---

[2] Please see the Infectious Diseases chapter for more information on CJD.

Red Neuron

 A red neuron is an extremely eosinophilic neuron with a nucleus that looks condensed and dark. It is due to hypoxic damage.

 Neurons that are particularly *vulnerable to hypoxia* (in adults) are:

- **P**yramidal neurons in the hippocampus (CA1)
- **P**yramidal neurons in layers 3 and 5 of the neocortex
- **P**urkinje cells in the cerebellum

3 cell types prone to damage from hypoxia all begin with the letter " P ".

Inclusions

Type of inclusion	Where found in cell	Type of cell
Bunina bodies	Cytoplasm	Neurons
Cowdry A	Nucleus	Neurons
Cowdry B	Nucleus	Neurons
Hirano bodies	Cytoplasm	Neurons
Lafora bodies	Cytoplasm	Astrocytes and neurons
Lewy bodies	Cytoplasm	Neurons
Lipofuscin	Cytoplasm	Neurons and glia
Marinesco bodies	Nucleus	Neurons, especially in substantia nigra and locus ceruleus
Negri bodies	Cytoplasm	Neurons, especially Purkinje cells, pyramidal cells (hippocampus), brainstem nuclei
Neurofibrillary tangle	Cytoplasm	Neurons
Pick bodies	Cytoplasm	Neurons and dentate granule cells of hippocampus
Rosenthal fibers	Cytoplasm	Astrocytes

Bunina Bodies

 Bunina bodies are intracytoplasmic eosinophilic inclusions, which can be a nonspecific finding, but are also found in motor neurons in patients with motor neuron disease such as Amyotrophic Lateral Sclerosis (ALS).[3]

To remember that ALS patients have **Bun**ina bodies: ALS patients become weak and have to sit on their **buns.**

Cowdry Inclusions

Both Cowdry type A and Cowdry type B inclusion bodies are intranuclear viral inclusions.

Cowdry bodies are **cowardly,** so they hide in the nucleus rather then venturing out into the cytoplasm where they may catch a virus.

Cowdry Type A Inclusions

Cowdry type A inclusion bodies are large and surrounded by a clear zone / halo. Only one is seen per cell.

The majority of viral intranuclear inclusions are type A e.g. CMV, HSV, VZV.

Cowdry type **A** inclusion bodies are **A**lone; only one is found in a cell. They are also **A**ngelic; they have a halo.

Cowdry Type B Inclusions

 Cowdry type B inclusions are small and multiple like bb's from a BB gun.

---

[3] For more information, please see the Neuromuscular Diseases chapter.

Cowdry type **B** inclusions are found in acute polio.

Change Polio to **B**olio to remember it is Type **B** inclusions that are associated with polio.

Glial Cytoplasmic Inclusions (GCIs)

GCIs are flame/sickle-shaped inclusions detected with silver stain that are **immunoreactive for alpha synuclein**.

GCIs are found in oligodendrocytes of patients with Multiple System Atrophy.

Granulovacuolar Degeneration (of Simchowicz)

Vacuoles containing a granule are seen in the cytoplasm of neurons in granulovacuolar degeneration.

Granulovacuolar degeneration is often found in pyramidal neurons in the hippocampus. It is associated with Alzheimer's disease.

Grannies with Alzheimer's disease have **"Granny"-vacuolar degeneration**.

Ground Glass Inclusions

Ground glass inclusions are intranuclear inclusions **found in oligodendrocytes in patients with PML**.

See also Bizarre Astrocytes above.

Lafora Bodies

Lafora bodies are PAS+ intracytoplasmic inclusions found in astrocytes and neurons in patients with Lafora body disease, a type of progressive myoclonic epilepsy with occipital seizures and **visual hallucinations**.

In Lafora body disease, Lafora bodies are found in the CNS, eccrine **sweat** glands, liver, cardiac muscle, and skeletal muscle.

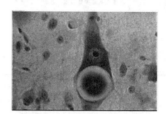

Lafora bodies are polyglucosan bodies → see photo, which looks like a "**Mercedes Benz** sign" →

Compared to **U**nverricht-**L**undborg Disease (**Cys**tatin B gene mutation), **Lafora**'s Disease progresses **faster**.

The new "**Lafora**" made by **Mercedes Benz** is much **faster** than **Ur Little Cys**'s car. It's so fast, you will **hallucinate** images going by and start to **sweat** profusely!

Lewy Bodies

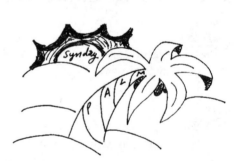

Lewy bodies are eosinophilic inclusions found in the cytoplasm that contain alpha-synuclein.

Yes, the test asks to differentiate the "*alpha-Synucleinopathies*" from the "*Tao-opathies*".
So, to remember the **alpha-Synucleinopathies**, think of "**PALM Synday**" –

      P is for **P**arkinson's disease,

      A is for **A**lzheimer's disease (but trickily, Alzheimer's can be both an "*alpha-Synucleinopathy*" and/or "*Tao-opathy*"),

      L is for **L**ewy Body dementia, and

      M is for **M**ultiple Systems Atrophy.

      Synday is for *Synucleinopathy*

The best thing about this mnemonic is that you don't need to recall all the *Tao-opathies* – if they're not there on **PALM Synday**, they're Tao!

Photo: Jeffrey A. Golden & Brian N. Harding. (2004). Developmental Neuropathology. *The International Society of Neuropathology*.

Lewy bodies are loose in the cytoplasm.

Lewy sounds like Louie, Donald Duck's nephew. Ducks like to swim, so Lewy bodies swim in the cytoplasm.

They look like this:

 In **idiopathic Parkinson's disease** Lewy bodies are found in the substantia nigra and locus ceruleus.

In **Dementia with Lewy Bodies**, Lewy bodies are more widespread. Not only are they in the substantia nigra and locus ceruleus but also the cortex, such as the entorhinal and cingulate cortices.

Lipofuscin

 Lipofuscin, which is found in neurons, is the most common inclusion associated with aging.

 As people age, they think about liposuction, and lipofuscin occurs with aging.

Marinesco Bodies

 Marinesco bodies are found in the nuclei of neurons, most often in pigmented brainstem nuclei e.g. substantia nigra and locus ceruleus. **Marinesco bodies** are in the **nucleus.**

 Marinesco bodies are the most common example of a Cowdry-type B inclusion. They can be multiple and are seen with aging.

 Marinesco bodies are eosinophilic/ **red** like **maraschino cherries.**

Lewy bodies are also eosinophilic and are found in neurons in the substantia nigra, but they are in the **cytoplasm**;

Neurofibrillary Tangles (NFTs)

Neurofibrillary tangles are intracytoplasmic neuronal inclusions that largely consist of **aggregates of tau proteins**.

They may be flame-shaped. The shape of neuron can affect the shape of the NFT.

NFTs are associated with Alzheimer's disease.

In Alzheimer's disease, one's thoughts become tangled, and neurofibrillary tangles form.

Pick Bodies

Pick bodies are spherical intracytoplasmic inclusions found in neurons in patients with Pick's disease. They are slightly basophilic, tau-positive, and can be seen well with silver-staining.[4]

Rosenthal Fibers

Rosenthal fibers are eosinophilic inclusions found in the cytoplasm of astrocytes that contain **O**paque, **T**ightly compacted "cigar-**S**haped" **E**osinophilic i**N**termediate filaments and **Glial Fibrillary Acidic Protein (GFAP)**.

Rosenthal fibers are found in many conditions. They can be:
- reactive (in tissue adjacent to a mass lesion)
- neoplastic (in pilocytic astrocytomas)
- degenerative (Alexander's disease).

Rosenthal fibers are a hallmark of Alexander's disease, a leukodystrophy characterized by developmental delay, macrocephaly, and seizures.

---

4 See also Ballooned Neurons section above and the Neurodegenerative Diseases chapter.

red hair
red ROSE-nthal
ed

Rosenthal fibers are also characteristic of Juvenile Pilocytic Astrocytomas.[5]

To remember the features of <u>ROSENTHAL</u> *fibers, think of your boring friend Rosenthal, who now has a <u>G</u>irl <u>F</u>riend with an <u>A</u>ctual <u>P</u>ersonality ! (GFAP = <u>G</u>lial <u>F</u>ibrillary <u>A</u>cidic <u>P</u>rotein).*

Also, the letters of his name spell out the important molecular features of the fibers:

<u>R</u>osenthal fibers

<u>O</u>paque

"cigar-<u>S</u>haped"

<u>E</u>osinophilic

i<u>N</u>termediate filaments

<u>T</u>ightly compacted

<u>H</u>omogeneous structures in

<u>A</u>strocytes and <u>A</u>lexander's disease;

<u>L</u>ow-grade (slow-growing) tumors like JPAs

Markers

Marker	What it Stains
Congo red	Amyloid
Desmin	Muscle
EMA (epithelial membrane antigen)	Arachnoid (meningioma)
GFAP (glial fibrillary acidic protein)	Astrocytes
NeuN	Nucleus of neuron
PAS (periodic acid-Schiff)	Carbohydrates
S100	Glia and Schwann cells
Synaptophysin	Synaptic vesicle protein (neuronal marker)
Transthyretin	Choroid plexus
Vimentin	Ependymal cells, intermediate filaments

---

[5] Please see the Neuro-oncology chapter.

Desmin

To remember that desmin stains muscle, remember that **Desmond Mason** with the New Orleans Hornets is **muscular.**

Alternatively, **desmin** and **decimate** begin with similar sounds. *Muscular people can decimate others in sports.*

EMA

Reminder: Meningiomas are EMA-positive because they arise from arachnoid cells.

PAS (Periodic Acid-Schiff) Stain

PAS stains glycogen/carbohydrate.

Some **diseases where PAS positivity is seen**:
- Adrenoleukodystrophy
- CADASIL
- Farber disease
- Glycogen storage diseases
    - Acid maltase deficiency
    - Muscle phosphorylase deficiency
- Krabbe's disease
- Lafora body disease

S100

S100 is a calcium channel binding protein. S100 stains act as a neural crest marker (Schwann cells, Melanocytes, and Glial cells), so S100 will stain schwannomas, melanomas, paraganglioma stromal cells, histiocytoma clear cell sarcomas, 50% of malignant peripheral nerve sheath tumors, astrocytes, oligodendroglia, ependyma, and choroid plexus epithelium. It is very sensitive for melanocytic tumors.

Synaptophysin

Synaptophysin is a synaptic vesicle protein. Antibodies to synaptophysin are used to identify synapses. They serve as a marker of neuronal differentiation.

 Think of synaptophysin as synapse findin'.

Keratin

Dry Keratin

Dry keratin is found in dermoid and epidermoid cysts.

 To remember **D**ry keratin is in **D**ermoid and epi**D**ermoid cysts, think of the letter D.

Wet Keratin

Wet keratin is seen in adamantinomatous craniopharyngioma.

 Adam never dries his hair so he always has a wet cranium mess -- you can remember wet keratin is seen in Adamantinomatous craniopharyngioma.

Axonal Spheroids

Axonal spheroids indicate diffuse axonal injury.

Diffuse Axonal Injury (DAI) is a type of head injury due to shearing forces, which can lead to a persistent vegetative state. It may be associated with petechial hemorrhages at the gray-white junction, involving the corpus callosum, or involving the rostral brainstem.

BUZZ WORDS If you are told about a patient who was in a car accident, had a **normal head CT in the ER, and is not waking up, think about diffuse axonal injury.**

Tips from the Authors

It's a good idea to review images on previous RITE exams in order to prepare for the RITE. Additional concise information about neuropathology can be found in Fuller and Goodman's textbook <u>Practical Review of Neuropathology</u>.

Neuropathology Quiz

(Answers on page 753)

1. Match the inclusion with the disease

    1) Cowdry A   A) ALS

    2) Cowdry B   B) Polio

    3) Bunina body   C) Rabies

    4) Negri body   D) CMV

2. Match the marker with what is stained.

    1) Desmin   A) Muscle

    2) EMA   B) Synapse

    3) Synaptophysin   C) Glycogen

    4) PAS   D) Arachnoid cells

    5) GFAP   E) Astrocyte

3. Which of the following is not a tauopathy?

    A. Alzheimer's disease

    B. Corticobasal ganglionic degneration

    C. Pick's disease

    D. Multiple system atrophy

    E. Progressive Supranuclear Palsy

4. Which of these is not found in Alzheimer's disease?

    A. Alzheimer type I astrocytes

    B. Amyloid deposition

    C. Granulovacuolar degeneration

    D. Hirano bodies

    E. Neuritic plaques

    F. Neurofibrillary tangles

Chapter 13

Neurophysiology

Autonomic Testing

Review of the Autonomic Nervous System

The autonomic nervous system is divided into the sympathetic nervous system (SNS), parasympathetic nervous system (PNS), and the enteric autonomic nervous system.

The Sympathetic and Parasympathetic Nervous Systems

 The SNS is responsible for the fight or flight response.

The PNS promotes homeostasis and digestion.

The SNS and PNS tend to have antagonistic effects.

- The SNS causes an <u>increase</u> in heart rate and blood pressure, pupil dilation, and bronchodilation.
- The PNS <u>decreases</u> heart rate, decreases pupil size, increases peristalsis, and causes bronchoconstriction.

 There are exceptions to this antagonistic relationship.

Activation of either the SNS or PNS can cause **secretion from the lacrimal**, **parotid**, and **submandibular glands**. However, activation of the PNS has a greater effect.

Also, the PNS and SNS have a complementary relationship as far as sexual function.

- The PNS causes erection.
- The SNS causes ejaculation.

To remember that the PNS is responsible for erection and the SNS is responsible for ejaculation: **P is before S in the alphabet, and erection (PNS) occurs before ejaculation (SNS).**

Or … P is for POINT (Parasympathetic) and S is for SHOOT (Sympathetic), so you **P**oint before you **S**hoot!

Some organs only receive **sympathetic innervation**:

· Sweat glands

· Piloerector muscles

· Most small blood vessels.

The PNS and SNS are organized similarly. There are cell bodies in the brain stem or spinal cord. Efferent axons leave these cell bodies and synapse on ganglia. Axons from these second order neurons then synapse on the target organ.

The exception is the **adrenal medulla**, which is **innervated directly by SNS preganglionic fibers**.

The cell bodies of the SNS are found in the intermediolateral (IML) cell column of the spinal cord from T1 to L2, also known as the **thoracolumbar system**.

The cell bodies for the PNS are cranial nerve nuclei 3,7,9, and 10 and the IML cell column at S2-S4, also known as the **craniosacral system**.

PNS Ganglia

Cranial Nerve	Ganglion	Destination
III (Oculomotor nerve)	Ciliary	Ciliary muscle and sphincter pupillae
VII (Facial nerve)	Sphenopalatine	Lacrimal gland
VII (Facial nerve)	Submandibular	Submandibular and sublingual glands
IX (Glossopharyngeal nerve)	Otic ganglion	Parotid gland
X (Vagus nerve)	(Multiple)	Heart, larynx, trachea, lungs, GI tract

To remember that the glossopharyngeal nerve is associated with the otic ganglion and is destined for the parotid gland, remember **GOP** for **Glossopharyngeal Otic Parotid**.

Sympathetic **preganglionic fibers are short** and the **postganglionic fibers are long**. The opposite is true for the parasympathetic system.

long pre

Acetylcholine is the neurotransmitter for **all preganglionic fibers** in the autonomic nervous system (parasympathetic and sympathetic nervous systems).

Also, all **postganglionic fibers** in the **PNS** and **sudomotor fibers** (postganglionic fibers which innervate sweat glands) **in the SNS** use **acetylcholine**.

Apart from the sudomotor fibers, the **SNS postganglionic** fibers use **norepinephrine**.

Bladder Function

There are **3 main actors**:

· Detrusor muscle of the bladder

· Internal sphincter

· External sphincter/ urogenital diaphragm.

The **detrusor muscle** and **internal sphincter** are composed of **smooth muscle**.

The **external sphincter** is **striated muscle**.

During micturition:

The **sphincters** relax.

The **detrusor muscle** contracts.

The *pontine micturition* center coordinates this through the *reticulospinal tracts to the spinal cord*.

To remember this, think of **PPQRSTU**: **P**ons **P**ees **Q**uickly via **R**eticulo-**S**pinal **T**ract **U**rination! (this mnemonic was made up on the "fly").

The external urethral sphincter is innervated by the **pudendal nerves**. The pudendal nerves carry somatic innervation to the external urethral sphincter from the motor neurons of **Onuf's nucleus (S2-S4)**. Activation of **nicotinic cholinergic** receptors causes this external sphincter to contract, promoting urine storage.

Type of Nerve	Nerve	Innervates		
Somatic	Pudendal	External urethral sphincter *contracts*	→ storage
Sympathetic	Hypogastric	Internal sphincter and detrusor muscle *contracts* *relaxes*	→ storage
Parasympathetic	Pelvic	Detrusor muscle *contracts*	→ pee

The **sympathetic nervous system** is responsible for **urine storage.**

Sympathetic preganglionic fibers originating from the IML travel to the bladder and urethra in the hypogastric nerves.

Norepinephrine causes **relaxation of the detrusor muscle** and **contraction of the internal sphincter** (smooth muscle).

 The **SNS** is responsible for urine Storage.

The PNS promotes urination.

The **p**reganglionic **p**arasympathetic fibers travel from the parasympathetic nuclei at S2-S4 to the bladder via the **p**elvic nerve.

Release of **acetylcholine results in bladder wall contraction allowing urination.**

 The **PNS**, via the **p**elvic nerve, **p**ushes out **p**ee.

Detrusor Reflex

Inhibition of the sympathetic fibers that cause bladder neck contraction

Voluntary relaxation of the external urethral sphincter

Activation of parasympathetic fibers that cause detrusor muscle contraction

The medial frontal lobes provide voluntary control of micturition. There is a cerebrospinopudendal pathway that allows volitional control of initiation and cessation of urination.

Tests of Autonomic Dysfunction

Sympathetic Sudomotor Testing

Recall that **sweat glands are innervated by sympathetic postganglionic** neurons that release **acetylcholine**.

Tests of sympathetic sudomotor function include:
- Quantitative Sudomotor Axon Reflex Testing (QSART)
- Sympathetic skin response
- Thermoregulatory sweat test

Quantitative Sudomotor Axon Reflex Testing (QSART)

QSART is a test of postganglionic sudomotor function.

This test can **identify postganglionic sympathetic failure**, which can be seen in small-fiber neuropathies.

It can also **identify excessive sweating**, which can be found with **reflex sympathetic dystrophy**.

Thermoregulatory Sweat Test

The thermoregulatory sweat test determines the distribution of sweating.

Sympathetic Vasomotor Testing

Tests of sympathetic vasomotor function:
- Tilt test (checking for heart rate [HR] and blood pressure [BP] changes)
- Valsalva (checking for changes in BP)
- Checking for BP changes with stressors such as exercise and cold.

Valsalva

Blood pressure changes with Valsalva: up, down, up, down, way up.

Blood Pressure in Valsalva Maneuver	Explanation
Phase 1: up	BP increases due to increased intrathoracic pressure. Heart rate decreases.
EARLY Phase 2: down	BP decreases due to less venous return. **Sympathetic dysfunction results in an exaggerated drop in blood pressure during the early stage of phase 2. This drop occurs due to lack of appropriate peripheral vasoconstriction.**
LATE Phase 2: up	BP increases due to increased sympathetic tone.
Phase 3 (Straining ends): down	BP decreases due to release of intrathoracic pressure
Phase 4: way up (overshoot)	BP overshoots the resting value due to increased venous return. **Absence of the usual blood pressure overshoot in phase 4 suggests sympathetic nervous system dysfunction.**

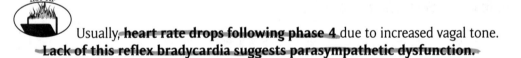

Usually, **heart rate drops following phase 4** due to increased vagal tone. **Lack of this reflex bradycardia suggests parasympathetic dysfunction.**

Parasympathetic Testing

Tests of parasympathetic function:

- HR changes with Valsalva
- HR response to standing
- HR response to deep breathing
- R-R interval variation

Heart Rate Response to Breathing

The response of the heart rate to breathing is a sensitive test for cardiovagal dysfunction.

Remember: Heart rate **in**creases with **in**spiration.

Diseases Associated with Autonomic Failure

Chagas' Disease

Chagas' disease is also known as **American trypanosomiasis.**

It is found in Central and South America.

It is due to *Trypanosoma cruzi,* which is a parasite.

It can cause an **autonomic neuropathy** characterized by **orthostatic hypotension, bradycardia, megaesophagus, megacolon,** and **congestive cardiomyopathy**.

To remember that Chagas' disease is associated with GI tract findings such as megaesophagus and megacolon, note that **Chagas** ends in **gas**.

Diabetes

Diabetic patients can have **postural hypotension, resting tachycardia, nocturnal diarrhea, delayed gastric emptying, impotence, distal anhydrosis, or miotic pupils** with a slow light reflex.

Dopamine β-Hydroxylase Deficiency

DOpamine β-**H**ydr**O**xylase **(which we will now affectionately call "DO-HO")** converts dopamine to norepinephrine, so patients with **DO-HO** deficiency have increased dopamine and lack norepinephrine.

$$\text{Dopamine} \xrightarrow[\text{DO-HO}]{} \text{Norepinephrine}$$

The gene for **DO-HO** deficiency has been mapped to chromosome 9q.

In **neonates, DO-HO** deficiency causes episodes of **hypothermia, hypoglycemia, and hypotension,** *which may be lethal.*

To recall the effects of DO-HO deficiency, think of this mnemonic: **"If no DO-HO, then BP go low, and so do gluco and tempo!"**

Adults have **ptosis** and **orthostatic hypotension.**

The postural hypotension can be treated with **L-Dops (DL-threo-dihydroxyphenylserine),** which is decarboxylated by dopa decarboxylase to norepinephrine

How L-Dops works:

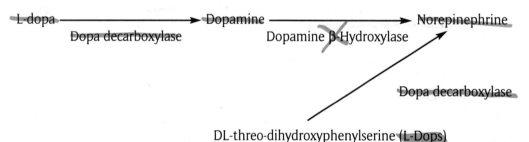

Fabry's Disease

Fabry's disease is an **X-linked recessive** sphingolipidosis due to **Alpha-galactosidase A deficiency** that causes a **small fiber neuropathy.**

Fabry's disease is associated with All **A**s: **A**lpha-galactosidase **A**, **A**croparesthesias, **A**utonomic dysfunction, **A**ngiokeratomas, **A**nhydrosis, **A**rrhythmia, **A**cute renal failure, and **A**bdominal pain. See page 174 for more details.

Familial Amyloid Polyneuropathy (FAP)

There are 4 types **Familial Amyloid Polyneuropathy (FAP)**.

FAP type 1, which is due to a defect in **TransThyRetin (TTR)**, causes a primarily **Small Fiber Neuropathy (SFN)**.

Patients initially have pain in the lower limbs. Pain and temperature sensation are lost.

Autonomic Nervous System (ANS) symptoms include orthostatic hypotension, impotence, and urinary difficulties.

FAP type 1 is also associated with **Carpal Tunnel Syndrome (CTS)**.

Congestive heart failure **(CHF)** may result in death.

To remember the features of Familial Amyloid Polyneuropathy, think of the **FACTS**:

> F = FAP
>
> A = ANS
>
> C = CTS and CHF
>
> T = TTR
>
> S = SFN

Hereditary Sensory and Autonomic Neuropathies (HSAN)

Lack of sensitivity to pain is common to HSAN.

Riley-Day Syndrome (Familial Dysautonomia)/ HSAN III

HSAN III is an autosomal recessive condition typically found in **Ashkenazi Jews**. It is due to a mutation in IKBKAP (IkappaB kinase complex-associated protein) on chromosome 9q.

HSAN III presents **at birth** with **hypothermia, hypotonia**, and **poor feeding.**

Patients have **severe postural hypotension, increased sweating**, episodes of **hypertension, skin blotching**, **recurrent emesis**, and **unexplained fever.**

The distinctive feature is **absence of fungiform papillae on the tongue**. They also **lack overflow emotional tears**.

Patients with Riley-Day syndrome/ Familial Dysautonomia/ HSAN III have *episodes where they appear riled up*; they have **intermittent hypertension, fever, and emesis**. Maybe they are upset *because they don't have fungiform papillae or overflow emotional tears.*

Lambert-Eaton Myasthenic Syndrome

Lambert-Eaton myasthenic syndrome is a neuromuscular junction disorder **due to antibodies directed against P/Q-type voltage-gated calcium channels**. It may be due to an **underlying malignancy such as small cell lung cancer**.

Lambert-Eaton syndrome usually presents in adults. Patients have a **dry mouth; constipation; proximal muscle weakness, especially the thighs; and decreased reflexes. Strength may improve temporarily after exercise**.

Please see the EMG findings below.

3,4-DiAminoPyridine

Although not a cure, therapy with **3,4-DiAminoPyridine** may help LEMS patients function better.

3,4-DAP inhibits **potassium-channels** which in turn permit calcium entry into the cell, despite the LEMS-antibodies produced against the voltage-gated **calcium channels**.

To remember the features, antibodies and treatment of LEMS, think of this *mnemonic*:
"A **small** (small cell lung cancer) **lamb** (LEMS) tries to escape a **Voltage Gate**, because he doesn't like getting **milked (calcium)**. He tries to jump the gate **3 or 4 times** (3,4-DAP) **repetitively** (rep stim), and his **muscle strength improves with this exercise**, so finally he **Kicks (K+=**potassium) the gate open to freedom."

EEG

What is an EEG?

An EEG (ElectroEncephaloGram) is the **summation of excitatory and inhibitory P̲ostsynaptic P̲otentials of P̲yramidal neurons**.

~~**6** cm² of cortex are needed to produce a field on the scalp.~~

To remember the answer to the question of *What is an EEG?* Think of the equation: **EEG** = (+/-) **PPP** + **6**.

EEG Terminology

Frequencies

	Frequencies
Delta	0 -<4
Theta	4 -<8
Alpha	8-13
Beta	>13

relaxed, drowsy. ↑c̄ cognition, stage I sleep.
↑ barb, benzo, chloral hydrate, antidepressants

To remember these in order, remember the phrase **D**ig **T**hat **A**wesome **B**eat.

PDR = α rhythm, posteriorly, during wakefulness, eyes closed, ↓c̄ eyes open and alerting

Polarity

Each EEG channel is a comparison of two inputs.

 When the **first input is positive** (or less negative) **compared to the second input**, the **deflection is downward**.

When the **first input is negative compared to the second input**, the **pen deflects upward**.

Positive (+) to negative (-) causes downward deflection:

Negative (-) to positive (+) is an upward deflection:

Montages

Bipolar Montage

 In a bipolar montage, inputs 1 and 2 are adjacent electrodes, and input 2 is input 1 in the next channel. Both inputs are active electrodes.

     For example,

     Channel 1: Fp1-**F3**

     Channel 2: **F3**-C3

     Channel 3: C3-P3.

Note that F3 is input 2 in the Channel 1 and input 1 in Channel 2.

Referential Montage

In a referential montage, input 2 is presumably inactive.

For example,

Channel 1: Fp1-Cz

Channel 2: F3-Cz

Channel 3: C3-Cz.

Here, Cz is used as the reference.

Activation Techniques

Hyperventilation

Hyperventilation is an activation procedure performed during EEG that is contraindicated in certain patients. **This can be remembered by: Hyperventilation is a SCAM and should not be performed in patients with:**

· **S**troke

· **S**ickle cell disease or trait

· **C**ystic fibrosis

· **C**ongenital heart disease

· **A**sthma

· **M**oyamoya

Generalized background slowing is a normal finding during hyperventilation.

Prolonged slowing can be seen if the patient is **hypoglycemic** or **hypoxic**.

Hyperventilation can elicit epileptiform discharges and seizures in childhood absence epilepsy.

Photic Stimulation

Photic stimulation is performed over 6 months of age.

non-cerebral

A **photomyogenic, or photomyoclonic, response** is when muscle contractions, such as contractions of the eyelids, occur during photic stimulation with the eyes closed.

frontal. ↑ amp c̄ continued stim.   ↑ in barb/EtOH w/D.   12-18Hz best.

A **photoparoxysmal response** is when photic stimulation results in epileptiform discharges. For example, this is seen in juvenile myoclonic epilepsy (JME).

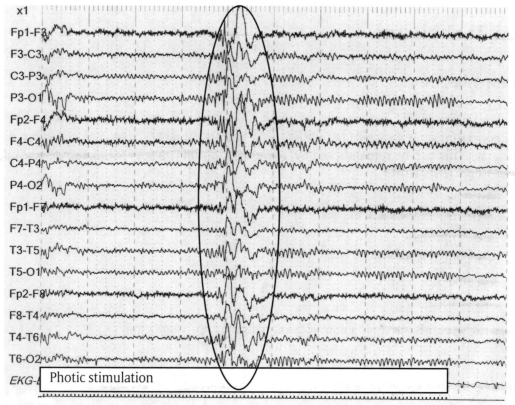

This is a photoparoxysmal response in a patient with JME.

A **photoconvulsive response** is when photic stimulation results in a seizure (usually seen with primary generalized epilepsies).

Normal EEG

Background Rhythm

At 3 months the posterior background rhythm should be 3 Hz, and at 5 months it should be 5 Hz.

The awake background/alpha rhythm should reach alpha frequency (at least 8 Hz) by age 3 years.

Benign EEG Findings

Kappa

Kappa is characterized by low amplitude waves in the temporal regions of alpha or theta frequency. They occur during cognitive tasks/thinking.

Phi Beta Kappa members have complex thoughts, and **kappa is seen during thinking.**

Lambda

Lambda waves are positive sharp transients in the occipital area seen during visual scanning.

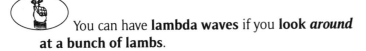

You can have **lambda waves** if you **look *around* at a bunch of lambs**.

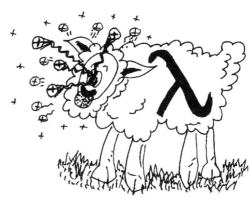

Mu Rhythm   *"rolandic alpha"*

arch

Mu is arciform 7 to 11 Hz activity seen best over the centroparietal regions. It is attenuated by movement or thoughts of movement of the contralateral body. (Eye opening has no effect on mu. This helps differentiate it from the patient's alpha rhythm.)

Slows c̄ aging

Mu activity is attenuated by **mu**vement/movement.

Benign Variant	Context	Appearance
Wicket spikes/wicket waves	Seen during drowsiness or light sleep in adults.	6-11 Hz activity in the temporal region. *arc-like, in a train, no bkgd distortion*
Posterior slow waves of youth	Seen in children and adolescents.	Delta activity with overriding alpha frequencies. Attenuate with eye opening. *SAIL WAVES*
14 and 6 positive bursts	Seen during drowsiness and light sleep, most common in adolescents.	Bursts of arciform activity at 14 or 6 Hz over posterior temporal head regions lasting for less than 3 seconds.
Six-hertz spike and wave bursts/ phantom spike and wave	Seen in teens and adults during wakefulness and drowsiness. Disappear in sleep.	Bursts of diffuse 6 Hz very small spike and higher amplitude wave discharges lasting up to a couple seconds.
Small sharp spikes of sleep *Benign Epileptiform transients of Sleep*	Seen in drowsiness and light sleep in adults	Brief, low voltage (< 50 microvolts) spikes, usually over the temporal region. *no background distortion*
Rhythmic temporal theta bursts of drowsiness/ psychomotor variant pattern	Seen in drowsiness in young adulthood.	5-7 Hz sharply contoured theta activity that occurs in bursts, maximal over the temporal regions.

To remember wicket spikes are 6-11 Hz and are seen during drowsiness in adults, think of this mnemonic: **Most adults are "wicked drowsy" at 6:11am!**

"temporal transients"
Sylvian theta   *Older than 40*   *episodic theta over*
(temporal)   *temporal region*

Artifact due to Eye Movement

Eyeblink Artifact

 The eye carries an electrical charge that can result in eyeblink artifact. Specifically, the **cornea is positive,** and the **retina is negative**.

When the **eye closes** (and rolls upward due to Bell's phenomenon), a positive deflection is seen in Fp1 and Fp2, which are directly above the eyes.

When the **eye opens**, a negative deflection is seen in these electrodes.

> Positivity = eyes closed (P=EC)
>
> Negativity= eyes open   (N=EO)

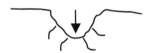 I'm **positive**, I'd **like to close my eyes and take a nap**.

For the girls: I like to look at **NEO** (Keanu Reeves in Matrix) because he has nice **PECs**.

To remember that a **positive deflection means the eyes are closed** and that **a negative deflection is seen when the eyes are open**, picture eyelashes on the wave. This represents the upper eyelid. It will look like the eye is closed when there's a positive deflection, and the eye is open when there's a negative deflection. (Remember that positive is downward and negative is upward in EEG.)

A positive deflection makes it look like eye is closed:

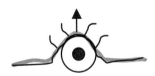

A negative deflection makes it look like the eye is open:

Lateral Eye Movements

 Lateral eye movements produce artifact primarily at F7 and F8.

When you **look left,** there is a **positivity at F7** and **negativity at F8.**

When you look **right, positivity is at F8** and **negativity is at F7.**

You are looking in the direction of the positivity.

A lateral rectus spike may precede lateral eye movements.

Abnormal EEG

Alpha Coma

Alpha coma is seen in certain coma patients.

There are **2 types of alpha coma.**

The **first type** is characterized by *posterior dominant alpha activity* that is *poorly reactive.* ^(Some reactivity)
This can be seen in certain brainstem lesions, for example **pontine strokes**.

The **second type** is characterized by *diffuse or frontal alpha activity* that is *poorly reactive.*
This can been seen **following anoxia**.

 Alpha coma can be seen with **a**noxia/**a**rrest.

Bancaud's Phenomenon

Bancaud's phenomenon is when the alpha activity over one hemisphere does not attenuate with eye opening. The nonreactive hemisphere is abnormal.

Anoxic Encephalopathy
- Burst Suppression
- Periodic Spike/Sharp waves, ⊕ myoclonus
- α coma
- bihemispheric PLEDs

Beta Coma

Beta coma is when coma patients have high-amplitude generalized beta activity.

This is seen with **encephalopathy secondary to medication** and some **acute brainstem lesion**s.

It has a **better prognosis than alpha coma**, *particularly if it is due to barbiturates or benzodiazepines.*

Patients may be in *beta* coma if they are extremely *buzzed.*

Alpha coma is *awful; beta* coma is *better.*

Breach Rhythm

Breach rhythm is due to a skull defect; the EEG activity may be higher in amplitude and spiky-looking.

Burst-suppression

Burst-suppression can be induced with **pentobarbital** or a **midazolam** drip for example.

In the setting of hypoxic injury, this carries a very poor prognosis.

Delta Activity

If it is *continuous and polymorphic,* focal delta activity may be due to *structural lesion.*

Epileptiform Discharges[1]

A **spike is less than 70 milliseconds** in duration.

A **sharp wave is 70 – 200 milliseconds** in duration.

---

[1] Please also see the Epilepsy chapter.

Finding the Maximum Voltage of an Epileptiform Discharge

In the bipolar montage, a phase reversal indicates the site of maximum voltage.

Phase reversals look like this:

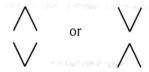

This EEG shows a phase reversal at P3:

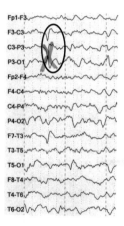

 To remember that phase reversals are seen in the bipolar montage, remember that a **bipolar patient's mood may reverse quickly**.

This phase reversal has positive polarity:

Positive sharp waves are rarely seen in adults.

This phase reversal has negative polarity:

Remember this by picturing the appropriate mathematical symbol:

The maximal potential is indicated by the location of the maximum amplitude in a referential montage.

 Attitudes can be reverential, and **amplitudes** mean **referential**.

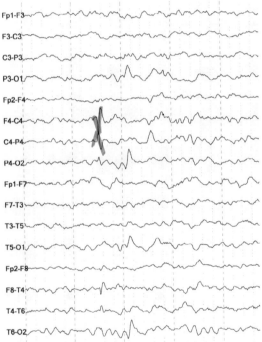

C4 spike in bipolar montage.

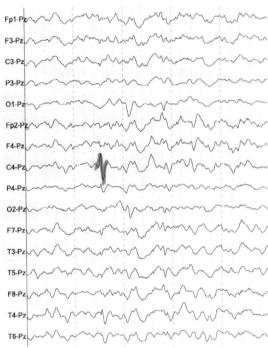

C4 spike in referential montage.

Frontal Intermittent Rhythmic Delta Activity (FIRDA)

 FIRDA is intermittent bisynchronous rhythmic delta activity over the frontal regions.

It is seen in **D**eep midline lesions, increased **I**ntracranial pressure, and **E**ncephalopathy (primarily in adults).

 To remember features of FIRDA, think of your poor **Aunt FIRDIE**, who is in a **D**eep **I**ntractible **E**ncephalopathy.

Occipital Intermittent Rhythmic Delta Activity (OIRDA)

 OIRDA is intermittent rhythmic bisynchronous delta activity occurring in the occipital regions. FIRDA tends to occur in adults, and OIRDA tends to occur in children with encephalopathy.

Periodic Lateralizing Epileptiform Discharges (PLEDs)

PLEDs are sharp activity occurring at fairly regular intervals over a hemisphere.

The most common cause is **stroke**, but classically PLEDs are associated with **Herpes encephalitis**.

If they give you a case of a person with **altered mental status, fever**, and **PLEDs**, think of Herpes.

PLEDs can evolve into seizures.

Triphasic Waves

Triphasic waves are frontally dominant, bisynchronous waves with three phases. There is an anterior-to-posterior lag.

These are classically seen in **hepatic encephalopathy**, but they can be seen in other encephalopathies as well.

Medication Effects

Barbiturates and benzodiazepines can cause beta activity.

Clozapine can cause **interictal discharges, generalized tonic-clonic seizures**, and **myoclonus.**

Clozapine causes Clonic activity.

In addition to clozapine, **meperidine (Demerol®)** and **bupropion (Wellbutrin®)** can cause seizures in people who don't have epilepsy.

Tramadol (Ultram®) and **diphenhydramine (Benadryl®)** can cause **seizures in patients with epilepsy.**

Lithium increases **interictal discharges** in patients with **seizures.**

To remember this, think of your friends **Ben**, **Tram**, and **Li** who have epilepsy and take **Ben**adryl, **Tram**adol and **Li**thium which makes their seizures worse. *BLT*

Then think of all the nonepileptics who must **CliMB** their way out of a seizure after they take

> **C**lozapine,
> **M**eperidine, and
> **B**upropion!

EEG Findings in Specific Diseases

Herpes Encephalitis

Patients with Herpes encephalitis have **fever, headache, behavior changes**, and **seizures**.

The classic **EEG finding** in Herpes encephalitis is **periodic lateralized epileptiform discharges (PLEDs). Sharp or sharp-and-slow wave complexes are seen every 1 to 3 seconds**. They may be seen bilaterally. If they are bilateral, they may be independent or synchronous.

Subacute Sclerosing Panencephalitis (SSPE)

 SSPE is a postinfectious encephalitis due to measles virus.

The age of onset is **5 to 15 years.**

Children who contract measles at an early age are at higher risk.

Stages of SSPE

Stage	Signs and symptoms
I	Personality changes and drop in grades
II	Myoclonic jerks and further intellectual deterioration
III	Stupor, extrapyramidal signs, autonomic instability, rigidity, hyperactive reflexes
IV	Chronic vegetative state

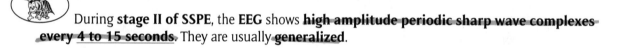

During **stage II of SSPE**, the **EEG** shows **high amplitude periodic sharp wave complexes every 4 to 15 seconds.** They are usually **generalized**.

For SSPE, remember the **5-15 Rule:** periodic sharp wave complexes are every ~**5-15 sec** in **kids age 5-15 yrs.**

Creutzfeldt-Jakob Disease (CJD)

There are **Four Forms** of CJD -- **all are fatal, and thus lead to "the end" (el Fin) -- so the mnemonic is FINS:**

· **F**amilial

· **I**atrogenic

· **N**ew variant

· **S**poradic

EEG Findings in Sporadic CJD: Generalized periodic sharp wave complexes that occur every 0.5-1.6 seconds.[2]

---

[2] Markand ON, Brenner RP. Organic Brain Syndromes and Dementias. In: Ebersole JS, Pedley TA eds. Current Practice of Clinical Electroencephalography, 3rd edition. Philadelphia: Lippincott Williams & Wilkins, 2003;396.

These EEG findings are ~~not seen~~ with New variant CJD.

Please see page 146 for more information on CJD.

EEG for Brain Death

 Requirements for assessing for brain death with EEG:

· At least **8 electrodes** should be used.

· **Sensitivity** should be set for **2 microvolts.**

· **Interelectrode distance** should be *at least* **10 cm.**

· **Impedance** should be **between 100 and 5000 ohms.**

· **Low-frequency filter** should be set for **< 1 Hz.**

· **High-frequency filter** should be set for **> 30 Hz.**

· **Duration** of study should be *at least* **30 minutes.**

 Brain death determination shouldn't result in **FITES** but sometimes it does because people don't know the requirements!

F for **F**ilter (low <1Hz, hi>30Hz), **I** for **I**mpedance (100-5000ohms) and **I**nterelectrode distance (>=10cm), **T** for **T**ime (>30min), **E** for **E**lectrode number (8 = Eight), and **S** for **S**ensitivity (Set to 2 microV).

Neonatal EEG

Neonatal EEG will be discussed only briefly, as it is beyond the scope of this book. This section is primarily for those studying for the Neurophysiology boards.

 EEG findings *vary depending on the gestational age.*

Development of the EEG

EEG Patterns of the Neonate

24-29 Weeks

Between **24 and 29 weeks gestation**, the **EEG looks the same when awake and asleep**. There are diffuse bursts of activity consisting of mixed frequencies followed by diffuse attenuation.

The EEG is **discontinuous**; epochs of higher amplitude activity are followed by periods of lower amplitude activity.

There is **interhemispheric synchrony**; at any point in time, the activity over both hemispheres looks similar.

30-36 Weeks

Between **30 and 36 weeks**, the interburst intervals become shorter during active sleep and wakefulness, and **a tracé discontinu (TD) pattern is seen during quiet sleep**.

Active sleep is analogous to rapid-eye movement (REM) sleep in adults. Unlike adults who go through all the other sleep stages before entering REM, neonates go straight into active sleep. See the sleep section below.

Quiet sleep (QS) is similar to non-rapid eye movement (NREM) sleep in adults.

TD looks similar to the EEG seen between 24 and 29 weeks; however, less synchrony is seen than between 24 and 29 weeks.

36-40 Weeks

At **36 weeks**, a pattern called **activité moyenne is seen in wakefulness and active sleep**, and a **tracé alternans pattern is seen in quiet sleep**.

Activité moyenne (AM) is a continuous pattern consisting of mixed frequencies. It is only seen during active sleep and while the patient is awake. It appears at 36 weeks.

Activité moyenne (AM) occurs while the patient is **A**wake and in **A**ctive sleep.

Tracé alternans (TA) is a discontinuous pattern that looks like tracé discontinu, but the amplitude of the interburst interval is greater in tracé alternans. The amplitude of the interburst interval in TD is less than 25 microvolts; whereas it is greater than 25 microvolts in TA. (To put it simply, the flat part is bumpier in tracé alternans.)

The **A**mplitude is **A**mplified in T**A** and **D**eflated in T**D**.

Discontinuity is limited to quiet sleep by 36 weeks. The background is continuous in active sleep and awake, where an AM pattern is seen. The background is discontinuous in quiet sleep, where a TA pattern is seen.

40-44 Weeks

At **40 weeks**, **continuous slow wave sleep** appears in quiet sleep. Continuous slow wave sleep (CSWS) is continuous delta and theta activity. It gradually replaces TA.

44-46 Weeks

At 44-46 weeks, sleep spindles appear.

48 Weeks

At 48 weeks (8 weeks post-term):
· Quiet sleep is seen at the onset of sleep (rather than active sleep/REM).
· CSWS is seen in QS; TA is gone.
· Sleep spindles become well organized.

Synchrony and Continuity

Synchrony refers to whether the **two hemispheres are producing a similar pattern at a given time.**

Synchrony and continuity develop in a similar pattern. First they are found in active sleep (AS), then they are found in awake, and last they are seen in quiet sleep (QS).

Development of synchrony and continuity:

Active sleep ⟶ Awake ⟶ Quiet sleep.

> **Summary of EEG Patterns in Neonates**
>
> · Activité moyenne (AM) is seen in active sleep and awake (beginning at 36 weeks).
>
> · TD, TA, and CSWS are seen in QS.
>
> Development of the EEG in quiet sleep:
>
> TD ➜ TA ➜ CSWS ➜ CSWS and spindles.

EMG/NCS

Definitions

Antidromic

Antidromic- the opposite direction from which the nerve usually conducts.

Recall that "anti" means against or opposite, so with antidromic stimulation the nerve is stimulated in the opposite direction from which it conducts.

Orthodromic

Orthodromic- the direction in which the nerve usually conducts.

Recall that "ortho" can mean correct, so the nerve is stimulated in the correct direction with orthodromic stimulation.

Orthopaedic surgeon **drones** think they're always **correct** and always headed in the **correct direction**.

Motor Unit

A motor unit is defined as an **A**nterior horn cell, its **A**xon, all the **M**uscle fibers innervated by the axon, and the neuromuscular **J**unctions.[3]

You can be a real **motor unit** in your department if you start reading the journal *JAMA* every week!

---

[3] Pryse-Phillips W. Companion to Clinical Neurology: 2nd edition. New York: Oxford University Press, 2003;609.

Nerve Conduction Studies (NCS)

Motor Conduction Studies

Supramaximal stimulation is used to obtain compound muscle action potentials (CMAPs).

 The **CMAP** is the **sum of all the individual muscle fiber action potentials**.

The latency, amplitude, duration, and area of the CMAP are measured.

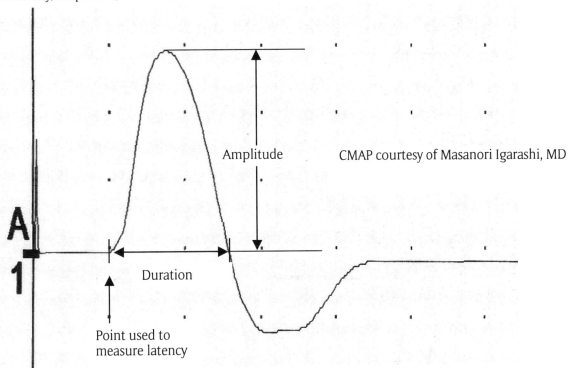

CMAP courtesy of Masanori Igarashi, MD

 Latency is the time from the stimulus to the initial CMAP deflection.

It reflects the fastest conducting motor fibers.

To calculate the latency and conduction velocity, distal and proximal stimulations are performed.

 The amplitude reflects the number of muscle fibers.

The duration reflects synchrony of muscle fiber firing.

Significant drops in area when comparing CMAPs with distal and proximal stimulation may indicate a conduction block.

Conduction block is a failure of action potential propagation. This is seen with contiguous focal demyelination.

Conduction block is indicated by a reduction of CMAP amplitude and area under the curve by more than 30% upon proximal stimulation and typically exceeds 50%.

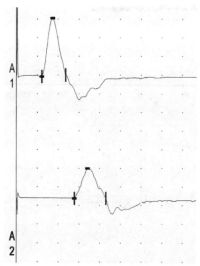

This is an example of conduction block in Guillain-Barré syndrome.

Courtesy of Masanori Igarashi, MD

Conduction block is seen in acquired demyelinating polyneuropathies, not in inherited demyelinating polyneuropathies.

An example of a disease where **conduction block** is seen is **multifocal motor neuropathy with conduction block**. This disease is associated with conduction blocks along motor fibers at sites where compression usually does not occur. It is characterized by **asymmetric weakness** and **atrophy** that typically **begins distally**. Patients may have **anti-GM1 antibodies**.

Conduction block is <u>not</u> seen in inherited demyelinating polyneuropathies, such as **Hereditary Motor Sensory Neuropathy Type 1 (HMSN-1)**. In HMSN-1, nerve conduction velocities are in the demyelinating range. Slowing is similar in all nerves.[4]

In **Martin-Gruber anastomosis it may look like there is a conduction block** between the wrist and below-elbow sites during ulnar nerve motor studies recording from the abductor digiti minimi.

---

[4] Please see the Neuromuscular Diseases chapter for more details.

In **Martin-Gruber** anastomosis fibers cross from the **Median** nerve and innervate (**Grab**) any of the following **4** muscles that are usually innervated by the **Ulnar** nerve:

- The **First** dorsal interosseous muscle
- The **AB**ductor digiti minimi
- The **AD**ductor pollicis
- The deep head of the **Flexor** pollicis brevis.

 In a **Martin-Gruber** anastomosis, the **Median Grabs FAB FAD 4 U**!

Sensory Conduction Studies

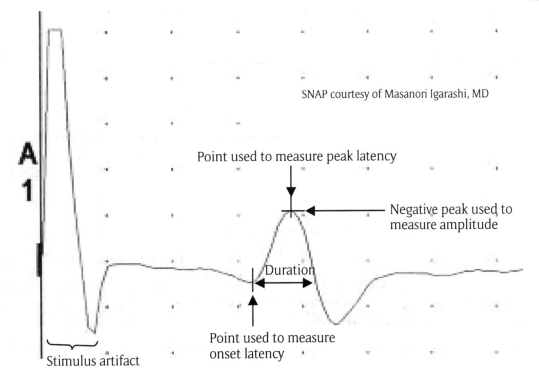 The sensory nerve action potential (SNAP) is the sum of individual sensory fiber action potentials.

SNAP courtesy of Masanori Igarashi, MD

Amplitude

The amplitude can be measured from the baseline to the negative peak or from positive peak to negative peak. The amplitude depends on the number of sensory fibers that depolarize.

Conduction Velocity

The conduction velocity is calculated by dividing the action potential onset latency by the distance from the stimulation point.

Conduction velocity is proportional to diameter. Larger diameter nerve fibers, which have more myelin and less resistance, have faster conduction velocities.

Measures of conduction velocity are of the fastest/largest diameter fibers.

In **demyelinating diseases**, the conduction velocity **is reduced by 20-30%**, measured from the lower limits of normal.

In **axonal diseases**, conduction velocity **is normal or slow** (less than a 20-30% reduction).

Onset Latency

The onset latency is the **latency between the stimulus and the onset of the negative potential**. It reflects the largest cutaneous sensory fibers, which are the fastest conducting fibers.

Peak Latency

The peak latency is the **latency from the stimulus to the peak of the negative potential**. It cannot be used to calculate conduction velocity.

Lower temperatures lead to **increased latency, duration, amplitude, and area of motor and sensory action potentials.**

↓ temp → slows Na⁺ⓒ inactivation → prolonged absolute refractory period ↓ velocity

Nerve Conduction Studies in Neuromuscular Conditions

NCS do not assess small myelinated (Aδ, B) or unmyelinated (C) fibers, which carry autonomic information and pain and temperature sensation.

NCS will be normal in small fiber neuropathies.

Findings in **demyelinating neuropathy**:

· Prolonged distal latency.

· Normal or reduced amplitude.

· Conduction velocity is reduced at least 20-30% from the lower limits of normal.

· Conduction block.

· Increased temporal dispersion may be seen.

Findings in **axonal neuropathy**:

· Decreased amplitude.

· Mild slowing (less than 20-30% from the lower limits of normal).

A **lesion proximal to the dorsal root ganglion** results in **loss of sensation with normal sensory nerve action potentials (SNAPs)**.

On the other hand, with a **plexus lesion, SNAPs are lost**.

In **carpal tunnel syndrome (CTS)**, routine NCS may be normal. Additional studies such as the median nerve palmar sensory response may provide electrophysiologic evidence of CTS.

Late Responses

F Response

F responses are recorded after the CMAP, when a motor nerve is stimulated antidromically with a supramaximal stimulus. The action potential travels in the antidromic direction to the anterior horn cell via the ventral root and then travels back down the motor nerve. Therefore, **F responses evaluate the integrity of the proximal motor pathway**. (The proximal motor axon is not tested in standard NCS.)

Loss of F responses is the earliest electrophysiologic finding of Guillain-Barré syndrome.

Since F responses are pure motor, they are not affected by conditions that only affect sensory nerves.

H Reflex

The H reflex is a monosynaptic reflex involving alpha motor neurons. The afferent limb is group Ia afferent fibers, which are the fastest conducting. Usually the H reflex is obtained by stimulating the tibial nerve with a submaximal stimulus in the popliteal fossa while recording over the gastrocnemius or soleus muscle.

absent/prolonged latency in S1 radic and gen. neuropathy

The H reflex tests the integrity of proximal sensory and motor pathways.

electrical correlate of ankle jerk

Differences between the F response and H reflex:

· The **H reflex** *involves a synapse*, the **F response** *does not.*
· **F responses** *involve motor nerves*, **H reflexes** *involve mixed nerves.*

EMG

Insertional Activity

To check insertional activity, the needle is moved quickly in a resting muscle in four quadrants. Movement of the needle causes muscle fibers to depolarize and produces a waveform.

If the waveform lasts more than 200 milliseconds, it is abnormal and indicates increased insertional activity.

Increased Insertional Activity

Increased insertion activity can be seen in neuropathic conditions such as **denervation** and **myopathic conditions** such as **polymyositis.**

Decreased Insertional Activity

Decreased insertional activity can be seen **when muscle is replaced by fat or connective tissue**.

Spontaneous Activity

After the initial insertional activity, the muscle should be silent if the needle is not moved (if one is not near the neuromuscular junction, where end-plate noise is heard). Any activity heard is abnormal.

 Spontaneous muscle discharges include:
- · Fibrillation potentials
- · Positive sharp waves
- · Fasciculations
- · Myotonia
- · Complex repetitive discharges
- · Myokymia
- · Neuromyotonia

Fasciculations, myokymia, and neuromyotonia originate from one or more motor units.

Multiple muscle fibers produce complex repetitive discharges.

Fibrillation potentials, positive waves, and myotonia are produced by single muscle fibers.

 To remember that fibrillation potentials are produced by a muscle fiber: **fi**brillations arise from a muscle **fi**ber.

 The **most common cause of fibrillations** and **positive sharp waves is denervation**.

If these are seen in paraspinal muscles, a lesion of the ventral nerve root is present (if there is not an indication of a necrotizing myopathy).

Myotonia

Myotonia is a motor fiber discharge that **waxes and wanes in amplitude and frequency**.

It sounds like a departing motorcycle or dive-bomber.

Electromyographic myotonia is found in many disorders including **myotonic dystrophy**, **acid maltase deficiency** (in the paraspinal muscles), **myotubular myopathy**, and **polymyositis**.[5]

Myokymia

Myokymia is characterized by **rhythmic grouped discharges** on EMG. The discharges arise spontaneously from the same motor unit or motor units.

Myokymia is seen in **radiation-induced plexopathy**, **multiple sclerosis**, and **pontine tumors**.

Recall from the Movement Disorders chapter that **Episodic Ataxia-1** is associated with myokymia and is due to a **potassium channel gene mutation**.

Neuromyotonic Discharges

Neuromyotonia is a **high frequency decrementing discharge** produced by a single motor unit, which sounds like a formula 1 car passing by.

Neuromyotonia is seen in **Isaac syndrome**.

Motor Unit Action Potentials (MUAPs)

Motor unit potentials are then assessed with increasing amounts of muscle contraction.

With **minimal muscle contraction**, the amplitude and duration of motor unit potentials are assessed.

Myopathic MUAPs are small (200 to 500 microvolts) and **short in duration**.
Neurogenic MUAPs are large (more than 5 millivolts) and **prolonged**.
Giant MUAPs may indicate **chronic reinnervation**.

Recruitment

Firing of the first motor unit action potential (MUAP) is seen at 5 Hz. The second begins to fire at 10 Hz.

The normal ratio of the firing frequency of the fastest firing MUAP to the number of motor unit action potentials is 5 to 1.

---

[5] Please see the Neuromuscular Diseases chapter.

This increase in motor units with increasing firing rates is called **recruitment.**

With maximal contraction, MUAPs overlap and individual MUAPs cannot be seen. This is called a **full interference pattern.**

A full interference pattern looks something like this:

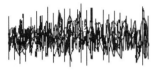

Decreased Recruitment

 Loss of MUAPs results in **decreased recruitment**. Fewer MUAPs are seen and they are firing at increased rates. This occurs with **axonal loss**, **conduction block**, or in **end-stage myopathy** where every muscle fiber of a MUAP has been lost.

Decreased recruitment is usually seen in **neuropathic processes**.

Decreased recruitment looks something like this:

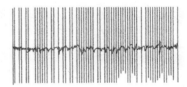

Early Recruitment

Early recruitment is seen in myopathies; a full interference pattern is seen with less than maximal contraction, but the amplitude of the motor unit potentials is reduced.

This is because there is a dropout of muscle fibers from the motor units in myopathies. The motor unit is smaller, and more motor units are needed to generate a given force.

Single-Fiber EMG (SFEMG)

In SFEMG, a needle records from a single muscle fiber or a pair of muscle fibers from the same motor unit.

This is the **most sensitive test for demonstrating impaired neuromuscular junction transmission.**

If the muscle is weak and SFEMG is normal, then there is no transmission defect.

Repetitive Nerve Stimulation Test

Neuromuscular transmission is assessed using trains of stimuli.

Repetitive nerve stimulation is **useful in the diagnosis of myasthenia gravis**, **Lambert-Eaton myasthenic syndrome**, and **botulism.**

Both Lambert-Eaton and myasthenia gravis patients have a CMAP decrement (greater than 10% drop) with repetitive stimulation at 2-5 Hz.

In Lambert-Eaton patients and botulism, the CMAP increases significantly with repetitive stimulation at 20-50 Hz.

Nerve Injury

Classification of Peripheral Nerve Injury

Neurapraxia

There is a loss of conduction but the axon is intact in neurapraxia. There is a conduction block with proximal stimulation.

Axonotmesis

The axon is disrupted but the sheath is intact in axonotmesis. This results in failure to conduct and wallerian degeneration of the part of the axon removed from the cell body.

Neuronotmesis

The axon and its associated connective tissues are disrupted in neuronotmesis. This is the most severe injury.

Projectile Injury –
(ie., bullet fragments from Gunshot Wound, GSW)

Kinetic Energy = **1/2 mass x Velocity^2** (squared)

Velocity is the single most important determinant of tissue injury from a projectile.

Tumble & fragmentation of the projectile can also alter the amount of damage but less than **Velocity**.

Blink Reflex

To test the blink reflex, the supraorbital branch of the trigeminal nerve is stimulated, and electrical responses are measured over the orbicularis oculi muscles.

Like the corneal reflex, the afferent limb is the ophthalmic division of the ipsilateral trigeminal nerve (V1), and the efferent limb is the facial nerves (CN VII).

Evoked Potentials

Evoked potentials are weak signals, so **averaging is used to increase the signal to noise ratio**.

Somatosensory Evoked Potentials (SSEPs)

SSEPs are generated by the **dorsal column-medial lemniscal system**.

Median Nerve

N9 = Brachial plexus = Erb's point

N11 = Cervical cord

P14 = Caudal brainstem (medial lemniscus)

N18 = Upper brainstem (with a contribution from the cuneate nuclei)[6]

N20 = Primary somatosensory cortex (contralateral to the stimulated hand)

Median nerve SSEPs help identify the central sulcus in preparation for epilepsy surgery. (Right median SSEPs are used to identify the central sulcus on the left and vice versa.)

Giant SSEPs are seen in progressive myoclonic epilepsy (PME), e.g. Unverricht-Lundborg disease.[7]

As mentioned above, median nerve SSEPs help identify lesions in the dorsal column-medial lemniscal system.

For example, an increase P14 –N20 latency suggests that there is a defect in the conduction between the brainstem and the somatosensory cortex.

Tibial Nerve

N8 = Tibial nerve

N19 = Cauda equina

N22 = Lumbar gray matter

P31 = Medial lemniscus[8]

N34 = Multiple brainstem generators[9]

P38 = Primary somatosensory cortex

Visual Evoked Potentials (VEPs)

Generators of VEPs: Brodmann areas 17 and 18.

A delay in P100 on one side indicates an ipsilateral lesion anterior to the optic chiasm.

Amplitude asymmetry may be normal.

normal latency = 100 MS

---

[6] Emerson R, Pedley TA. Somatosensory evoked potentials. In Ebersole JS, Pedley TA (eds): Current practice of clinical electroencephalography: 3rd edition. Philadelphia: Lippincott William & Wilkins, 2003;904.

[7] Please see the epilepsy chapter for more information about PME.

[8,9] Emerson R, Pedley TA. Somatosensory evoked potentials. In Ebersole JS, Pedley TA (eds): Current practice of clinical electroencephalography: 3rd edition. Philadelphia: Lippincott William & Wilkins, 2003;912.

Brainstem Auditory Evoked Potentials

The well-known mnemonic to remember the peaks is **NCSLIMA.**

I	**Nerve** (Acoustic / 8th)
II	**Cochlear** nuclei (medulla)
III	**Superior** olivary complex (pons) + trapezoid body
IV	**Lateral** lemniscus (pons)
V	**Inferior** colliculus (midbrain)
VI	**Medial** geniculate (thalamus)
VII	**Auditory** radiations (thalamocortical)

The latency of peaks I, III, and V are identified and the interpeak latency between the peaks are calculated. These are obligate waveforms that should be seen in normal subjects.

Waveform V is usually the most prominent. It is the last waveform to disappear as the stimulus intensity is decreased.

BAEP Findings in Specific Conditions

Acoustic Neuromas

An acoustic neuroma may cause the interpeak latency between waveforms I and III to be prolonged.

Brain Death

All the waveforms may be absent or only wave I will be seen bilaterally in the setting of brain death.

Multiple Sclerosis (MS)

The III-V interpeak latency may be prolonged or wave V may be decreased in amplitude or absent in patients with MS.

BAEP Abnormalities	Significance
Increase in I-III IPL	Conduction defect between distal acoustic nerve and lower pons.
Increase in III-V IPL	Conduction defect between lower pons and midbrain.
Only waveform I seen	Conduction defect involving the proximal acoustic nerve or the pontomedullary junction.
No wave I, III-V IPL normal	Peripheral auditory dysfunction.

IPL= Interpeak latency

Sleep

Anatomy[10]

The **suprachiasmatic nucleus of the hypothalamus** is responsible for **circadian rhythms**.

Wakefulness

The following **promote wakefulness:**

- **DopAmine** (from the ventral tegmental area)
- **NorEpinephrine** (from the locus coeruleus)
- **HistAmine** (from the tuberomammillary nucleus of the posterior hypothalamus)
- **SeroTonin** (from the medial and dorsal raphe nuclei)
- **Orexin/ hypocretin** (from the posterior and lateral hypothalamus)
- **Acetylcholine** (from the pedunculopontine and laterodorsal tegmental areas) is *increased during wakefulness and REM*.

To list the awakening neurotransmitters, think of this: **DA NE HA S T O AWAKEN!**

---

[10] For more information see these articles:

Baumann C, Bassetti C. Hypocretins (orexins) and sleep-wake disorders. Lancet Neurol 2005;4:673-82.
España RA, Scammell, TE. Sleep neurobiology for the Clinician. Sleep 2004;27:811-820.

Deficient orexin (also known as hypocretin) causes narcolepsy.

Sleep

Adenosine promotes sleep. Caffeine and **theophylline** *block adenosine receptors*, which promotes wakefulness. We assume that your adeonsine receptors are adequately blocked if you are actually awake while reading this.

Neurons of the basal forebrain and anterior hypothalamus are important for sleep onset.

Inhibition of hypocretin neurons by GABA from preoptic and basal forebrain neurons is important in the initiation of sleep.

Neurons in the ventrolateral preoptic (VLPO) area of the anterior hypothalamus, which produce GABA and galanin, inhibit the arousal systems during non-rapid eye movement (NREM) sleep.

REM sleep is a result of activation of neurons in the lateral dorsal/pedunculopontine tegmental area (LDT/PPT area). These neurons produce atonia by activating the medial medulla, which inhibits motor neurons.

It's interesting that gait abnormalities in Parkinson's disease have been correlated with loss of neurons in the pedunculopontine nucleus (PPN), which is important for production of REM and atonia during REM, and that patients with Parkinson's disease are at increased risk for REM behavior disorder, which is due to loss of atonia during REM.

Normal Sleep

Sleep Stages

Sleep Stage	EEG Findings
I	Vertex waves, slowing of background.
II	Sleep spindles and K complexes are first seen.
III	20-50% delta activity
IV	Greater than 50% delta activity
REM	Looks similar to awake EEG but there's no muscle artifact, the background is slightly slower, and there are rapid eye movements and irregular respirations.

Stages I-IV are **non-rapid eye movement (NREM)** sleep.
NREM predominates in the first third of sleep, and REM predominates in the last third.

Stages I-II are also referred to as **light sleep**.

Stages III-IV are also referred to as **deep sleep/ slow wave sleep**.

Drowsiness

During drowsiness, bursts of bisynchronous theta/delta activity can be seen, particularly in children. This is called **hypnagogic hypersynchrony**, but it can be seen when waking up as well, in which case it is called **hypnopompic hypersynchrony.** So this is what you are expreriencing while reading this.

To remember **hypnopompic** means **awakening** (pompic) **from sleep** (hypno), think of the volcano **awakening** the city of **Pompeii** (remember that from history class or were you sleeping?); to remember **hypnagogic** means **while falling asleep**, think of how **groggy** (gogic) you get when it's your bedtime!

Over age 10 years, slow lateral eye movements are the first sign of drowsiness, but they are not always seen.

Positive occipital sharp transients (POSTs) are waves found in the occipital regions that have positive polarity. They tend to look like checkmarks and occur in runs. They appear in drowsiness and light sleep. POSTs are maximal in adolescence.

Stage I

Benign Epileptiform transients of Sleep - small sharp spikes in drowsiness & background distortion

Vertex waves are waves with negative polarity seen over the vertex. They first appear in stage I sleep.

POSTS - pos. occ. sharp. transients of Sleep - monophasic triangular

Stage II

Sleep spindles and/or K complexes are first seen during stage II sleep.

Sleep spindles are thought to arise from neurons in the **reticular nucleus of the thalamus**. They are maximal over the central head regions. The duration and frequency of spindles vary with age. In adults, spindles have a frequency of about 12-14 Hz. *1st c 2mo. synch c 2yrs. + c age*

K complexes are complexes that first appear during stage II sleep. There is a high amplitude negative component followed by a positive component. They last 0.5 seconds and can be followed by sleep spindles.

K spindle

K complexes can be elicited by noise during sleep.

"**K**" Complexes can be created by **too** much (**stage II**) noise (**K**langity **C**lang) during sleep.

Stages III-IV

Stages III and IV are known as **slow-wave-sleep**.

REM

Sawtooth waves are theta-frequency waves that resemble saw teeth and are found in brief runs over the frontocentral regions during REM.

1. We are more likely to wake from REM sleep than from NREM sleep. Animals that awaken from REM periodically scan the environment for possible predators!

2. Studies suggest that REM is important for consolidation of procedural and spatial memories. Declarative memory is consolidated during slow wave sleep.

3. Medications that can suppress REM sleep include tricyclic antidepressants and monoamine oxidase inhibitors.

Sleep Changes with Age

In the neonate, quiet sleep is equivalent to NREM and active sleep is like REM in adults.

Quiet sleep is associated with a *tonic chin EMG, regular respirations*, and *absence of eye and body movements.*

Active sleep is characterized by *phasic chin EMG, irregular respirations* and *limb movements, rapid eye movements,* and *sucking.*

At **birth, half of total sleep** time is spent in **REM**.

Infants **less than 2-3 months** of age often **enter REM directly from drowsiness**.

Sleep spindles are present by **2 months.**
Vertex waves appear at **3-4 months** but are not **well-formed** until **5 months.**

Sleep spindles appear *before vertex waves* in the development of the EEG.

Sleep spindles are present by **2 months**, and **vertex waves** appear at **3-4 months**.

Synchronous spindles are seen at age 2 years.

Sleep spindles first appear in stage 2 sleep, appear by age 2 months of age, and are synchronous by 2 years of life.

REM decreases to 30% of total sleep time at **1-2 years of age**.

Percentage of time spent in each sleep stage in adulthood:

Stage 1	< 5%
Stage 2	40-60%
Stages 3-4	10-20%
REM	18-25%

The **elderly** have:

· An **increase** in stage 1 sleep

· A **decrease** in slow-wave sleep.

Sleep Disorders

Sleep Disorder	Sleep stage
Cluster headaches	REM
Confused Arousals	Slow-wave sleep
Night Terrors	Slow-wave sleep
Nightmares	REM
Periodic limb movements	Stage I and Stage II sleep (Light sleep)
Rhythmic movement disorder (e.g. head banging)	Light sleep and transitions between sleep and wakefulness
Sleep walking (Somnambulism)	Slow-wave sleep

MNEMONIC

To remember the 3 sleep disorders associated with Slow-wave sleep, think of this: She **SAT** up **SLOWLY**: **S**omnambulism, confused **A**rousals, and Night **T**errors all occur in **SLOW**-wave sleep.

Somnambulism, night terrors, and confused arousals tend to occur in the first half of the night. (Recall that NREM predominates in the first third of sleep, and REM predominates in the last third.)

Cluster Headaches

Cluster headaches can **arise out of REM**.

They are **brief, severe, Unilateral headaches** that occur in the **distribution of V1** and are accompanied by **autonomic signs** such as **L**acrimation, **C**onjunctival injection, **E**yelid Edema, **S**tuffiness / **S**not (rhinorrhea), or p**T**osis.

Cluster headaches respond to oxygen by face mask.

Similar to nightmares, **cluster headaches**, which are a **nightmare for the patients** who have them, **occur in REM**.

To remember all the important features of cluster headaches, think of the name, CLUSTER:

- **C** = Conjunctival injection
- **L** = Lacrimation
- **U** = Unilaterality
- **S** = Stuffiness / Snot (rhinorrhea)
- **T** = pTosis (hey, the p is silent anyway)
- **E** = Eyelid Edema
- **R** = REM sleep

Night Terrors versus Nightmares

Night terrors are a **parasomnia** that occurs during **slow-wave sleep.** A person, usually a child, awakens from sleep, looks frightened, and may cry out. He/she is **difficult to arouse and is disoriented**. The child has **no memory of the event the next morning**. Night terrors usually occur during **the first half of the night**.

Nightmares tend to occur in the **second half of the night**, since REM is more prominent in the second half of the night.

A nightmare is a dream which causes one to wake up in REM and experience a negative emotion, such as fear, on average once per month. They are uncommon in children under five, yet about 25% of older children get a nightmare weekly. The incidence rises somewhat in teenagers, but drops by 30% in adulthood.

Restless Leg Syndrome (RLS)

Patients with restless leg syndrome (RLS) have an unpleasant sensation in the limbs, such as a crawling feeling, resulting in the desire to move them. Sensations are worse in the evening and when sitting or lying down. They are relieved by leg movement.[11]

Patients with RLS may also have **Periodic Limb Movement Disorder (PLMS)**, which is a distinct condition that is diagnosed with objective testing. RLS may be primary (idiopathic) or secondary. Causes of **secondary RLS** include *pregnancy, kidney failure* (ARF), *and abnormalities of iron* (Fe+++), *calcium* (Ca++), *potassium* (K+), or *magnesium* (Mg++).

To remember the causes of secondary RLS, think about your father (Pa) who suffers from this disease:

PA Can't Move, Kick, or Feel his legs!

Pregnancy, ARF, Ca++, Mg++, K+, Fe+++

Treatments for primary RLS include dopaminergic medications (ropinirole, pramipexole, pergolide, bromocriptine, Sinemet); benzodiazepines such as clonazepam; and opiates.

Periodic Limb Movement Disorder (PLMD)

Periodic limb movement disorder is a sleep disorder **diagnosed with polysomnography**. Patients with PLMD have **daytime sleepiness** or **insomnia** and **excessive periodic limb movements (PLMS)**.

Specifically, patients with PLMD have greater than 5 PLMS per hour of sleep.

Periodic limb movements (PLMS) are involuntary, stereotyped movements that meet specific criteria on polysomnography. They usually involve the legs and resemble a triple-flexion response. They tend to last 0.5 – 10 seconds[12] and occur in a cluster of at least four movements separated by 5 to 90 seconds (usually 20 to 40 seconds).[13]

Periodic limb movements occur in light sleep.

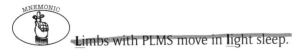

Limbs with PLMS move in light sleep.

---

[11] Please see the Movement Disorders chapter for more details about RLS. [12] The old criteria used 5 seconds as the maximum.

[13] Zucconi M, Ferri R, Allen R, et al. The official World Association of Sleep Medicine (WASM) standards for recording and scoring periodic leg movements in sleep (PLMS) and wakefulness (PLMW) developed in collaboration with a task force from the International Restless Legs Syndrome Study Group (IRLSSG). Sleep Medicine 2006;7:175-183.

REM Sleep Behavior Disorder (RBD)

Due to a lack of muscle paralysis during REM, people with RBD can act out their dreams. This usually occurs **during second half of the night when REM is more prevalent.**

Patients with **Parkinson's disease, Multiple system atrophy, Alzheimer's disease**, and **dementia with Lewy bodies** are at *increased risk for this disorder.*

Case presentation for RBD:
An elderly gentleman tackles the dresser or tries to slam-dunk his wife.

 Patients with **RBD** may act **RaBiD**.

 Patients with **RBD** may knock over the **LAMP** next to the bed! (LAMP=dementia with **Lewy** bodies, **Alzheimer's** disease, **Multiple** system atrophy, **Parkinson's** disease).

PALM Synday = Synucleinopathies

RBD can be treated with **clonazepam**.

Sleep-Related Eating Disorder (SRED)

SRED is a **parasomnia** characterized by involuntary eating and drinking during sleep. The foods most frequently consumed are high in calories, sugars, and salt. SRED is more common in women than men.

Episodes occur during **partial arousals** from sleep, sometimes in the setting of with somnambulism, with spotty recall the next day. Rarely, **inedible or even toxic substances** are ingested.

To remember **SRED**, think of a **woman** half-asleep, wearing a **S**carf that is **RED** and eating **S**alty **RED** potato chips and **S**weet **RED** strawberries (which do have a high glycemic index!)

Narcolepsy

 Narcolepsy is characterized by a tetrad (and a brilliant mnemonic): **Every Cat Sleeps Here, Here, or Here!**

· Excessive daytime sleepiness
· Cataplexy
· Sleep paralysis
· Hypnagogic or Hypnopompic Hallucinations

Clinical Features

Cataplexy

Cataplexy is characterized by brief episodes (a few seconds) of loss of muscle tone without loss of consciousness, often due to emotion.

Cataplexy causes one to be **cat**apulted to the ground when certain emotions occur.

Hypnagogic and Hypnopompic Hallucinations

Narcolepsy can be associated with **Hypnopompic** (while awakening) or **Hypnagogic** (while falling asleep) **Hallucinations**.

To remember **hypnopompic** means **awakening** (pompic) **from sleep** (hypno), think of the volcano **awakening** the city of **Pompeii** (remember that from history class or were you sleeping?); to remember **hypnagogic** means **while falling asleep**, think of how **groggy** (gogic) you get when it's your bedtime!

A solid mnemonic for those narcoleptics out there (or those who have acquired narcolepsy reading this drivel).

Sleep paralysis

Sleep paralysis is the inability to move upon awakening and/or going to sleep. It lasts up to 10 minutes.

Risk Factors for Narcolepsy

Narcolepsy is associated with specific HLA types: **DQ**B1*0602, **DQ**AI*0102 (DQ 1), **DR**2.

DQ (**D**airy **Q**ueen) makes you a **Narcoleptic** doctor (**DR**) because the ice cream is so yummy!

Low levels of orexin/hypocretin, which is produced by the lateral hypothalamus, **have been found in the CSF of patients with narcolepsy**.

Diagnosis of Narcolepsy

Narcolepsy is diagnosed by doing a PolySomnoGram (PSG) *FIRST* to rule out other sleep disorders and to ensure that the patient has slept at least 6 hours. Then, a **multiple sleep latency test (MSLT)** is done the next day.

Multiple sleep latency test (MSLT):

> Patients take four or five 20-minute naps during the day, spaced 2 hours apart.
>
> Average sleep latency is determined. Normal is = 10 minutes.

MSLT findings consistent with narcolepsy:

> Mean sleep latency (average of minutes to fall asleep) is <5 minutes.
>
> Onset of REM within 10-15 minutes of sleep during = 2 naps during MSLT.

Treatment of Narcolepsy

Treatments for excessive daytime somnolence:

> · Modafinil
>
> · Stimulants (such as methylphenidate, pemoline, or dextroamphetamine).

Treatments for **cataplexy, sleep paralysis, and hypnagogic hallucinations**:

> · **Sodium oxybate/GHB** (Xyrem)
>
> · SSRIs
>
> · TCAs, such as Imipramine (Tofranil)

Treatment of Insomnia

Over-the-counter:

- **Antihistamines (Benadryl®)** – has anticholinergic, antitussive, antiemetic, and sedative properties, but it lowers the seizure threshold.
- **Melatonin** - entrains the suprachiasmatic nucleus to environmental cycles, helps in circadian rhythm sleep disorders, shift-worker sleep disorder, Seasonal Affective Disorder, and is a possible geroprotector!

Prescription:

- **Benzodiazepines (Halicon®, Restoril®, Valium®, clonazepam etc.)** – also treat sleepwalking and night terrors. However, these drugs may cause dependence.
- **Zolpidem (Ambien®)** – agonist at benzodiazepine binding site on GABAA neurons; original version helps sleep initiation, but patients awoke in the middle of the night; Ambien CR (extended release) lasts >6 hrs. **Zolpimist** oral spray contains Ambien's active ingredient.
- **Zaleplon (Sonata®)** – for "middle of night insomnia"; also agonist at GABAA benzo binding site.
- **Eszopiclone (Lunesta®)** – short-acting hypnotic; also agonist at GABAA benzo binding site.
- **Ramelteon (Rozerem®)** – binds to MT1 and MT2 receptors in the suprachiasmatic nucleus; no abuse or dependence.
- **Trazodone (Desyrel®), amitriptyline (Elavil®),** and **Doxepin (Silenor®)** – antidepressants; since insomnia is a common symptom of depression, these may treat "sleep anxiety".
- Gabapentin

Side Effect Warnings

The FDA warned in 2007 that some prescription sleep medications may cause complex sleep-related behaviors, such as "sleep driving."

Systemic Diseases with Sleep Abnormalities

Fatal Familial Insomnia

Fatal familial insomnia is an autosomal dominant prion disease characterized by insomnia followed by dementia.

Patients also may present around age 50 years and symptoms last about 15 months before death occurs. Symptoms include **ataxia, dementia, dysautonomia**, and of course, severe **insomnia** refractory to treatment. MRI may reveal degeneration of **thalamic subnuclei** (specifically the **VA and MD**).

Families in **VA** and **MD can't sleep** with all the **demented** congressmen arguing nearby at the capitol!

Kleine-Levin Syndrome (also known as Sleeping Beauty Syndrome)

Kleine-Levin Syndrome (KLS) is a condition found most often in teenage boys that is characterized by recurrent episodes of excessive sleep **(hypersomnolence lasting >18 hours per day)**, **excessive food intake (hyperphagia), and hypersexuality** (more common in men than women, and associated with a longer disease course).[14] Symptoms are cyclical, often lasting days or months, and then followed by asymptomatic stages of months or years.

Patients with **Kleine-Levin Syndrome** are **recline-lovin'**.

Etiology

Unknown, perhaps a hereditary predisposition or an autoimmune disorder (or both) are to blame, causing hypothalamic dysfunction.

A deficiency of dopamine transporter density in the lower striatum may be the biochemical abnormality.

---

[14] Yeah, this does sound like the average teenager, but it is beyond normal.

Hyperphagia = Polyphagia = Metaphagia

Other disorders besides KLS that cause hyperphagia (compulsive hunger) include **Prader-Willi Syndrome** and **Bardet Biedl Syndrome**, as well as **diabetes**, of course.

Myotonic Dystrophy

Patients with myotonic dystrophy may have **excessive daytime sleepiness that responds to Modafinil**.[15]

Sleeping Sickness (African Trypanosomiasis)

Sleeping sickness is due to a bite from the **tsetse fly infected** by the protozoan, ***Trypanosoma brucei***.

There are 2 stages to **African Trypanosomiasis**:

· **1st stage "hemolymphatic phase"** – fever, headaches, joint pains, itching, and lymph node swelling due to circulatory/lymphatic parasite invasion.
· **2nd stage "neurologic phase"** – confusion, incoordination, and extreme fatigue alternating with night-time insomnia and mania as the parasite passes through the blood-brain barrier.

Treatment

· Pentamidine or Suramin for 1st stage only
· Eflornithine and/or Melarsoprol for 2nd stage

Prognosis

Untreated, African Trypanosomiasis leads to mental deterioration, coma, and is invariably fatal.

---

[15] Please see the Neuromuscular Diseases chapter for more information about myotonic dystrophy.

Neurophysiology Quiz

(Answers on page 755)

1. Match the condition with the EEG.

    1) Triphasic waves with anterior to posterior lag.

    2) Burst-suppression

    3) High amplitude generalized periodic sharp wave complexes every 4 to 15 seconds.

    4) Generalized periodic sharp wave complexes that occur every 0.5- 1.6 seconds.

    A. SSPE

    B. CJD

    C. Hepatic encephalopathy

    D. Severe anoxic injury

2. Match the description with the EEG finding.

    1) Attenuated by movement or thoughts of movement of the contralateral body.

    2) Delta activity with overriding alpha frequencies

    3) 6-11 Hz activity in the temporal region during drowsiness or light sleep in adults

    4) Positive sharp transients in the occipital area seen during visual scanning.

    A. Lambda

    B. Mu

    C. Posterior slow waves of youth

    D. Wicket spikes

3. Which of these nerves is not involved in Martin-Gruber anastomosis?

    A. The first dorsal interosseous muscle

    B. The abductor digiti minimi

    C. The abductor pollicis longus

    D. The adductor pollicis

    E. The deep head of the flexor pollicis brevis.

4. Narcolepsy has been associated with low levels of which of the following?

  A. Adenosine

  B. GABA

  C. Glutamate

  D. Orexin/hypocretin

Chapter 14

Pediatric Neurology

Neonatal Neurology

Extracranial Hemorrhage

Caput Succedaneum

 Caput succedaneum is scalp soft tissue swelling that usually affects the presenting portion of the head. It usually occurs at the vertex and is associated with molding of the head. It can cross suture lines and may be associated with ecchymosis.

Caput succedaneum **succ**eeds in crossing suture lines, but then the baby's head modeling career goes **caput**!

Cephalohematoma

A cephalohematoma is a hemorrhage in the subperiosteal space.

Large cephalohematomas can cause anemia and hyperbilirubinemia.

Subgaleal Hemorrhage

Subgaleal hemorrhage is a hemorrhage beneath the aponeurosis. It crosses suture lines and can cause significant blood loss.

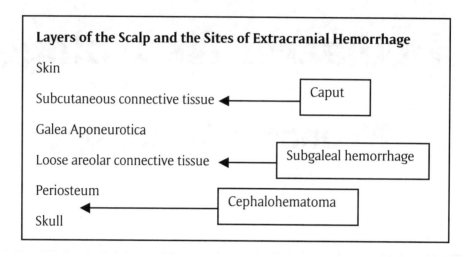

Layers of the Scalp and the Sites of Extracranial Hemorrhage

Skin

Subcutaneous connective tissue ← Caput

Galea Aponeurotica

Loose areolar connective tissue ← Subgaleal hemorrhage

Periosteum

Cephalohematoma →

Skull

Intraventricular Hemorrhage (IVH)

Grade	Radiologic Finding
I	Localized to the germinal matrix
II	In the ventricle but less than 50% of the ventricular volume
III	Blood distends the ventricle
IV	Blood extends into the surrounding parenchyma

In general, **IVH arises from the germinal matrix in premature babies and from the choroid plexus in full-term neonates**.

Congenital Hydrocephalus

Fetal hydrocephalus is most often due to:

· Aqueductal stenosis

· Communicating hydrocephalus

· Dandy-Walker malformation

· Myelomeningocele.

MASA Syndrome

There is an X-linked recessive form of aqueductal stenosis associated with adducted thumbs, agenesis of the corpus callosum, and mental retardation. This is called **MASA syndrome**, which stands for **M**ental retardation, **A**phasia, **S**huffling gait, and **A**dducted thumbs.

MASA syndrome is due to mutation in the **L1CAM gene**. (L1CAM is a neural cell adhesion molecule.)

There are additional X-linked syndromes due to mutations in the L1CAM gene: X-linked hydrocephalus (HSAS), X-linked complicated spastic paraparesis (SP1), and X-linked corpus callosum agenesis (ACC). In addition to MASA syndrome, these are grouped together under the name **CRASH syndrome**, which stands for **C**orpus callosum hypoplasia, **R**etardation, **A**dducted thumbs, **S**pastic paraparesis, and **H**ydrocephalus.

To remember that MASA is associated with **CRASH** syndrome: **It's better for MASA to be associated with CRASH than NASA.**

To remember that MASA is associated with <u>aque</u>ductal stenosis, link MASA and AQUA.

Picture a **Cam**aro crashing to remember that L1**CAM** is associated with CRASH syndrome. With **adducted thumbs** and **spastic paraparesis**, of course these patients crash.

Dandy-Walker Syndrome

The 3 guys in the **A.V.** club in high school were all **dandy walkers,** so…

Dandy-Walker syndrome is characterized by a triad – A.V., A.V., and A.V.:

1) **A**genesis of the cerebellar **V**ermis
2) **A**bnormal (Cystic dilatation of the) 4th **V**entricle
3) **E**nlarged posterior fossa with elevation of the tentorium (**A**dvancing **V**ossa)

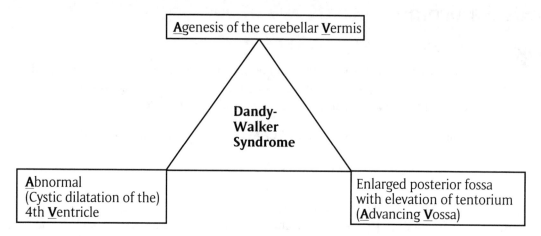

Patients may have congenital hydrocephalus, but it often develops postnatally.

Patients may have agenesis of the corpus callosum, an occipital encephalocele, developmental delay, cortical malformations, seizures, polycystic kidneys, or cardiac anomalies.

 Dandy-Walker is a misnomer; their walking is not dandy. Dandy-Walker patients tend to have ataxia.

*Dandy-Walker syndrome can be seen as part of **PHACES syndrome**, which is characterized by **P**osterior fossa malformations, **H**emangiomas of the face, **A**rterial anomalies, **C**oarctation of the aorta and other cardiac defects, **E**ye abnormalities, and **S**ternal clefting or **S**upraumbilical raphe.*

Seizures

 Seizures on the **first day of life** are often due to **Hypoxic-Ischemic Encephalopathy (HIE)**.[1]

The **first** thing these newborns want to do is **Seize the day** and **HIE**-tail it outa the womb!

Recall from the Epilepsy chapter that **benign familial neonatal seizures** are due to mutations in **voltage-gated potassium genes**.

Don't forget about metabolic causes.

---

[1] There is a list of causes of neonatal seizures in Fenichel's textbook <u>Clinical Pediatric Neurology: a Signs and Symptoms Approach.</u>

Glucose Transporter Type 1 Deficiency (DeVivo Syndrome)

Glucose transporter type 1 deficiency is due to a mutation in SLC2A1 gene, which encodes the protein Glut 1, a glucose transporter.

Patients with glucose transporter type 1 deficiency may present with **neonatal seizures**, but seizures usually develop **between one and 4 months of age** and are **difficult to control**.

They may have **apnea** and **eye movements resembling opsoclonus**.

These patients are also developmentally delayed and develop microcephaly, spasticity, and ataxia.

Glucose transporter type 1 deficiency is diagnosed by lumbar puncture. Patients have a **low CSF Glucose** (< 40), a **low ratio of CSF glucose to blood glucose** (about 1/3), and a **normal CSF lactate**.[2]

Glucose transporter type 1 deficiency is treated with the **ketogenic diet**.

> ### What is the ketogenic diet???
>
> - It is high in fats, low in carbs, and adequate in protein.
>
> - It **mimics starvation** and forces the body to burn fats instead of the regular carbohydrate load. Usually, carbs from food are converted into glucose, but in a low-carb (or zero-carb) diet, the liver converts fat into fatty acids and ketone bodies (which replace glucose as the CNS energy source).
>
> - Thus, the ketogenic diet promotes **ketosis**, which acts a surrogate antiepileptic medication.

Nonketotic Hyperglycinemia (Glycine Encephalopathy)

Nonketotic hyperglycinemia is an autosomal recessive condition due to a defect in glycine cleavage.

6-8hrs old

Neonates with nonketotic hyperglycinemia are **lethargic** and **hypotonic**. They have **multifocal myoclonus**, **hiccups**, and **apnea**.

When you are given a case of a neonate with **hiccups, seizures,** and a **burst-suppression pattern** on the EEG, think of nonketotic hyperglycinemia. Another clue would be a mother noticing hiccups or movements suggestive of myoclonus in utero.

Nonketotic hyperglycinemia is diagnosed by an **elevated CSF glycine** and **elevated CSF-to-plasma glycine** ratio.

Treatments for nonketotic hyperglycinemia include sodium benzoate, diazepam, and dextromethorphan (NMDA receptor antagonist).

---

[2] Check the blood glucose just prior to the lumbar puncture.

Pyridoxine Dependency

Pyridoxine dependency causes seizures that are difficult to control. They may present on the first day of life, but it is recommended that this diagnosis be **considered in children less than 18 months with refractory seizures.**

Recall that pyridoxine is a cofactor for glutamic acid decarboxylase, which is required for GABA synthesis.

$$\text{Glutamate} \xrightarrow[\text{Glutamic acid decarboxylase (GAD)}]{\text{pyridoxine}} \text{GABA}$$

Pyridoxine dependency is diagnosed by giving intravenous pyridoxine during an EEG. Also, an oral trial for several days may be used to diagnose it.

Some patients with pyridoxine-dependent seizures were found to have mutations in the *ALDH7A1* gene on 5q, which encodes **antiquitin**.[3]

Mutations in *ALDH7A1* also can cause folinic acid-responsive seizures.

Both pyridoxine and folinic acid are recommended if patients have α-aminoadipic semialdehyde (α-AASA) dehydrogenase deficiency due to *ALDH7A1* mutations.[4]

Hypotonia

Hypotonia is divided into **central** and **peripheral** hypotonia; some diseases, however, can cause both.

Central hypotonia is due to a *lesion in the* **brain or spine** and may be associated with **encephalopathy, seizures, dysmorphic features, or organ malformations. Reflexes are normal or brisk.**

Peripheral hypotonia is due to a *lesion of the* **motor unit**. These patients tend to be **alert but may be weak or have decreased reflexes**.

---

[3] Mills PB, Struys E, Jakobs C, et al. Mutation in antiquitin in individuals with pyridoxine-dependent seizures. Nat Med 2006; 12:307-309.

[4] Gallagher RC, Van Hove JL, Scharer G, et al. Folinic acid–responsive seizures are identical to pyridoxine-dependent epilepsy. Ann Neurol 2009;65:550–556. Please see the Metabolic Diseases chapter for more information.

Motor Unit

A motor unit is defined as an **A**nterior horn cell, its **A**xon, all the **M**uscle fibers innervated by the axon, and the neuromuscular **J**unctions.[5]

You can be a real **motor unit** in your department if you start reading the journal *JAMA* every week!

Bilirubin Encephalopathy/Kernicterus

Acute bilirubin encephalopathy first causes hypotonia and stupor. Then hypertonia with opisthotonus is seen. Then hypotonia may again be seen.

Chronic bilirubin encephalopathy results in bilateral high-frequency hearing loss and abnormal movements such as *chorea or dystonia.*

To remember the features of chronic bilirubin encephalopathy, think of your friend Billy Rubin who despite his high-frequency hearing loss, he could still hear the bass rhythms and therefore was a pretty good dancer (chorea).

Congenital Hypothyroidism

Clinical findings of congenital hypothyroidism include **prolonged neonatal jaundice**, **an umbilical hernia**, **large fontanelles**, **macroglossia**, and **constipation**.

Patients with congenital hypothyroidism have **hypotonia** and **delayed development**.

TORCH Infections

TORCH stands for **T**oxoplasmosis, **R**ubella, **C**ytomegalovirus, and **H**erpes simplex.[6]

---

[5] Pryse-Phillips W. Companion to Clinical Neurology: 2nd edition. New York: Oxford University Press, 2003;609.
[6] Please see the Infectious Diseases chapter.

Birth Injuries

Erb-Duchenne Paralysis/Erb's Palsy

Erb's palsy is a brachial plexus injury at birth involving the upper trunk or C5-C6 roots.

This is the most common brachial plexus injury in newborns.

It results in weakness of the deltoid, biceps, brachioradialis, and supinator muscles.

Therefore, the arm is adducted, internally rotated, and extended, and the forearm is pronated. This is called the **waiter's tip position**.

To remember that Erb-Duchenne paralysis/**Erb's** palsy is associated with a waiter's tip position, and that it results in weakness of the **D**eltoid, **BR**achioradialis, **B**iceps, and **S**upinator muscles, remember this request, "Waiter, **D**o **BR**ing **B**ack **S**ome h**ERB**s."

Klumpke's Paralysis

Klumpke's paralysis is a brachial plexus injury involving the lower trunk (C8-T1).

This is a rare plexus injury.

Patients with Klumpke's paralysis have weakness of the forearm extensors, wrist and finger flexors, and intrinsic hand muscles.

The hand has a **clawlike deformity**, the elbow is flexed, the forearm is supinated, and the wrist is extended.

Picture somebody holding a "Klump" of sand.

Horner's syndrome may be seen because sympathetic fibers accompany T1.

Complete Brachial Plexus Palsy

Patients with a complete brachial plexus palsy have a **flail arm** that is **areflexic**.

Like patients with Klumpke's paralysis, the patient may have a Horner's syndrome.

Congenital Malformations

Cardiofacial Syndrome/ Cayler Syndrome

 In cardiofacial syndrome, also known as Cayler syndrome, hypoplasia of the depressor anguli oris causes an **asymmetric face** that is particularly **noticeable when the patient is crying**.

Cayler syndrome is associated with **c**ardiac anomalies. You can also change it to "**Crier**" **syndrome** to remember that it is noticeable when the **depressed** baby is **crying** his **heart** out.

CHARGE Syndrome

See Genetic conditions below.

Duane Syndrome

Duane syndrome is a congenital disorder due to hypoplasia of the abducens nucleus and nerve with aberrant innervation of the lateral rectus by branches of CN III.

During adduction, narrowing of the palpebral fissure, and globe retraction are seen.

Klippel-Feil Syndrome

Patients with Klippel-Feil syndrome have **abnormal fusion of the cervical vertebrae** or a **reduction in the number of cervical vertebrae.**

 They also have a **short neck, a low hairline posteriorly**, and **reduced neck movement**.

Other congenital anomalies may be present such as Sprengel deformity (see below) or genitourinary malformations.

 Patients with **Klippel-Feil** have their neck **Klipped** due to fewer vertebrae and they also **Feil** like they have to Urinate frequently due to GU malformations. Because of these deficits, they can't just **Spreng** out of bed anymore.

Marcus Gunn Syndrome

 This is different than a Marcus Gunn pupil.[7]

In **Marcus Gunn syndrome**, the **eyelid lifts when the mouth opens and falls when the mouth closes** or vice versa. It is thought to be due to aberrant innervation.

Sprengel Deformity

Sprengel deformity is characterized by scapula elevation.

It may be associated with Klippel-Feil syndrome.

 Patients with **Klippel-Feil** can't just **Spreng** out of bed anymore.

Vein of Galen Malformation

A vein of Galen malformation is an arteriovenous malformation that results in shunting of arterial blood into an enlarged cerebral vein. Specifically, the median prosencephalic vein of Markowsky becomes dilated.

---

[7] Please see the Neuro-ophthalmology for information about the Marcus Gunn pupil.

This is a **misnomer. The vein of Galen is not involved in the vascular malformation**. The normal vein of Galen does not form due to this vascular malformation.

A vein of Galen malformation **can cause congenital hydrocephalus**.

Think of a vein of Galen malformation if a case describes **high output congestive heart failure** and a **cranial bruit** in a neonate.

Craniosynostosis

Craniosynostosis is premature closure of one or more of the sutures. The head does not grow perpendicular to the closed suture resulting in an abnormal skull shape.

Recall that the anterior fontanelle closes at 9-18 months, and the posterior fontanelle closes at 3-6 months.

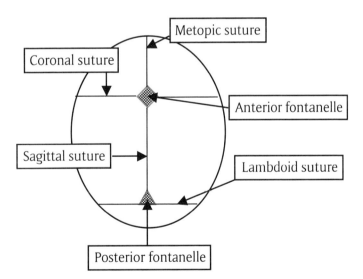

Types of Craniosynostosis

Sagittal Synostosis

Premature fusion of the sagittal suture causes a **scaphoid head shape** (*scaphocephaly*); the head is long and narrow. This is also known as **dolichocephaly**.

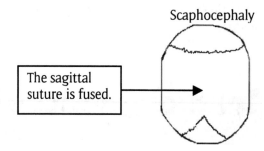

Scaphocephaly

The sagittal suture is fused.

A **s**caphoid head shape is due to **s**agittal suture synostosis.

This is the most common form of craniosynostosis.

Coronal Synostosis

Premature closure of the **coronal sutures** *causes* **brachycephaly**. The skull is **short and wide**.

Brachycephaly

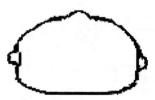

(View from above)

Think of a **short, wide** fellow who drank too many **Corona** beers and **Brayched** his Cephaly (head) against a wall, making it look like the head above.

Lambdoid Synostosis

Unilateral lambdoid synostosis results in ipsilateral occipitoparietal flattening and contralateral frontal and parietal bossing. The ipsilateral ear is displaced posteriorly, toward the flattened area.[8]

Looking down from above, the head is a trapezoid shape due to flattening on one side and frontal and parietal bossing on the other.[9]

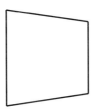

 Lambd**oid** suture synostosis causes head to be shaped like trapez**oid**.

 This can be distinguished from deformational plagiocephaly, which is due to positioning.

Deformational plagiocephaly results in <u>anterior</u> displacement of the ear ipsilateral to the flattening. (Imagine the bed pushing the ear forward.) There is <u>ipsilateral</u> frontal bossing and contralateral occipital bossing.

If viewed from above, the head looks like a parallelogram due to flattening and frontal bossing on one side and occipital bossing on the other.[10]

 Positional **p**lagiocephaly causes the head to be shaped like a **p**arallelogram.

---

8 Kabbani H and Raghuveer TS. Craniosynostosis. American Family Physician 2004;69:2863-2870.

9 Sheth RD, Iskandar BJ. Craniosynostosis. Emedicine January 9, 2007.

10 Sheth RD, Iskandar BJ. Craniosynostosis. Emedicine January 9, 2007.

Metopic Synostosis

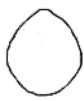

Premature closure of the metopic suture causes **trigonocephaly**. The forehead is pointed with a **prominent ridge in the middle.**

(View from above. Note pointed forehead.)

Trigonocephaly starts with **Tri** like **Tri**angle, and this pointed head looks like a Triangle from above.

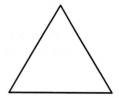

Conditions Associated with Craniosynostosis

Apert's Syndrome (Acrocephalopolysyndactyly Type I)

Patients with Apert's syndrome have multiple synostoses; the **coronal suture is the most often affected**.

Patients with Apert's syndrome also have **syndactyly, proptosis**, and **hypertelorism.**

Patients with **Apert's** syndrome wish that they could get their fingers **apart**, but they have syndactyly. Although it's hard to tell, Apert's patients really do have **10** fingers and the gene defect is on chromosome **10**.

It is due to a mutation in **fibroblast growth factor receptor-2 (FGFR2)** on 10q and is autosomal dominant.

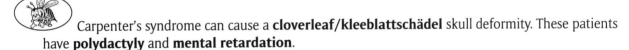 To remember **FGFR2**, know that Apert's patients are all **F**or **G**etting **F**inger **R**eductions, **too**!

Carpenter's Syndrome (Acrocephalopolysyndactyly Type II)

Carpenter's syndrome results in closure of multiple sutures. It is **autosomal recessive**.

 Carpenter's syndrome can cause a **cloverleaf/kleeblattschädel** skull deformity. These patients have **polydactyly** and **mental retardation**.

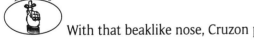 **Polydactyly** may **help a carpenter** who needs to hold more tools.

Crouzon's Disease (Craniofacial Dysostosis)

Crouzon's disease is associated with **closure of the coronal** and **basal skull sutures** and with **malformation of facial bones.**

Patients with Crouzon's disease have **hypertelorism, proptosis**, a **beaklike nose**, and **maxillary hypoplasia**.

Like Apert's syndrome, Crouzon's disease has been mapped to 10q, and some of these patients have mutations in FGFR2. However, patients with **Crouzon's disease don't have syndactyly**.

With that beaklike nose, Cruzon patients are Crusin for a bruisin!

Patients with **Crouzon's** disease can *pick up* **croutons** because they **don't have syndactyly** but they still have 10 fingers (chromosome 10).

Pfeiffer's Syndrome (Acrocephalopolysyndactyly Type 5a)

Patients with the classic form of Pfeiffer's syndrome have mutation in FGFR2, like patients with Apert's syndrome, or a mutation in FGFR1 (chromosome 8p).

Pfeiffer's syndrome **affects the coronal** and **basal skull sutures**.

 Polydactyly differentiates Pfeiffer's syndrome from Apert's syndrome.

 Polydactyly occurs in **P**feiffer's syndrome.

Patients with Pfeiffer's syndrome also have **broad thumbs**.

Development

Head Growth

The average FOC at birth for a **term infant is 35 cm**.

 Head growth in first year of life:
- · 2 cm per month for the first 3 months
- · 1 cm per month for the next 3 months (4-6 months of age)
- · 0.5 cm per month from 7 to 12 months of age.

Developmental Milestones

Motor

At **4 months**, babies can **reach for objects** and **automatic sucking disappears**.

 Babies can reach **for** objects at **four** months. *Babies need to stop automatically sucking on fingers so that they can reach.*

At **6 months**, babies **sit** and can **transfer objects from one hand to the other**.

 Babies s̲it at s̲ix months and can s̲witch hands.

At 2.5 years, most toddlers are toilet trained.

 Totally Toilet Trained Toddlers at Two.

Since girls are typically toilet trained before boys...

 Females Flush First!

At **3 years** of age, children can **throw overhand** and **ride a tricycle**.

 Children th̲row overhand at th̲ree and ride a tricycle. (**Th**ree wheels at 3 years.)

Language

At **9 months of age**, infants can say **mama/dada**.

 It takes **9 months to be a mama/dada**, and at **9 months babies can say "mama"/ "dada"**.

At **2 years** of age, a **child speaks in phrases**.

At **3 years** of age, a child can **recognize 3 colors** and **speak in sentences**.

At **6-8 years of age**, a child can **name the days of the week**.

 Around **7 years**, kids can name the **7 days of the week**.

Drawing

 A child can **copy a line at 2-3 years**.

At **36 months**, a child can **draw a circle (360 degrees)**.

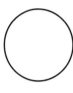

A child can **copy a cross at 3.5-4.5 years**.

 A child can copy **one line at around 2**, and **2 intersecting lines (a cross) at about age 4**.

Alternatively, one can remember that at **age 4,** a child can draw **a cross**, which **has 4 quadrants** and **looks a bit like a 4.**

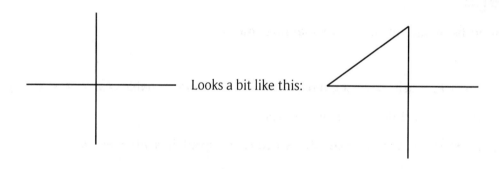

Looks a bit like this:

A child can **copy a square** at **4 – 4.5 years**.

 A child can **copy a figure with 4 sides** at **4 years**.

 A child can **draw a man with six parts by age six**.

At **7**, a child can **copy a diamond**.

The **top half of the diamond looks like a seven (7) turned counter-clockwise**.

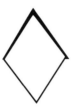

Card sharks may remember **7 of diamonds**.

At **age 12,** a child **can copy a cube**, which is **made from 12 lines**.

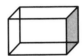

Genetic Conditions

Angelman Syndrome

Angelman syndrome is also known as "Happy Puppet Syndrome".

Multiple mutations may cause this:

- Deletion of maternally derived 15q11-13.
- Duplication of paternal chromosome 15 (uniparental disomy).
- Mutation in the **ubiquitin-protein ligase E3A (UBE3A) gene** (15q11-13).
- Mutation in the imprinting center (15q11-13).

This is an example of genomic imprinting; the phenotype depends upon whether the mutation is in the chromosome from the mother or father.

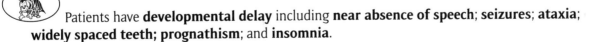Patients have **developmental delay** including **near absence of speech; seizures; ataxia; widely spaced teeth; prognathism**; and **insomnia**.

Children with Angelman syndrome may have **epilepsy** as a result of a deletion of the region of chromosome 15 that codes for the β3 subunit of the GABA A receptor.

 Absence of <u>paternally derived</u> 15q11-13 causes Prader-Willi syndrome, which is described below.

Prader-Willi Syndrome

 Prader-Willi syndrome is a cause of **neonatal hypotonia**.

Patients **feed poorly initially**. Later, they **develop an insatiable appetite and become obese**.

They have **small hands and feet**, **almond-shaped eyes**, **hypogonadism**, and **mental retardation**.

Prader-Willi syndrome is due to the deletion of paternal 15q11-13 or maternal disomy. Like Angelman syndrome, this is an example of imprinting.

Prader has no **Father** (paternal chromosome is deleted), while Angel**Man** has no Angel**Mama** (maternal chromosome deleted) – remember this it is crucial!!

Cri-du-chat Syndrome

Due to problems with the **larynx and nervous system**, infants affected with this syndrome have a characteristic cry like a meowing kitten (French = "Cry of the Cat").

Severe cognitive, speech, and motor delays, excessive drooling, feeding problems (difficulty swallowing and sucking) all can result in poor growth and development. Often these patients also have hypotonia, microcephaly, hypertelorism, micrognathia, short fingers, and cardiac defects.

The genetic abnormality is a 5p chromosomal **deletion**.

To remember the genetics of Cri-du-chat, think about why the cat is crying – **because she's missing her "p"**.

CHARGE Syndrome

CHARGE stands for **C**oloboma of the eye, **H**eart anomaly, choanal **A**tresia, **R**etardation of mental and somatic development, **G**enital abnormalities (microphallus), and **E**ar abnormalities/deafness.

CHARGE syndrome is autosomal dominant. A mutation in the chromodomain helicase DNA-binding protein-7 (*CHD7*) gene on chromosome 8q is responsible for most cases.

CHARGE syndrome is associated with **CHD** (congenital heart disease) and **CHD7** (chromodomain helicase DNA-binding protein-7).

DiGeorge's Syndrome

DiGeorge's syndrome is characterized by **hypoplasia of** organs derived from the third and fourth pharyngeal pouches such as the **thymus, parathyroid gland**, and **great vessels**.

DiGeorge's syndrome may present with **seizures, jitteriness, tetany, hypocalcemia**, or a **heart defect**.

It is due to a microdeletion of chromosome 22q.

Both DiGeorge's syndrome and velocardiofacial syndrome are CATCH syndromes. CATCH stands for **C**ardiac **A**bnormality, **T**-cell deficit, **C**lefting, and **H**ypocalcemia.

DiGeorge Washington and his **22,000** queasy soldiers were **q**uite **jittery** in the American revolution because they knew if the British were to **CATCH** them they would cut out their **thymus** and **heart**!

Fragile X Syndrome

Fragile X is characterized by **mental retardation, large ears, a long face, and macroorchidism**.

It is due to a **triplet repeat (CGG) in the FMR1 gene**, which is on the X chromosome.

Remember: in Fragile X you see **(C) Giant Gonads**, and the condition is due to expansion of the **CGG** repeat in the FMR1 gene.

Rett Syndrome

Rett syndrome is a neurodegenerative disease that primarily affects girls. It is **X-linked dominant** and can be lethal in males.

Classic Rett syndrome is due to a mutation in the **MECP2 gene**, which maps to **Xq**. Mutations in the **CDKL5** (cyclin-dependent kinase-like 5) gene, which is also known as **STK9**, have been found to cause an early-onset form of Rett syndrome that is associated with seizures.

Patients with classic Rett syndrome are normal until 3 or 6 months of life.

Clinical stages of Rett syndrome:

- **Stage I Early Onset (3-6 months):** Head growth decelerates, developmental delay is seen, autistic-like behavior begins, and patients develop hand wringing.
- **Stage II Regression (1 to 4 years):** There is loss of purposeful hand movements and loss of speech. Seizures, abnormal breathing, stereotypic hand movements, and hypotonia are seen.
- **Stage III Stabilization**
- **Stage IV Late Motor Deterioration**: The patient loses the ability to walk.

The Three Trisomy's: 13, 18, and 21

To remember that **P**atau is trisomy **13**, **E**dwards is **18** and **D**own's is **21**, think of this:

You hit **P**uberty at **13**, you can vote in an **E**lection at **18**, and you can **D**rink at age **21**.

Trisomy 13 (Patau's Syndrome)

The major neurological findings in Trisomy 13 are **holoprosencephaly** and **developmental delay.** The patients also have **episodes of apnea in early infancy**.

To remember **P**atau (trisomy **13**) is associated with apnea, recall that when you realized what **P**uberty was at age **13**, you became out of breath (apneic)!

Trisomy 18 (Edward's Syndrome)

Patients with Trisomy 18 have **mental retardation, flexion deformities** and **overlapping of the fingers**, and **rocker bottom feet**.

To remember **E**dwards (trisomy **18**) is associated with **rocker** bottom feet, recall that when you cast your first ballot in an **E**lection at age **18**, you **rocked** the vote!

Both Trisomy 13 and Trisomy 18 are associated with **omphalocele, polycystic kidneys**, and **cardiovascular abnormalities**.

Trisomy 21 (Down Syndrome)

Patients with Down syndrome have **brachycephaly, epicanthal folds, Brushfield spots** (white speckles on the iris), **simian creases, late closure of fontanelles, hypotonia**, and **heart defects** most commonly involving the atrioventricular septum.

There is an increased **risk for leukemia, Hirschsprung's disease**, and **duodenal atresia**.

Atlanto-axial instability results from laxity of the transverse ligaments that bring that the odontoid process near to the anterior arch of the atlas.

A risk factor for developing Down Syndrome is Advanced Maternal Age (AMA>35 years). Decreased alpha-fetoprotein and unconjugated estriol are also associated with Down Syndrome. Down Syndrome usually results from Nondisjunction during maternal meiosis.

Patients with Down syndrome develop Alzheimer's disease at an early age. Recall that amyloid precursor protein is on chromosome 21.

Velo-Cardio-Facial Syndrome (VCFS)

Like DiGeorge's syndrome, VCFS is due to a deletion at 22q and is a CATCH syndrome. As mentioned above, CATCH stands for **Cardiac Abnormality, T**-cell deficit, **Clefting, and Hypocalcemia**.

Patients with velocardiofacial syndrome have **cleft palate, hypernasal speech** due to velopharyngeal insufficiency, a **bulbous nose**, and **micrognathia**.

Williams Syndrome

Williams syndrome is due to a mutation at 7q. This includes the gene that encodes **elastin**, which leads to cardiovascular and connective tissue abnormalities.

Patients with Williams syndrome often have **supravalvular aortic stenosis**.

Hypotonia and **hyperextensible joints** may lead to **delayed milestones**.

Patients also have **elfin facies**, a **stellate iris pattern**, **hypercalcemia**, a **friendly personality**, and **musical talent.**

To remember the features of Williams syndrome, think of a **friendly elf** named **William Elastin**, who plays "body **music**" with his **hyperextensible joints** for his **stellar friend Iris**. William has **7** letters and the mutation is on chromosome **7**.

Wolf-Hirschhorn Syndrome

Patients with Wolf-Hirschhorn syndrome are said to have **Greek helmet facies**; they have a **High hairline, frontal bossing**, and **hypertelorism**. They may also have a **cleft lip and palate**.

Neurological features include **mental retardation** and **microcephaly**.

It is due to a deletion at 4p.

To remember features of Wolf-Hirschhorn Syndrome, think of your **boss**, Mr. **Wolf**, who had a small head (**microcephaly**) and widely spaced eyes (**hypertelorism**). For Halloween one year, he wore a **Greek Helmet** but came in **4th p**lace in the costume contest (chromosome 4p) at work so therefore he was **fired** (**deleted**).

Brain Development

The nervous system arises from the **ectoderm**.

Primary Neurulation

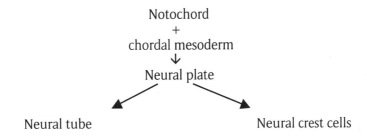 Primary neurulation refers to formation of the neural tube except the part caudal to the lumbar region.

It occurs in the 3rd and 4th weeks of gestation.

Primary Neurulation:

Notochord
+
chordal mesoderm
↓
Neural plate

Neural tube   Neural crest cells

The notochord and chordal mesoderm lead to the formation of the **neural plate** at 18 days gestation.

The neural plate bends at the midline, forming a **neural fold**.

The margins of the neural fold fuse at the midline and result in the formation of the **neural tube**.

The central nervous system (brain and spinal cord) arises from the neural tube.

Cells at the edge of the neural folds are excluded from the neural tube and form neural crest cells.

The neural crest cells give rise to the dorsal root ganglia, sensory ganglia of the cranial nerves, Schwann cells, cells of the pia and arachnoid, melanocytes, adrenal medulla, and postsynaptic autonomic neurons.

The ventral half of the neural tube is the *basal plate.*

The dorsal half of the neural tube is the *alar plate.*

The **sulcus limitans** is the boundary between the alar and basal plates.

The **basal plate** gives rise to motor neurons such as motor neurons of the cranial nerves and the anterior horn of the spinal cord.

The **alar plate** gives rise to sensory neurons such as the sensory nuclei of the thalamus, the posterior horn of the spinal cord, and the sensory neurons of the cranial nerves. It also gives rise to the prosencephalon, other parts of the thalamus, the cerebellum, the inferior olives, the red nucleus, and the quadrigeminal plate.

To remember that the alar plate is the dorsal half of the neural tube and is associated with sensory neurons, remember **SAD** for **Sensory Alar Dorsal**.

To remember that the basal plate is the ventral half of the neural tube and is associated with motor neurons, remember **BMV** for **Basal Motor Ventral**.

Folate is a regulator of neural tube closure. That is why it is recommended that pregnant women take folate to prevent neural tube defects.

Segmentation

The neural tube divides along the rostral-caudal, dorsal-ventral, and medial-lateral axes. This is called **segmentation** or **regionalization**.

Embryonic divisions of the brain are the forebrain (prosencephalon), the midbrain (mesencephalon), and the hindbrain (rhombencephalon).

The **prosencephalon** develops into the *diencephalon and telencephalon.*

The **mesencephalon** develops into the *midbrain.*

The **rhombencephalon** develops into the *metencephalon and the myelencephalon.*

Embryonic divisions and the structures to which they give rise:

Prosencephalon (Forebrain)
    Diencephalon
        Thalamus
        Hypothalamus
        Subthalamic nucleus
        Globus pallidus
        Substantia nigra
    Telencephalon
        Striatum (caudate and putamen)
        Cerebral cortex

Mesencephalon= Midbrain

Rhombencephalon (Hindbrain)
    Metencephalon
        Pons
        Cerebellum
    Myelencephalon
        Medulla

The prosencephalon consists of the diencephalon and telencephalon.

The prosencephalon undergoes cleavage in the fifth and sixth weeks of gestation:

    1) Horizontal cleavage results in formation of the optic vesicles and olfactory bulbs and tracts.

    2) Transverse cleavage results in separation of the diencephalon from the telencephalon.

    3) Sagittal cleavage results in formation of the cerebral hemispheres, lateral ventricles, and basal ganglia.

The diencephalon consists of words containing "thalamus", the globus pallidus, and the substantia nigra.

The glob**us** pallid**us**, like the structures ending with thalam**us**, arises from the diencephalon.

Recall that nigra means black, and the color black is associated with death, in order to remember that the substantia nigra is part of the diencephalon (**die**ncephalon).

Formation of the Cortex

Overview of formation of the cortex:

Neuronal proliferation (8-16 weeks gestation) → Migration (10-20 weeks gestation)→ Differentiation (from 20 weeks on)

Neuronal Proliferation

Neuronal proliferation occurs between 8 and 16 weeks gestation. This occurs in the ventricular zone.

Neuronal Migration

Post-mitotic neuroblasts move away from the **ventricular zone** and form the **preplate**.[11]

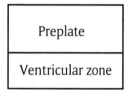

Between 6-20 weeks gestation, neuroblasts migrate from the ventricular zone into the preplate and form the **cortical plate**.

The cortical plate splits the preplate, which creates a **marginal zone** and **subplate**.

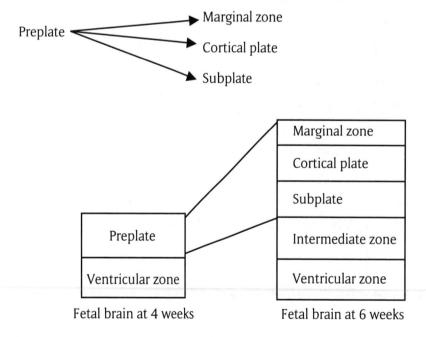

Fetal brain at 4 weeks   Fetal brain at 6 weeks

---

[11] Ellison D, Love S, Chimelli L, et al. Neuropathology. Barcelona: Harcourt Publishers Limited, 2000;3.19.

Migrating neurons follow an **inside-out pattern**. Neurons that arrive early take deep positions, and later arriving neurons take more superficial positions in the cortex.

Neurons migrate along **radial glia**.

Layers 2- 6 of the mature cortex arise from the cortical plate.

Layers of the mature cerebral cortex:

I.	Molecular Layer
II.	External granular layer
III.	External pyramidal layer
IV.	Internal granular layer
V.	Internal pyramidal / ganglionic layer
VI.	Multiform layer

By 27 weeks gestation, all 6 layers are present.
(Layer I is closest to the pia; layer VI is closest to the ventricle.)

Brain Malformations

Disorders of Primary Neurulation

Anencephaly
anterior

Anencephaly is absence of the cerebral hemispheres due to failure of anterior neural tube closure. It usually occurs at 24 days gestation.

Myeloschisis

Myeloschisis is a failure of posterior neural tube closure. The neural structures protrude, and the spinal cord is exposed (there is no skin or membrane covering).

Encephalocele

  An encephalocele is due to a failure of anterior neural tube closure; intracranial contents herniate through a midline skull defect.

Most encephaloceles are occipital.

An encephalocele is one cause of an **elevated alpha-fetoprotein** on the triple screen.

Encephaloceles are found in **Meckel-Gruber syndrome**, also known as **Meckel's syndrome**.

Meckel's Syndrome is also characterized by **microcephaly, microphthalmia, cleft lip, polydactyly, polycystic kidneys**, and **ambiguous genitalia**.

The letters in MECKEL'S can be used to remember the clinical findings:

Microcephaly

Encephalocele

Cleft lip

Kidneys polycystic

Eyes small (microphthalmia)

Lots of fingers (polydactyly)

Sex ambiguous

Myelomeningocele

A myelomeningocele is a protrusion of spinal contents due to failure of posterior neural tube closure. There is a membrane covering (unlike myeloschisis).

Arnold-Chiari Malformation

Type I

Chiari Type I malformations are characterized by displacement of the cerebellar tonsils at least 5 mm through the foramen magnum. Syringomyelia may be present in up to 50% of cases.

Patients with Chiari I malformations report **suboccipital headaches**. Severe cases may be associated with lower cranial nerve findings and/or spinal cord involvement and may require surgical decompression.

Type II

In Chiari Type II malformations, the cerebellar tonsils are displaced into the cervical canal; the medulla is inferiorly displaced, appears long and thin, and may be kinked; and there is a lumbosacral myelomeningocele. The tectum appears beaked.

Hydrocephalus and cortical malformations may be seen.

Type III

A Chiari Type III malformation is a Type II malformation plus an occipital encephalocele.

Type IV

Cerebellar hypoplasia occurs in Chiari Type IV.

Disorders of Secondary Neurulation / Caudal Neural Tube Formation

Secondary neurulation refers to formation of the caudal neural tube (the lower sacral and coccygeal segments).

Disorders of secondary neurulation result in occult dysraphic states. There is a layer of skin covering the lesions.

There may be a clue such as a **dimple, hair tuft,** or **lipoma**. The conus and filum are abnormal. **Tethering of the cord** and **vertebral anomalies** are frequently associated with these conditions.

Caudal Regression Syndrome

Patients with caudal regression syndrome have malformations of the structures arising from the caudal region of the embryo such as the hindgut, urogenital system, caudal spine, spinal cord, and lower limbs.

Infants of diabetic mothers are at risk for this.

Diastematomyelia

 Diastematomyelia refers to a **bifid spinal cord**. A septum may divide the spinal cord longitudinally.

Meningocele

A meningocele is characterized by protrusion of the meninges but not neural tissue through a vertebral defect. Most often this occurs in the lumbosacral region.

Myelocystocele

A myelocystocele is a dilation of the central canal of the caudal neural tube.

Myelocystocele may be associated with *gastrointestinal* or *genitourinary anomalies* such as **bladder or cloacal extrophy, imperforate anus,** or **omphalocele**.

Disorders of Segmentation

Schizencephaly

Schizencephaly is characterized by a cleft in the cortex that extends from the ventricle to the surface of the brain and is lined in gray matter. It is called **open-lipped** *if the walls of the cleft do not approximate and* **closed-lipped** *if they do.*

It is due to mutations in the EMX2 gene on 10q.

It has been considered a migration abnormality.

To remember the disorders of abnormal neuronal migration, think of little **Lisa** who says: "She who **migrates, HoPPS** away!"
Lissencephaly, **H**etero**t**opia, **P**olymicrogyria, **P**achygyria, and **S**chizencephaly.

Prosencephalic Malformations

Disorders of Prosencephalic Formation

Aprosencephaly

Aprosencephaly is absence of the prosencephalon, which consists of the diencephalon and telencephalon.

Recall that the telencephalon includes the striatum and cerebral cortex, and the diencephalon includes the thalamus, hypothalamus, subthalamic nucleus, globus pallidus, and substantia nigra.

Atelencephaly

Atelencephaly is absence of the telencephalon.

Disorders of Prosencephalic Cleavage

Holoprosencephaly

Holoprosencephaly is characterized by failure of the prosencephalon to divide into two cerebral hemispheres and for the telencephalon and diencephalon to separate.

Holoprosencephaly is associated with absence of the olfactory bulbs and tracts. Patients tend to have **midline facial defects**. **Cyclopia** can be seen. Organ malformations may occur.

Alobar Holoprosencephaly

Alobar holoprosencephaly is the most severe form of holoprosencephaly. There is no separation of the hemispheres and there is a single ventricle, which often is associated with a cyst. The corpus callosum is absent. The thalamus and basal ganglia are fused.

Semilobar Holoprosencephaly

Semilobar holoprosencephaly is less severe. The posterior hemispheres are separated to some degree, although the anterior hemispheres are fused. The splenium of the corpus callosum is present.

Lobar Holoprosencephaly

Lobar holoprosencephaly is associated with near normal separation of the hemispheres and lateral ventricles, but the septum pellucidum is absent, and there is incomplete formation of the interhemispheric fissure and cerebral falx.

Multiple genes have been identified. The first gene identified codes for sonic hedgehog (Shh) on 7q. Shh is one of the signals that promote prosencephalic cleavage. Recall from above that holoprosencephaly is seen in Trisomy 13. It can also be seen in Trisomy 18.

Holotelencephaly

 The telencephalon is a single-sphered structure, but the diencephalon is not as involved.

Disorders of Midline Prosencephalic Development

Agenesis of the Corpus Callosum

Agenesis of the corpus callosum is found in multiple conditions, one of which is **Aicardi syndrome**.

 AICardi Syndrome is an *X-linked* **dominant** condition that is characterized by a triad:

    1) **A**genesis of the corpus callosum
    2) **I**nfantile spasms
    3) **C**horioretinal lacunae

Aicardi syndrome starts with AIC and the 3 major features of it also start with A, I and C!

Agenesis of the Septum Pellucidum

Agenesis of the septum pellucidum is often found with other anomalies. An example is the syndrome of absence of the septum pellucidum with schizencephaly.

Septo-optic Dysplasia (DeMorsier Syndrome)

Septo-optic dysplasia is characterized by **optic nerve hypoplasia, absence of the septum pellucidum, and hypopituitarism**. Some patients have a mutation in the homeobox gene HESX1 on 3p.

S.O.D has 3 letters, so it is due to a defect on chromosome 3.
(Von Hippel-Lindau is similar. VHL has 3 letters and is on chromosome 3.)

Disorders of Neuronal Proliferation

Some forms of microcephaly and megalencephaly are due to abnormal proliferation.

Disorders of Neuronal Migration

To remember the disorders of abnormal neuronal migration, think of little **Lis**a who says:
"She who **migrates, HoPPS** away!"
Lissencephaly, **H**eterotopia, **P**olymicrogyria, **P**achygyria, and **S**chizencephaly.

Lissencephaly-Pachygyria

Lissencephaly, which means **smooth brain**, is due to impaired neuronal migration. The cortex is thick and lacks gyri and sulci. It occurs during the third or fourth month of gestation.

Pachygyria refers to **thick gyri** that are decreased in number.

Think of a **Pachyderm** (i.e., elephant) which has **thick skin**!

There are a number of conditions associated with lissencephaly including:
- · Miller-Dieker syndrome (MDS)
- · Lissencephaly due to a LIS1 mutation
- · Lissencephaly due to a DCX mutation
- · Lissencephaly with agenesis of the corpus callosum
- · Lissencephaly with cerebellar hypoplasia

These conditions are associated with a **fewer than normal number of layers of cortex.**

Miller-Dieker Syndrome

Heads Up

Miller-Dieker and isolated lissencephaly sequence cause microcephaly due to lissencephaly and are found on chromosome 17.

Neurofibromatosis type 1, Alexander's disease, and **Canavan's disease** (aspartoacylase deficiency) all cause **macrocephaly** and are also found on **chromosome** 17.

Patients with Miller-Dieker syndrome have lissencephaly, microcephaly, seizures, craniofacial abnormalities, and cardiac defects. Their prognosis is worse than patients with isolated lissencephaly.

Miller-Diecker syndrome is due to a **17p deletion**. This includes the **LIS1 gene**, which is responsible for isolated lissencephaly. The deletion also includes the 14-3-3 gene.

17 Miller beers will give LISa a LISp.

The deletion also includes the 14-3-3 gene.

Isolated Lissencephaly

One form of isolated lissencephaly is due to a mutation in the LIS1 gene on 17p. The gene encodes PAFAH1B1 (platelet activating factor acetylhydrolase isoform 1B, alpha subunit).

LIS1 gene mutations are seen in isolated lissencephaly sequence, Miller-Dieker syndrome, and subcortical band heterotopia (see below).

Another form of isolated lissencephaly is due to a mutation in the DCX gene, which encodes doublecortin, at Xq. Males develop lissencephaly, and heterozygous females have subcortical band heterotopia, also known as double cortex syndrome.

Double cortin has **double standards**.

The **females** have **subcortical band heterotopia**. (women wear headbands!)

The **males** have **lissencephaly**. (men love Lisa!)

Mutations in the LIS1 gene on 17p can cause lissencephaly or subcortical band heterotopia. Also, mutations in DCX on Xq can cause lissencephaly (in males) or subcortical band heterotopia (in females).

Lissencephaly due to a **DCX** mutation tends to be more severe **anteriorly**.
Lissencephaly due to a **LIS1** mutation tends to be more severe **posteriorly,** if there is a difference in the anterior and posterior regions.

Lissencephaly with Agenesis of the Corpus Callosum

There is an X-linked form of lissencephaly that is due to a mutation in the ARX gene on Xp. It is also known as **X-linked lissencephaly with abnormal genitalia (XLAG)**.

These patients have **lissencephaly, absence of the corpus callosum, epilepsy, hypothalamic dysfunction (especially hypothermia),** and **ambiguous genitalia**.

Since it causes ambiguous genitalia, **ARX mutations** make one ask, **AR**e you **XX** or XY?

Lissencephaly with Cerebellar Hypoplasia

There is a lissencephaly associated with cerebellar hypoplasia. It is due to a mutation in the *RELN* gene at 7q, which encodes **reelin**.

To remember that lissencephaly with cerebellar hypoplasia is due to a mutation in reelin:
-A patient with **lissencephaly and cerebellar hypoplasia** will be **reelin' from unsteadiness.**

Cobblestone Lissencephaly (type II)

In cobblestone lissencephaly, the cortex lacks recognizable layers. The neurons are present on the brain surface and in the meninges because they migrate too far. [12]

Syndromic congenital muscular dystrophies (CMD) are associated with cobblestone lissencephaly, eye abnormalities, and muscle weakness.

mild **Fukuyama CMD**, which is found primarily in Japan, is associated with a mutation in the gene on 9q that encodes fukutin.

med **Muscle-eye-brain disease**, which is found common in Finland, is due to a defect in POMGnT1 on 1p.

severe **Walker-Warburg syndrome** is due to a mutation in POMT1 on 9q.

H ydrocephaly
A gyria
R etinal
D ysplasia
E ncephalocele

---

[12] Please see the Neuromuscular Diseases chapter for more information.

Polymicrogyria

Patients with polymicrogyria have small gyri that are increased in number. The most common location is surrounding the Sylvian fissure. This is another disorder of neuronal migration. Genetic, metabolic, and environmental causes, such as intrauterine infection, have been identified.

Different subtypes of polymicrogyria correlate with the brain region affected:
- Bilateral Frontal Polymicrogyria (BFP)-Motor delay, spastic quadriparesis
- Bilateral Fronto-Parietal Polymicrogyria (BFPP)-Motor delay, dysconjugate gaze, cerebellar signs. (Brainstem and cerebellum are also abnormal, and patients have ventriculomegaly.) Associated with gene defects in *GPR56*.
- Bilateral Perisylvian Polymicrogyria (BPP)- Motor delay, pseudobulbar signs, arthrogryposis, lower motor neuron disease
- Bilateral Parasagittal Parieto-Occipital Polymicrogyria (BPPOP)
- Bilateral Generalized Polymicrogyria (BGP)-Motor delay

All of the above are associated with varying degrees of cognitive delay and seizures.

Patients with polymicrogyria have small gyri that are increased in number.

Heterotopia

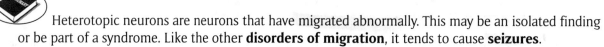

Heterotopic neurons are neurons that have migrated abnormally. This may be an isolated finding or be part of a syndrome. Like the other **disorders of migration**, it tends to cause **seizures**.

Again, to remember the disorders of abnormal neuronal migration, think of little **Lisa** who says:

"She who **migrates, HoPPS** away!"

Lissencephaly, **H**eter**o**topia, **P**olymicrogyria, **P**achygyria, and **S**chizencephaly.

Periventricular Nodular Heterotopia

In periventricular nodular heterotopia, nodules of gray matter line the walls of the ventricle.

Some cases are due to mutations in the FIL-1 gene, which is on Xq and encodes filamin-1. Most cases of this are found in females; it can be a lethal mutation in males.

actin-binding protein

 Mutations in **FIL**-1 cause heterotopic neurons to start to **fill** in the ventricle.

Subcortical Band Heterotopia/Double Cortex Syndrome

A band of heterotopic gray matter is seen in the subcortical region in patients with subcortical band heterotopia/ double cortex syndrome.

Recall that subcortical band heterotopia is found in females with mutations in DCX on Xq; whereas males have lissencephaly. Also, mutations in the LIS1 gene on 17p can cause subcortical band heterotopia or isolated lissencephaly.

To remember that subcortical **band** heterotopia is found in **females** and **lis**sencephaly is in **men**, think of this: **women** wear head**band**s and men love **Lis**a!

Cerebellar Hypoplasia

Hemispheric Cerebellar Hypoplasia

A number of conditions are associated with hemispheric cerebellar hypoplasia. This includes lissencephaly with cerebellar hypoplasia due to reelin mutations, which was mentioned above.

Cerebellar Vermis Hypoplasia

A number of conditions are associated with hypoplasia of the cerebellar vermis. One of these conditions is Dandy-Walker malformation, which was mentioned above. Another is Joubert syndrome.

Joubert Syndrome

Patients with Joubert syndrome have **oculomotor apraxia, hyperpnea alternating with central apnea in neonates,** and **vermal agenesis**.

The midbrain-hindbrain junction looks like a **molar tooth** in Joubert syndrome.

Pontocerebellar Hypoplasia

Pontocerebellar hypoplasia is also found in a number of conditions, some of which are neurodegenerative.

One example is **congenital disorder of glycosylation Ia,** which is associated with **inverted nipples** and **abnormal fat pads**.

Migraine Variants/Migraine Equivalents

To remember the major features of migraines, think of this:
If you get a migraine, you just want to **PUNT** it away!
Phono/Photophobia, **U**nilaterality, **N**ausea, **T**hrobbing

Here is the International Headache Society (IHS) diagnostic criteria for **cOmmon vs. clAssic migraines**:

"cOmmon Migraine" (withOut aura) –

Diagnostic criteria[14]:

A. At least 5 headaches, > 4 - 72 hours in adults and 1-72 hours in children (untreated or unsuccessfully treated), with at least 2 out of 4 items:

1. **U**nilaterality (May be bilateral in young children)
2. **T**hrobbing/Pulsating quality
3. Moderate or severe intensity
4. Aggravation by or avoidance of routine, physical, "Activities of Daily Living"

---

[13] Please see the Metabolic Diseases chapter for more details.

[14] Headache classification committee of the IHS. Classification and diagnostic criteria for headache disorders, cranial neuralgias and facial pain. *Cephalalgia* 1988 8: 1-96.

B. During each headache, at least 1 of the 2 symptoms must occur:

　1. **P**honophobia **and** **P**hotophobia

　2. **N**ausea **and/or** vomiting

"cl**A**ssic migraines" (with **A**ura) –

Diagnostic criteria[15]:

A. At least 1 of the following Aura features:

1. Language difficulty (i.e., aphasia)

2. Unilateral paresthesias or anesthesias (numbness)

3. Unilateral weakness

4. Homonymous visual disturbance

B. At least 2 headaches with at least 3 of the 4 items:

1. At least 1 **fully reversible** Aura

2. Aura lasts > 4 minutes

3. Aura lasts < 60 minutes, unless multiple Auras arise

4. Migraine **follows** Aura after an "asymptomatic stage" > 60 minutes, unless Migraine starts with the Aura

Abdominal Migraine

Patients with abdominal migraines have intermittent attacks of abdominal pain, vomiting, and anorexia.

Acute Confusional Migraine

Acute confusional migraine typically affects children 10 years old or older but may be seen as young as 5 years. The child is disoriented, agitated, and may appear to be in pain. It usually lasts for a few hours and often resolves after the child sleeps.

---

[15] Headache classification committee of the IHS. Classification and diagnostic criteria for headache disorders, cranial neuralgias and facial pain. *Cephalalgia* 1988 8: 1-96.

Alice In Wonderland Syndrome (AIWS)

Patients with Alice In Wonderland Syndrome experience **spatial distortion** and **illusions** before a migraine. For example, objects may appear small or large (**micropsia** or **macropsia**, respectively).

Similarly, patients with AIWS may also lose a sense of time, which seems to pass very slowly.

Consequently, velocity is also misperceived – making movement seem frighteningly distorted.

Other possible causes of AIWS are brain tumors, seizures, hallucinogenic drugs, and infectious mononucleosis. Often, objects can appear small and distant (teliopsia) or large and close (peliopsia). Another symptom of AIWS is sound distortion, with any tiny noise being perceived as a clattering sound!

 To remember the features of this syndrome, just think of the book "Alice in Wonderland" written by Lewis Carroll. The main character Alice says: "It was much pleasanter at home when one wasn't always growing larger and smaller, and being ordered about by mice and rabbits."

Benign Paroxysmal Vertigo

Benign paroxysmal vertigo is characterized by **intermittent episodes of unsteadiness** that may be accompanied by **nystagmus** and/or **vomiting.**

It tends to occur in **young children**.

Basilar Artery Migraine (BAM)

Patients with **BAM**, which is also called **Bickerstaff's Syndrome** or **Brainstem Migraine**, or **Basilar-Type Migraine**, have episodes of **vertigo, ataxia,** dysarthria, tinnitus, and **vision changes** such as **diplopia**.

This may be associated with **nausea** and **vomiting**. An **occipital headache** may precede, occur with, or follow the symptoms. Until it goes away, it may be severely disabling, unsurprisingly!

Aborting BAM with triptans or other vasoconstrictors is **<u>contraindicated!!</u>**

Cyclic Vomiting

Cyclic vomiting is characterized by **intermittent episodes of vomiting**, which can be severe enough to cause dehydration.

It tends to occur in **infants and children**.

Other conditions such as metabolic disease and intermittent bowel obstruction should be ruled out.

Hemiplegic Migraine

Hemiplegic migraine is a type of migraine with aura. Patients with hemiplegic migraine have a **transient hemiparesis** followed by a headache. Hemisensory changes, visual field defects, and aphasia may accompany the weakness.

There are sporadic and familial forms.

Familial Hemiplegic Migraine

Familial Hemiplegic Migraine-1 (FHM1)

FHM1 is due to a mutation in the *CACNA1A* gene on 19p.

Recall that mutations in the CACNA1A (voltage-dependent P/Q-type calcium channel alpha-1A) gene also cause spinocerebellar ataxia-6 (SCA 6) and episodic ataxia-2 (EA2).

To remember that gene *CACNA1A* on chromosome 19p causes FHM1, EA2, and SCA6, think of this:

Have a <u>FEAST</u> on route <u>A1A</u> for <u>19</u> people!

The disorders in this mnemonic are <u>in order</u>: FHM-**1**, EA-**2**, and SCA-**6**. Route **A1A**=CACN**A1A**; 19 people = 19p.

Familial Hemiplegic Migraine-2 (FHM2)

FHM2 is due to a mutation in the *ATP1A2* (the alpha-2 subunit of the sodium/potassium pump) gene on 1q.

Mutations in this gene also cause alternating hemiplegia of childhood, which shares clinical features with FHM.

Alternating hemiplegia of childhood, which presents at less than 18 months of age, causes episodes of paralysis and involuntary movements lasting minutes to days.

Familial Hemiplegic Migraine-3 (FHM3)

FHM3 is due to a mutation in the *SCN1A* gene.

Recall that mutations in the SCN1A gene also cause generalized epilepsy with febrile seizures plus and Dravet syndrome.

Familial Hemiplegic Migraine-4 (FHM4)

FHM4 is due to a mutation on 1q.

Menstrual Migraine (Catamenial Migraine)

Interestingly, the ratio for Women:Men for migraine is 3:1.

>50% of women with migraines have them around their menstrual cycle.

>10% of women migraineurs had them start at menarche.

>65% of women migraineurs had them disappear while pregnant (not menstruating).

Nearly all do not have Aura. Migraine with Aura is likely unrelated to the menstrual cycle.

Pure Menstrual Migraine Without Aura

Diagnostic criteria[16]:

A. Attacks, in a menstruating woman, fulfilling the criteria for Migraine without Aura

B. Attacks that occur exclusively from days -2 to +3 of menstruation in at least 2 out of 3 menstrual cycles and at no other times of the cycle.

---

[16] Headache Classification Subcommittee of the International Headache Society (2004). "The Classification of Headache Disorders, 2nd Edition". *Cephalagia* (Oxford, England, UK: Blackwell Publishing) 24 (Supplement 1).

Menstrually-Related Migraine Without Aura

Diagnostic criteria[17]:

> A. Attacks, in a menstruating woman, fulfilling the criteria for Migraine without Aura
>
> B. Attacks that occur exclusively from days -2 to +3 of menstruation in at least 2 out of 3 menstrual cycles, and additionally at other times of the menstrual cycle. (Note: There is no day 0.)

Treatment

The reason for the distinction between pure menstrual and menstrually-related migraines is that women with migraines within that 5-day period (-2 to +3) benefit more from hormone therapy than from vasoconstrictors or triptans.

Pathophysiology

Menstrual migraines may be due to Estrogen withdrawal. However, women taking Oral Contraceptive Pills (OCPs) or Hormone Replacement Therapy (HRT), which suppress the regular hormonal changes leading to menstruation from withdrawal of Progesterone concentrations, could have these migraines from Progesterone withdrawal.

Ophthalmoplegic Migraine

Ophthalmoplegia and **orbital pain** characterize ophthalmoplegic migraine. Patients may also have **ptosis** and a **dilated pupil**.

During events, **MRI may show thickening of CN III with enhancement**.

Paroxysmal Torticollis

Patients with paroxysmal torticollis have **episodes of head tilt**, **vomiting**, and **ataxia** that last for **hours to days**.

It tends to occur in **young children**.

Often, there's a **family history of migraine**.

---

[17] Headache Classification Subcommittee of the International Headache Society (2004). "The Classification of Headache Disorders, 2nd Edition". *Cephalagia* (Oxford, England, UK: Blackwell Publishing) 24 (Supplement 1).

Retinal Migraine/Ophthalmic Migraine

Patients with retinal migraines have **positive or negative visual phenomenon in association with a headache** (before, during, or after the headache). This migraine variant tends to occur **during adolescence**.

Triggers for migraine

Many triggers may provoke a migraine attack, including:
- hunger
- caffeine
- nitrates in some foods
- alcohol
- hormonal changes
- emotional or physical stress, or over-exertion
- environmental factors (i.e., weather, altitude)
- sleep deprivation
- medications
- bright lights

Concussion vs. Contusion

Concussion

Acute confusion or Loss Of Consciousness (LOC) after Traumatic Brain Injury (TBI), often with decreased reflexes, paralysis, bradycardia, and even respiratory distress, and later, post-traumatic amnesia. Neuroimaging, EEG, and CSF are usually normal.

Grades of Concussion with Durations and Symptoms, as per the **American Academy of Neurology** (AAN):

	Grade I	**Grade II**	**Grade III (a/b)**
Symptoms	Confusion, but no LOC	Confusion, but no LOC	Yes, LOC
Duration	lasts <15 minutes	lasts >15 minutes	IIIa: lasts seconds IIIb: lasts minutes

Contusion (contusio cerebri)

A brain tissue "bruise" that occurs in 20–30% of TBI patients, resulting in microhemorrhages (or even worse, like SDH) on neuroimaging and residual hemosiderin-laden macrophages (orange/yellow tinged) on autopsy. Frontal contusion can cause anosmia from injury to the cribriform plate and the Olfactory Nerve (CN I).

The top causes of TBI are: Motor Vehicle Collisions (MVC), falls, sports injuries, and bicycle accidents, in that order.

The Most

Sydenham's chorea is the most common **acquired chorea of childhood**.

Intraventricular hemorrhage is the most common **neonatal intracranial hemorrhage**.

The most common cause of **facial asymmetry at birth** is **weakness/aplasia of the depressor anguli oris muscle**.

Pediatric Neurology Quiz

(Answers on page 757)

1. When you are given a case of a neonate with hiccups, seizures, and a burst-suppression pattern on the EEG you should think of which condition?

    A. Maple syrup urine disease

    B. Nonketotic hyperglycinemia

    C. Glucose Transporter Type 1 Deficiency

    D. DiGeorge's syndrome

2. A neonate with high output congestive heart failure and a cranial bruit may have this condition.

    A. A subdural hematoma

    B. Grade II IVH

    C. Holoprosencephaly

    D. Vein of Galen malformation

3. Match condition and the gene with which it is associated.

    1) Angelman syndrome   A. CACNA1A gene

    2) Rett syndrome   B. UBE3A

    3) Familial Hemiplegic Migraine-1   C. MECP2

    4) Periventricular Nodular Heterotopia   D. FIL-1

4. Pregnant women should take which of the following to prevent neural tube defects?

    A. Iron

    B. Vitamin K

    C. Folate

    D. Vitamin B12

5. Cobblestone lissencephaly is associated with

    A. Trisomy 13

    B. Trisomy 18

    C. Congenital muscular dystrophy

    D. LIS1 mutations

6. Link the lissencephaly with its gene mutation. An answer may be used more than once.

      1) Miller-Dieker syndrome   A. Reelin

      2) Isolated lissencephaly   B. LIS1

      3) Lissencephaly with agenesis of the corpus callosum   C. ARX

      4) Lissencephaly with cerebellar hypoplasia   D. Filamin-1

7. Match the syndromes.

      1) Dandy-Walker syndrome   A. CATCH

      2) DiGeorge's syndrome   B. CRASH

      3) MASA syndrome   C. PHACES

      4) Velocardiofacial syndrome

8. Which of the following disorders do NOT involve a migration abnormality?

      1) Heterotopia

      2) Polymicrogyria

      3) Pachygyria,

      4) Schizencephaly.

      5) All of the above involve migration abnormalities

9. Which chromosome is affected in Cri-du-chat Syndrome?

      1) 8q duplication

      2) 5p deletion

      3) 1p duplication

      4) 18q deletion

10. The top cause of TBI in the USA is:

      1) Motor Vehicle Collisions (MVCs)

      2) Falls

      3) Sports injuries

      4) Bicycle accidents

      5) Studying too hard for the Neurology Boards

Chapter 15

Stroke

National Statistics

#4 CAUSE OF MORTALITY in the USA

Every year 150,000 people die from stroke.

- *Stroke accounts for **1:18 deaths** in the US annually.*
- *The stroke death rate fell 45%, and the actual number of stroke deaths fell 15% in the past decade.*

Stroke was the third leading cause of death until recently but stroke doctors are doing such a bang up job these days keeping stroke patients alive, reversing strokes entirely, and treating stroke risk factors that stroke itself has just slipped below pulmonary diseases, now the new #3. Nevertheless, stroke is still a major public health burden nationwide and worldwide.

#1 CAUSE OF MORBIDITY (disability) in the USA

Every year 800,000 people have a stroke, 600,000 1st attacks, 200,000 recurrent.

- *Every **40 seconds**, someone in the US has a stroke.*
- ***HALF** of all hospitalizations for acute neurologic disease are for stroke.*
- *The cost is > $30 Billion / year for medical and physical/occupational therapy for stroke survivors.*

Vascular Anatomy

The Internal Carotid arteries supply the anterior circulation, and the Vertebral arteries and Basilar artery supply the posterior circulation.

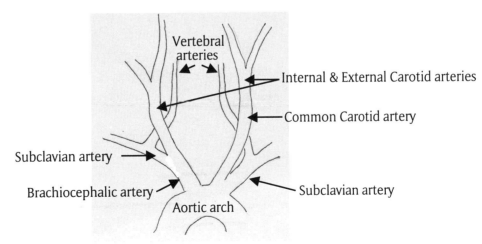

The **right common carotid** arises from the brachiocephalic artery.

The **left common carotid** arises from the aorta.

The **vertebral arteries** arise from the subclavian arteries.

The **left subclavian artery** arises from the aorta; the **right subclavian arises** from the brachiocephalic artery.

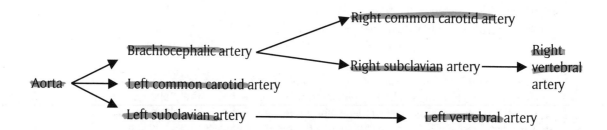

The aorta gives off the brachiocephalic, left common carotid, and left subclavian arteries.

The aorta gives off the brachiocephalic, left common carotid, and left subclavian arteries.

The aorta gives off **Common B.S.**: the left **Common** carotid, the **B**rachiocephalic, and the left **S**ubclavian arteries.

The brachiocephalic copies off the aorta and gives off a common carotid and a subclavian (the right common carotid and subclavian).

The subclavians give off the vertebrals, which give rise to the basilar artery.

Anterior Circulation

Internal Carotid Artery (ICA)

The 7 segments of the ICA are:
Cervical (C1), **Petrous** (C2), **Lacerum** (C3),
> – *Note: C2 and C3 comprise the "Petrous portion"*

Cavernous (C4), **Clinoid** (C5), **Ophthalmic** (C6), and **Communicating** or terminal segment (C7).
> – *Note: C6 and C7 comprise the "Supraclinoid portion"*

Mnemonic for ICA segments (in order): **Cer**tain **Pe**ople **L**ike **Cave**s **Cl**eaned **O**n **Comm**ission!!

After the C7 segment, arise the five Major branches of the ICA:
· **Ophthalmic** artery (first major branch)
· **Posterior** communicating artery
· **An**terior choroidal artery
· **Middle** cerebral artery (MCA)
· **An**terior cerebral artery (ACA)

 Mnemonic for ICA branches (in order): **O**h, **Po**lish **An**y **M**uddy **A**rea!!
· **O**phthalmic artery (first major branch)
· **Po**sterior communicating artery
· **An**terior choroidal artery
· **M**iddle cerebral artery (MCA)
· **An**terior cerebral artery (ACA)

Ophthalmic Artery

As mentioned above, the ophthalmic artery is the first major branch of the internal carotid artery.

Amaurosis fugax is due to emboli causing temporary occlusion of the retinal artery, which is a branch of the ophthalmic artery.[1]

Posterior Communicating Artery

The posterior communicating artery supplies the hypothalamus, optic tract, and anterior and medial thalamus.

An aneurysm here can cause a CN III palsy.

The posterior communicating arteries connect the anterior and posterior circulation.

To remember the brain territories supplied by the posterior communicating arteries, think of the **Posterior COM**pany (**PCOM**) supplying **O**ld **T**ime **HAM** on **Th**ursdays, meaning the posterior communicating arteries supply the **O**ptic **T**ract and the **H**ypo-, **A**nterior, and **M**edial **Th**alami.

---

[1] For more information, please see the Neuro-ophthalmology chapter.

Anterior Choroidal Artery

The anterior choroidal artery supplies the medial globus pallidus, tail of the caudate, genu and posterior limb of the internal capsule, uncus, hippocampus, portions of the thalamus (ventral anterior, ventral lateral, and lateral geniculate nuclei), optic tract, origin of optic radiations, cerebral peduncle, red nucleus, subthalamus, substantia nigra, and choroid plexus.

A stroke in the anterior choroidal artery territory causes contralateral hemisensory loss, hemiparesis (due to involvement of the posterior limb of the internal capsule), and a **homonymous hemianopia that spares the horizontal meridian**.

The visual field defect with a stroke in the **right** anterior choroidal artery distribution, which causes a lateral geniculate body lesion, looks like this:

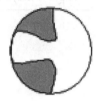

 The anterior choroidal supplies **HOT CROSS GUCCI**:

> **H**ippocampus
> **O**ptic tract
> **T**halamus (ventral anterior, ventral lateral, and lateral geniculate nuclei)
>
> **C**audate (tail of the caudate)
> **R**ed nucleus
> **O**ptic radiations
> **S**ubthalamus
> **S**ubstantia nigra
>
> **G**lobus pallidus (medial)
> **U**ncus
> **C**erebral peduncle
> **C**horoid plexus
> **I**nternal capsule

Anterior Cerebral Artery (ACA)

The ACA supplies the medial cortex of the frontal lobes and anterior parietal lobes.

Clinical Findings with ACA Strokes

ACA infarction causes contralateral **weakness and sensory loss** primarily involving the leg **(Leg > Arm > Face)**.

Alien hand syndrome can be seen due to damage to the supplementary motor area.[2]

Left arm apraxia is seen with involvement of the anterior corpus callosum.

If the dominant hemisphere is infarcted, patients may have **transcortical motor aphasia.**

On the **TCM** channel (Turner Classic Movies), you can watch **reruns** of **silent** films (TCM patients can repeat but not speak).

Bilateral medial frontal lobe damage can cause **lower extremity weakness, incontinence,** and **akinetic mutism.**

Akinetic mutism may occur with bilateral medial frontal damage e.g. to the **cing**ulate gyrus. Patients with Akinetic mutism won't be able to **cing**, either!

The recurrent artery of Heubner (also known as the medial striate artery) is a major branch of the ACA.

The recurrent artery of Huebner supplies the head of the caudate, anterior limb of the internal capsule, and anterior putamen.

Infarction in the territory of the artery of Heubner causes contralateral face and arm weakness.

The letter A recurs in ACA, so the recurrent artery of Heubner is a branch of the ACA.

Infarction of the anterior cerebral artery causes contralateral lower extremity weakness and sensory loss; however, infarction of the recurrent artery of Heubner, which is a branch of the ACA, causes contralateral face and arm weakness.

---

2 Please see the Behavioral Neurology chapter for more information.

Middle Cerebral Artery (MCA)

Branches of MCA:

Divisions of MCA

Superior division

Supplies lateral cortex above the Sylvian fissure.

Inferior division

Supplies lateral cortex below the Sylvian fissure (that is not supplied by the posterior cerebral artery).

Lenticulostriate penetrators

Medial lenticulostriate arteries

Supply lateral segment of the globus pallidus.

Lateral lenticulostriate arteries

Supply putamen, superior internal capsule, caudate, corona radiata.

Clinical Syndromes Seen with MCA Strokes

Infarction at the **MCA stem** causes global aphasia, contralateral hemiplegia, contralateral sensory loss, and contralateral homonymous hemianopsia.

Patients may have a gaze preference toward the side of the lesion in the acute period.

If the dominant hemisphere is affected, the patient will have aphasia.

If the nondominant hemisphere is affected, the patient will have neglect and may have anosognosia (denial of impairment).

Handedness / Dominance / Laterality

~95% of RIGHT-handers process speech in the LEFT hemisphere.

Only ~50% of **LEFT**-handers process speech in their **LEFT** hemisphere, like most right-handers.

However, ~25% of left-handers process speech **EQUALLY IN BOTH** hemispheres,

And ~25% process speech in the **RIGHT** hemisphere.

Amaurosis fugax differentiates the ICA syndrome from the MCA syndrome.

Infarction of the **superior division MCA** resembles MCA stem infarction, except the weakness involves the face and arm more than the leg. Also, if the lesion involves the dominant hemisphere, Broca's aphasia is seen rather than global aphasia.

If the nondominant hemisphere is affected, the patient will have neglect.

Wernicke's aphasia is seen with **inferior division MCA** syndromes involving the dominant hemisphere. If the nondominant hemisphere is affected, the patient will have neglect. Patients may have a visual field cut.

A **lenticulostriate** infarction causes a contralateral **pure motor hemiparesis.**

Arterial supply to the internal capsule:
- Anterior limb: recurrent artery of Heubner (branch of the ACA)
- Genu and middle and inferior part of posterior limb: Anterior choroidal artery (off the ICA)
- Superior aspect of anterior and posterior limbs: Lenticulostriates (branches of the MCA)

Circle of Willis

The anterior and posterior circulations are connected in the Circle of Willis.

Circle of Willis

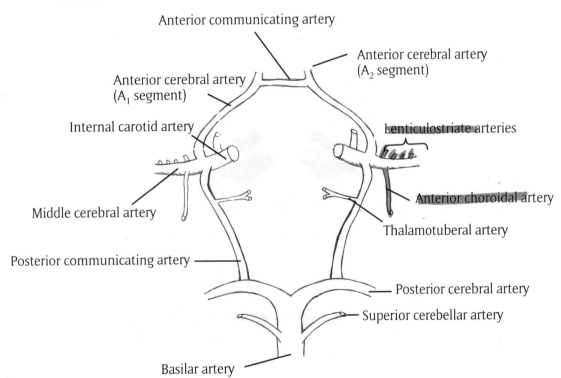

Posterior Circulation

Vertebral Artery

The vertebral artery arises from the subclavian artery.

Branches of the vertebral artery:

PICA

Anterior spinal artery

Posterior spinal artery

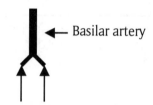

Vertebral arteries

 The vertebral arteries form an upside-down V when they meet to form the basilar artery.

Posterior Inferior Cerebellar Artery (PICA)

The PICA is the largest branch of the vertebral artery.

It supplies the inferior cerebellum and dorsolateral medulla.

Occlusion of the PICA can cause the lateral medullary (Wallenberg) syndrome. See below.

Anterior Spinal Artery

The anterior spinal artery supplies the anterior 2/3 of the cord.

This includes the lateral corticospinal tracts, lateral spinothalamic tracts, and anterior horns.

Therefore, infarction causes paralysis and loss of pain and temperature sensation below the lesion.

The dorsal columns are supplied by the posterior spinal arteries, so **vibration and position sense are preserved**.

Posterior Spinal Artery

The posterior spinal arteries, of which there are two, supply the dorsal aspect of the cord. They may arise from the vertebral or posterior inferior cerebellar arteries.

Basilar Artery

The basilar artery is formed when the left and right vertebral arteries merge.

Branches:

· Paramedian and circumferential perforators

· AICA (Anterior Inferior Cerebellar Arteries)

· SCA (Superior Cerebellar Arteries)

· IAA (Internal Auditory Artery – can be branch of AICA)

· PCA (Posterior Cerebral Arteries)

Posterior Circulation

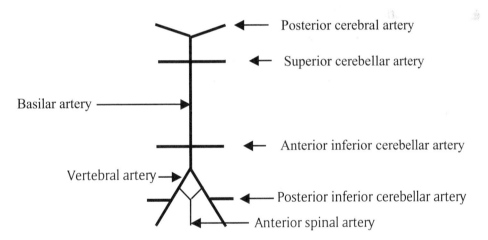

Posterior cerebral artery

Superior cerebellar artery

Basilar artery

Anterior inferior cerebellar artery

Vertebral artery

Posterior inferior cerebellar artery

Anterior spinal artery

Anterior Inferior Cerebellar Artery (AICA)

The AICA supplies the caudal lateral pons tegmentum and ventrolateral cerebellum.

Occlusion of the AICA can cause the Lateral Inferior Pontine Syndrome (LIPS). It may also cause the Medial Inferior Pontine Syndrome (MIPS) if the occlusion is near the origin of the artery. Please see below.

An occlusion of the AICA can cause unilateral deafness.

Think of the **AI** in **AICA** as standing for **A**uditory **I**mpairment.

To remember that **Lateral Inferior Pontine Syndrome** is due to an occlusion of the AICA, remember that you use your **LIPS** when eating **ACAI** berries.

Superior Cerebellar Artery (SCA)

The **S**CA **S**upplies the **S**uperior cerebellum, **S**uperior cerebellar peduncle, the **S**uperior pons, the **S**ympathetic tract, and **S**pinothalamic tracts.

The **S**CA **S**upplies **5** **S**uperior **S**tructures (and **5** looks like an **S**, surprisingly!)

Occlusion of the SCA results in nystagmus, ipsilateral ataxia, contralateral loss of pain and temperature (spinothalamic involvement), and an ipsilateral Horner's (due to involvement of the sympathetic tract). Patients may have also partial deafness or palatal myoclonus.

Internal Auditory Artery (IAA)

The IAA may arise from AICA or the basilar artery.

It supplies the auditory, vestibular, and facial nerves.

Posterior Cerebral Artery (PCA)

The PCA supplies the inferomedial temporal lobes, occipital lobes, midbrain, and thalamus.

Branches of the PCA:

Mesencephalic artery

This gives rise to **interpeduncular branches** which supply the red nuclei, substantia nigra, medial lemnisci, medial longitudinal fasciculi, medial cerebral peduncles, and oculomotor and trochlear nerves and nuclei.

Thalamoperforate branches/ paramedian thalamic arteries

These supply the inferior, medial, and anterior thalamus.

The **artery of Percheron** is a variant of these branches. In this situation, an artery from one PCA supplies the medial thalami bilaterally. **Occlusion of this vessel causes bilateral lesions of the medial thalami**.

Each Thalamus looks like a golf ball. **Where do you put your golf ball? Perch-her-on Bil's Tee! (Percheron Bilateral Thalami)**

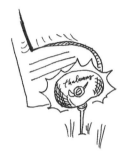

Thalamo-**Geniculate** branches

These supply the Lateral **Geniculate** Body (LGB) and central and posterior thalamus.

Posterior choroidal artery

Supplies posterior thalamus, posterior hippocampus, and choroid plexus.

Recall that the anterior choroidal artery is a branch of the ICA and also supplies the thalamus, hippocampus, and choroid plexus.

Cortical branches

Inferior temporal arteries

These supply the inferior aspect of the temporal lobes.

Parieto-occipital artery

Calcarine artery

This supplies occipital cortex.

To remember the Posterior Cerebral Artery branches think of **P**oliticians **C**oasting **A**long (**PCA**) like **MITT** (**M**esencephalic artery, **I**nterpeduncular artery, **T**halamoperferator branches, **T**halamogeniculate branches), who was **P**olitically **C**orrect **In Pa**sadena, **Cal**ifornia (**P**osterior **C**horoidal artery, **In**ferior temporal artery, **Pa**rietal occipital artery, **Cal**carine artery).

PCA infarcts cause a number of the conditions from the Behavioral Neurology chapter.

Alexia without Agraphia

PCA infarcts involving the occipital cortex and splenium of the corpus callosum of the dominant hemisphere can cause alexia without agraphia.

Without your spleen, you'll have alexia **without** agraphia: you can write a book without your spleen, but you can't read what you've written!

Anton's syndrome

Anton's syndrome is denial of cortical blindness. It is due to bilateral occipital lobe damage, which can occur with bilateral PCA infarcts.

Bálint syndrome

Balint syndrome is characterized by oculomotor-apraxia, optic ataxia, problems with depth perception, and simultagnosia.

It is due to bilateral parietal-occipital damage.

Korsakoff syndrome

Korsakoff syndrome can be seen with a lesion of both mediodorsal nuclei of the thalamus or the dominant mediodorsal nucleus due to occlusion of the paramedian thalamic branch(es).

Prosopagnosia

The inability to recognize familiar faces. This can be seen with bilateral mesiotemporal-occipital lesions.

Ischemic Stroke

Thalamic Strokes

Thalamus

The thalamus is supplied primarily by the posterior communicating arteries and the perimesencephalic branch of the posterior cerebral artery (PCA). The anterior choroidal artery (off the ICA) supplies the ventral anterior, ventral lateral, and lateral geniculate nuclei.

Thalamic infarctions tend to occur in these distributions: anterior, dorsal, paramedian, and posterolateral.[3]

Region of Thalamus	Arterial Supply	Clinical Syndromes
Anterior	Pol**A**r or tubero-thalamic artery*	**A**bulia, **A**pathy, **A**phasia and **A**ffect (Neuropsychological) changes
Dorsal	Posterior choroidal artery†	Visual field defect
Paramedian	Posterior thalamoperforating arteries (paramedian thalamic arteries)†	Altered mental status and vertical gaze abnormalities
Posterolateral	Thalamo-**Geniculate** artery†	Pure sensory stroke, sensorimotor stroke, or Dejerine-Roussy syndrome

*The polar artery is a branch of the posterior communicating artery.
†These are branches of the PCA.

---

[3] Brazis PW, Masdeu JC, Biller J. Localization in clinical neurology: 4th edition. Philadelphia: Lippincott Williams & Wilkins, 2001;407-410.

The Thalamus

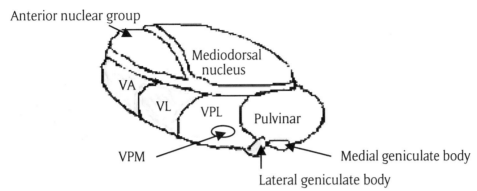

VA= ventral anterior nucleus, VL = ventral lateral nucleus, VPL = ventral posterior lateral nucleus, VPM= ventral posterior medial nucleus

Anterior Thalamus

 Occlusion of the pol**A**r or tubero-thalamic artery results in a stroke in the **A**nterior thalamus.

 Abulia and **A**pathy are seen with **A**nterior thalamic strokes, as is **A**phasia and **A**ffect changes (below).

Recall from the Behavioral Neurology chapter that patients with **A**bulia lack initiative and have delayed, slowed responses. They **A**re **A**ble but lack initiative to **A**ct.

 Bi**polar** disorder is an **Affect**ive disorder, and strokes in the **polA**r artery affect one's **Affect**.

Thalamic Aphasia

Typically, a fluent speech, with intact repetition, but with a comprehension deficit, including **N**eologisms (making up new words), **A**ttention fluctuations, **P**araphasias (word substitution), and **P**erseverations (word repetition despite lack of stimulus).

Patients with Thalamic Aphasia want to take a **NAPP** – **N**eologism, **A**ttention fluctuation, **P**araphasia, and **P**erseveration.

Infarcts in the dominant hemisphere can cause "Thalamic Aphasia"; whereas, lesions in the nondominant hemisphere cause hemineglect.

Dorsal Thalamus

Occlusion of the posterior choroidal artery causes a dorsal thalamic lesion.

 This results in visual field defects such as a **homonymous quadrantanopia or homonymous horizontal sectoranopias.**

Paramedian Thalamus

A stroke in the paramedian thalamus results from occlusion of the posterior thalamoperforating arteries.

 Initially patients may be **somnolent** and have a **vertical gaze paresis.**

Later, **disinhibition** may be seen because this lesion results in disconnection of the thalamus from the frontal lobe.

Amnesia may also occur.

As mentioned above, **Korsakoff syndrome** can be seen due to an occlusion of the paramedian thalamic branch(es).

Posterolateral Thalamus

Lesions of the posterolateral thalamus are due to an occlusion of the thalamogeniculate artery. This can result in a pure sensory stroke, sensorimotor stroke, or Dejerine-Roussy syndrome.

Dejerine-Roussy syndrome is characterized by:

· Contralateral hemianesthesia and hemiataxia.
· Dysesthesia.
· Transient hemiparesis.
· Choreoathetoid movements.

Brainstem Strokes

Cranial Nerves and Brainstem Level

	Midbrain	**Pons**	**Medulla**
Medial	CN III nucleus and nerve (rostral midbrain), CN IV nerve and nucleus (caudal midbrain), mesencephalic trigeminal tract.	CN VI nucleus and nerve and CN VII (which wraps around the nucleus of CN VI)	CN XII nucleus and nerve
Lateral	————	————	Spinal trigeminal nucleus, vestibular nucleus, nucleus ambiguus, nucleus tractus solitarius, dorsal motor nucleus of CN X, and CN X

Brainstem: Midbrain

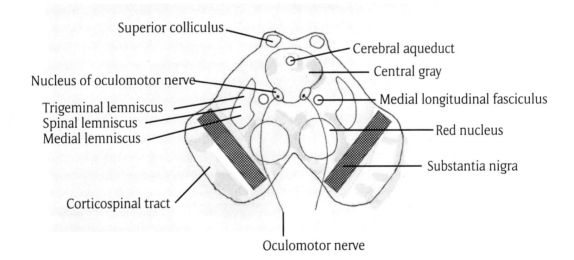

Medial Midbrain

	Cranial Nerves	Other Structures	Blood Supply
Rostral	CN III nerve and nucleus, mesencephalic trigeminal tract	MLF, Edinger-Westphal nucleus, superior colliculus, red nucleus, substantia nigra, corticospinal tract	PCA
Caudal	CN IV nerve and nucleus, mesencephalic trigeminal tract	MLF, decussation of the superior cerebellar peduncles, red nucleus, substantia nigra, corticospinal tract	PCA

MLF= medial longitudinal fasciculus, PCA = posterior cerebral artery.

Lateral Midbrain

	Cranial Nerves	Other Structures	Blood Supply
Rostral	—	Corticospinal tract, substantia nigra, medial lemniscus, medial geniculate body	PCA
Caudal	—	Corticospinal tract, substantia nigra, medial lemniscus	PCA

CN = Cranial nerves

Weber's Syndrome

In Weber's syndrome, the lesion is in ventral midbrain, involving CN III and the cerebral peduncle.

Patients have an ipsilateral CN III palsy and contralateral weakness.

MNEMONIC

Weber's syndrome is associated with **we**akness.

Claude's Syndrome

Claude's syndrome is due to a lesion of the midbrain tegmentum affecting the red nucleus, CN III, and the brachium conjunctivum.

Patients have an ipsilateral CN III palsy and contralateral ataxia and tremor.

To remember that Claude's syndrome is due to a lesion of the red nucleus, think of Santa Claus in a red suit.

 To remember that Claude's syndrome is associated with ataxia and tremor, remember **Cl**aude is **cl**umsy.

Benedikt's Syndrome

Benedikt's syndrome is due to a lesion of the midbrain tegmentum affecting the red nucleus, CN III, the corticospinal tract, and the brachium conjunctivum (decussation of superior cerebellar peduncles).

Patients have an ipsilateral CN III palsy and contralateral weakness, ataxia, and tremor.

 Benedikt's syndrome involves the **B**rachium.

 Benedikt involves symptoms of **B**oth Weber syndrome and Claude syndrome.

Parinaud's Syndrome

Parinaud's syndrome is due to a lesion compressing the dorsal midbrain and pretectal area.

 A **CRUEL** constellation of eye findings are seen in Parinaud's syndrome:

1. **C**onvergence-**R**etraction nystagmus on attempted up-gaze
2. Paralysis of **U**pgaze and accommodation
3. **E**yelid retraction (Collier sign)
4. **L**ight-near dissociation

Think of Parinaud's syndrome as paralyzed syndrome due to paralysis of voluntary vertical gaze, especially upgaze, and paralysis of accommodation.

The patients with Parinaud's syndrome and paranoia should be pitied, because they can't look to see if someone is dropping something on them.

 To remember that Parinaud's syndrome is associated with the **pretectal area**, remember that *when one is paranoid, one **protects** oneself.* **When one is paranoid (Parinaud's), one protects (pretectal) oneself.**

Brainstem: Pons

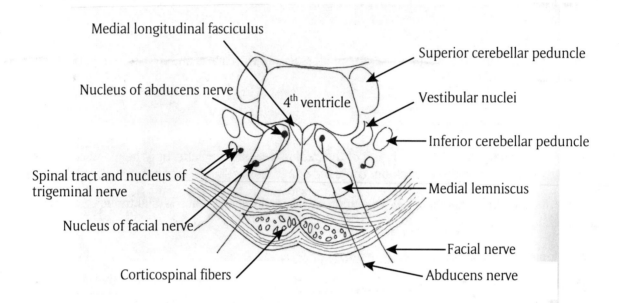

	Cranial Nerves Affected	Other Structures	Blood Supply
Medial pons	CN VI nucleus and nerve, CN VII nerve	Pyramidal tract, MLF, ML	Basilar artery
Lateral pons	Nuclei of CN VII and VIII, spinal trigeminal nucleus and tract, CN V.	MCP, sympathetic tract, ST tract	Basilar artery (rostral pons) and AICA (caudal pons)

AICA= anterior inferior cerebellar artery, ML= medial lemniscus, MLF= medial longitudinal fasciculus, MCP= middle cerebellar peduncle, ST= spinothalamic tract.

Millard-Gubler Syndrome "Hemiparesis Alternans"

Millard-Gubler syndrome is due to a lesion in the ventral pons. It involves CN 6 and 7 and the corticospinal tract.

Patients have an **ipsilateral lateral rectus palsy, ipsilateral peripheral 7th nerve palsy**, and a **contralateral (facial sparing) hemiparesis**. Because one hemi-face is weak and yet the contralateral hemi-body is weak, this **Millard-Gubler Syndrome** is also known as **"Hemiparesis Alternans"**.

Millard has 7 letters, and Gubler has 6. Therefore the syndrome involves cranial nerves 6 and 7.

Millard-Gubler was the **V**ice **P**residential (**V**entral **P**ons) **C**andidate **S**eeking **T**raction (**CST**= **C**ortico**S**pinal **T**ract) in **'67** (CN **6** & **7**).

Millard sounds like Mallard. Mallard ducks are found in ponds, so **Millard-Gubler involves the pons**.

Locked-in Syndrome

Locked-in syndrome is due to bilateral **v**entral **p**ontine lesions. It is a nightmare, and survivors are often **dead** in weeks/months.

It can occur with central pontine myelinolysis, due to rapid correction of hyponatremia, but also from an acute clot in the Basilar Artery resulting in a devastating stroke.

Patients with locked-in-syndrome are quadriparetic due to **C**ortico**S**pinal **T**ract involvement and can't speak due to **C**ortico-**B**ulbar **T**ract involvement. Face and horizontal eye movements are also impaired, due to CN **6** & **7** involvement, but **patients can blink and move their eyes vertically. Despite such dramatic face and limb weakness, the patient is alert and awake as cortex is spared.**

> Eye deviation in frontal versus pontine strokes:
>
> With pontine strokes, the eyes look at the hemiparesis.
>
> With pontine strokes, the eyes ponder the paresis.
>
> With frontal lobe strokes, the eyes look toward the lesion and away from the paresis.
>
> With frontal lobe strokes, the eyes focus on the infarct.

The two (bilateral) **V**ice **P**residential (**V**entral **P**ons) **C**andidates **S**eeking **T**raction (**CST**= **C**ortico**S**pinal **T**ract) in **'67** (CN **6** & **7**) were **locked-in** a **dead** tie because their votes **C**ouldn't **B**e **T**allied (**C**ortico **B**ulbar **T**ract).

Lateral Inferior Pontine Syndrome (LIPS)

The Lateral Inferior Pontine Syndrome (LIPS) involves CN 5, 7, 8 (nerve and nucleus); the PPRF; the spinothalamic tract; the middle cerebellar peduncle; and the cerebellum. **It can be seen with occlusion of the AICA.**

- Involvement of the main sensory nucleus and descending tract of CN V results in decreased **facial** sensation.
- Ipsilateral **facial** paralysis is due to facial nerve or nucleus involvement.
- Nystagmus, vomiting, and vertigo results from involvement of the **V**estibular nerve or nucleus.
- **E**ar deafness and tinnitus is due to involvement of the auditory nerve or cochlear nuclei.
- PPRF lesion causes gaze paresis to the side of the lesion.
- Decreased pain and temperature of the contralateral body is due to **S**pino**T**halamic tract involvement.
- Ipsilateral ataxia results from involvement of the middle cerebellar peduncle, **R**eticular Nucleus, and cerebellar hemisphere.

To remember the features of The Lateral Inferior Pontine Syndrome (**LIPS**), think of this exclamation: "**AICA**!!! His **LIPS** are the **VERST**! I just can't **face** him!"

V- **V**estibular nucleus/nerve

E - **E**ars (deafness/tinnitus, auditory nerve, cochlear nuclei)

R - **R**eticular Nucleus, MCP, PPRF

ST - **S**pino**T**halamic tract

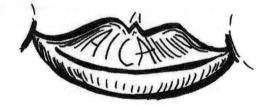

face – CN V and VII (ipsilateral facial numbness and weakness)

Medial Inferior Pontine Syndrome (MIPS)

The medial inferior pontine syndrome (MIPS) is also known as Foville syndrome. The pontine structures affected include the corticospinal tract, the medial lemniscus, and the abducens nerve. Depending on the size of the infarct it can also involve the facial nerve. It has many similarities to medial medullary syndrome, but because it is located higher up in the brainstem, in the pons, it involves higher cranial nerve nuclei (CN VI instead of CN XII). It occurs as a result of stroke from paramedian branches of the Basilar artery or proximal AICA.

Brainstem: Medulla oblongata

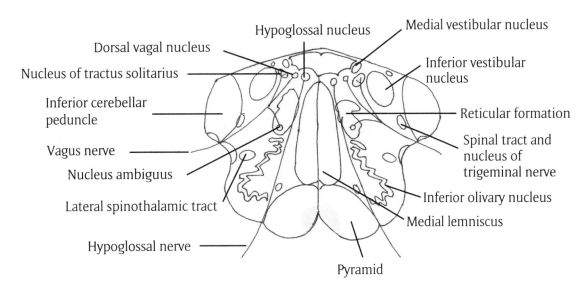

	Cranial Nerves Affected	Other Structures	Blood Supply
Medial medulla	CN 12 nucleus and nerve	ML, CS tract, MLF	**Pa**ra**M**edian branches of the Vertebral artery and Anterior Spinal arteries
Lateral medulla	Nucleus ambiguus, spinal trigeminal nucleus, nucleus tractus solitarius, dorsal motor nucleus of CN X, vestibular nucleus, CN X	ICP, sympathetic tract, ST, inferior olivary nucleus	PICA via vertebral artery

CS= corticospinal tract, ICP = inferior cerebellar peduncle, ML = medial lemniscus, MLF = medial longitudinal fasciculus, PICA = posterior inferior cerebellar artery, ST = spinothalamic tract.

Medial Medullary Syndrome

The medial medulla is supplied by **Pa**ra**M**edian branches of the vertebral and anterior spinal arteries.

- Involvement of the hypoglossal nucleus and CN **XII** causes ipsilateral weakness of the tongue.
- Involvement of the **pyramidal** tract causes contralateral limb weakness.
- Involvement of the medial lemniscus (**D**orsal **C**olumns) causes contralateral decreased vibration and position sense.

To recall features of **Medial Medullary Syndrome**, think of this appointment: "**Me**et **Me** at **12 P.M.** by the **pyramid** in **D.C.**"

Medial Medulla, CN **12** (XII and hypoglossal nucleus), **P.M.** = **P**ara**M**edian arteries, **pyramidal** tract, and **D**orsal **C**olumns.

Wallenberg's Syndrome/ Lateral Medullary Syndrome

Wallenberg's syndrome can be due to vertebral artery stroke or posterior inferior cerebellar artery (PICA) stroke.

Involvement of the:

· Trigeminal nucleus and tract results in ipsilateral decreased facial pain and temperature sensation.

· **V**estibular nucleus causes vertigo, nystagmus, and nausea/vomiting.

· Nucleus solitarius leads to decreased taste ipsilaterally.

· **A**mbiguus Nucleus or fibers of CN 9 and 10 produces ipsilateral paralysis of palate, vocal cord, and pharynx; hoarseness; dysarthria; and dysphagia.

· **S**pino**T**halamic tract results in decreased contralateral body pain and temperature sensation.

· **S**ympathetic fibers cause an ipsilateral Horner's syndrome.

· Inferior cerebellar peduncle leads to ipsilateral ataxia/dysmetria

Wallenberg sounds like **movie star** "Marky Mark" **Wahlberg**. To recall features of Wallenberg syndrome, think of: **Wahlberg's VASST** **L**ibrary of **M**ovie **S**cenes (**Lateral Medullary Syndrome**)

V- **V**estibular nucleus/nerve

A - **A**mbiguus Nucleus

S - **S**ympathetic Fibers

ST - **S**pino**T**halamic tract

Classic Lacunar Stroke Syndromes

Tthere are 5 major/common ones:

1. Pure Motor

Weakness is the same in the face, arm, and leg.

Possible site of infarct:

        Posterior limb of internal capsule

        Basis pontis (ventral pons)

        Corona **R**adiata

 Pabst **B**lue **R**ibbon® is a very **pure** beer that gets the **motor** running.

2. Pure Sensory

Pure hemisensory loss is due to an infarct involving the contralateral **ventral posterior lateral (VPL)** nucleus of the thalamus.

3. Sensorimotor

Same possible sites of infarct as motor, but also includes the thalamus.

4. Dysarthria-Clumsy Hand Syndrome

Acute onset of dysarthria and a clumsy hand may be due to a lesion in any of these 3 locations:

       · **B**asis pontis

       · **I**nternal capsule

       · **C**erebral peduncle

 With a clumsy hand, you can't hold on to a **BIC** pen!

5. Ataxic Hemiparesis (AH)

Contralateral weakness, especially the lower extremity and ipsilateral limb ataxia may be due to a lesion in either of these locations:

· Posterior limb of the internal capsule

· Basis pontis

Stroke Subtypes, Mimicks, and Risk Factors

Do NOT use the term **"CVA"** for **"Cerebral Vascular Accident"** – stroke doctors hate it, and nickname those who use it **"Confused Vascular Analysts"**. Instead of CVA, use the word Stroke, and if possible, identify which Subtype of Stroke it is (i.e., Ischemic Stroke versus Hemorrhagic Stroke, and then even further, Lacunar versus Cardioembolic Ischemic Stroke, etc…)

Stroke is defined as **sudden focal neurological deficit of a vascular cause.**

· **Very few non-vascular neurologic disorders will cause _sudden onset of focal_ brain dysfunction.**

· Stroke Mimics: In one study, 78/411 patients (19%) had other conditions:

1. Seizure with post-ictal paralysis (17%)

2. Systemic infection (17%)

3. Brain tumors (15%)

4. Toxic/metabolic derangement (13%)

5. Other (Migraine, Transient Global Amnesia/TGA, Multiple Sclerosis, BPPV, Psychiatric disease)[4]

Increased age is the strongest risk factor for stroke.

Hypertension, Smoking (tobacco), Hypercholesterolemia, Obesity, physical inactivity, and Diabetes are is the most common modifiable risk factors for stroke.

80% of all strokes are Ischemic, while 20% are Hemorrhagic.

Ischemic strokes are due to **vessel occlusion or vessel dissection, thrombosis, intra- or extra-cranial atherosclerosis, embolism (from the heart, aortic arch, or another vessel like the carotid artery),** or **systemic hypotension.**

---

4 Libman RB, Wirkowski E, Alvir J, Rao TH. Conditions that mimic stroke in the emergency department. Implications for acute stroke trials. Arch Neurol 1995 Nov;52(11):1119-22.

On MRI, **Diffusion Weighted Imaging,** or DWI, concurring or "matching" with Advanced Diffusion Coefficient, or ADC, is the most sensitive imaging technique for detecting acute ischemic stroke.

Ischemic stroke can be divided into **embolic** and **thrombotic strokes** and **watershed infarcts**.

Watershed Stroke

Systemic hypotension can produce watershed infarcts, which result in **specific clinical syndromes.**

Transcortical aphasias can occur due to watershed infarcts.

Ischemia between the ACA and MCA bilaterally can cause a **man in the barrel syndrome** (proximal arm and leg weakness).

MCA-PCA watershed infarcts cause **difficulties with visual processing**

Embolic Stroke vs. Thrombotic Stroke

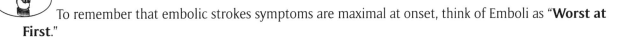 **Embolic strokes** usually are of **sudden onset** and **symptoms** are maximal **near the onset.**

To remember that embolic strokes symptoms are maximal at onset, think of Emboli as **"Worst at First."**

Emboli usually **originate from the heart**, but can be **intra-arterial**, **arise from the aorta**, or be **paradoxical.** (Via a Patent Foramen Ovale or PFO, a Deep Vein Thrombosis in the leg could in theory embolize through the heart and then eject arterially into the brain – although recent data in the "CLOSURE I Trial" suggest percutaneous closure of PFOs does not have any statistical benefit for cryptogenic stroke patients.)

Thrombotic strokes may be abrupt in onset but **tend to evolve over time**.

Thrombotic stroke may be due to **large artery occlusive disease** or **disease in small penetrating arteries**.

Stroke due to Atrial Fibrillation

· Most common cardiac dysrhythmia, prevalence increases with age

· Can last minutes to days ("paroxysmal") or be permanent

· Can be valvular (ie, from rheumatic valve disease) or non-valvular

· Symptoms include syncope, palpitations, chest pain or nothin' (asymptomatic)

· The irregularly irregular rhythm seen in AFib causes stasis of blood in the Atria, especially the Left Atrial Appendage, which in turn leads to the formation of a mural thrombus that can dislodge into the arterial circulation, reach the brain, cut off blood supply to brain parenchyma, and **cause an ischemic stroke**.

  ○ Risk of stroke with AFib is SEVEN TIMES (7X) general population, depending on associated conditions, and this risk can be estimated by the $CHADS_2$ score – a higher number corresponds to a greater risk of stroke

  ○ Treatment is typically an oral **anticoagulant** (ie, warfarin, dabigatran, rivaroxaban, apixaban, etc.), or at least an **antiplatelet** (aspirin, clopidogrel, etc), but anticoagulation offers significantly more risk reduction if tolerated

  ○ $CHADS_2$ score has been validated by many studies and now has been expanded to the CHA_2DS_2-VASc score:

	Condition	Points
C	Congestive heart failure	1
H	Hypertension (BP>140/90 or on antihypertensive medication)	1
A_2	Age ≥ 75 years	2
D	Diabetes Mellitus	1
S_2	Prior Stroke/TIA or thromboembolism	2
V	Vascular disease (peripheral artery disease, MI, aorta plaque)	1
A	Age 65–74 years	1
Sc	Sex category (woman)	1

CHA_2DS_2-VASc Score	Stroke Risk % per year
0	0
1	1.3
2	2.2
3	3.2
4	4.0
5	6.7
6	9.8
7	9.6
8	6.7
9	15.2

The CHA₂DS₂-VASc can be balanced by (or at least compared with) a patient's HAS-BLED score for bleeding risk on oral anticoagulation

Each feature gets one point

- **H**ypertension (systolic ≥ 160mmHg)
- **A**bnormal renal or liver function tests
- **A**ge ≥ 65 years
- **S**troke in past (risk for hemorrhagic transformation)
- **B**leeding
- **L**abile INRs (difficulty with Coumadin use)
- **E**toh use
- **D**rugs that "thin the blood" such as NSAIDs, etc

Lip GY, et al. (Dec 2010) "Identifying patients at high risk for stroke despite anticoagulation." *Stroke 41(12):2731-8.*

HAS-BLED score of >3 indicates increased one-year anticoagulation bleeding risk – such as intracranial hemorrhage, any bleed requiring hospitalization, or hemoglobin drop > 2g/L (or requiring transfusion of blood products).

Transient Ischemic Attack (TIA)

A transient ischemic attack (TIA) is an episode of neurological signs and symptoms due to ischemia lasting for less than 24 hours.

Most TIAs are just 10-15 minutes in duration.

To remember that a TIA must last <24 h, think of **"Tia en un Dia."** *(Dia is day in Spanish)*

ABCD² score:

The ABCD² score determines severity of TIAs, need for hospitalization, and risk for future Stroke:

Points	Age	Blood Pressure	Clinical Features of TIA	Duration of TIA	Diabetes
0	<60 yrs	Normal, <140/90	Other	<10 minutes	Absent
1	**≥60** yrs	High, ≥140/90, or taking BP pills	Speech disturbance (dysarthria or aphasia); No weakness	10 to 59 minutes	Present
2			Weakness (unilateral)	**≥60** minutes	

*Stroke risk at 1 wk: Score 1-3 (low = 1.2%), Score 4-5 (moderate = 5.9%), Score 6–7 (high = 11.7%).

Johnston SC, *et al.* (January 2007). "Validation and refinement of scores to predict very early stroke risk after TIA". Lancet 369 (9558): 283–92.

Hemorrhage

Intracerebral Hemorrhage (ICH)

ICH may present with signs of **increased intracranial pressure, vomiting**, **headache** and **altered mental status.** Headache occurs in 40% of ICH patients, compared with 17% of ischemic stroke patients. Seizures occur in 7% of ICH patients (more commonly lobar than deep).

20% of all strokes are Hemorrhagic, while 80% are Ischemic.

ICH is more than twice as common as Subarachnoid Hemorrhage (SAH) and is more likely to result in death or disability than SAH or even ischemic stroke.

At this time, clinical trials are still trying to uncover what's the optimal management of ICH -- either surgical or medical, or both -- in various patient population subtypes.

Some causes of intracerebral hemorrhage:

- · Amyloid angiopathy
- · Angioinvasive fungal infections (e.g. *Aspergillus*)
- · Aneurysm
- · Coagulation disorders, Hemophilia, or other bleeding diathesis
- · Cocaine
- · Hypertension
- · Neoplasms

The mnemonic (in order) for metastatic cancers that tend to bleed intracranially: *My Cranium Really Bleeds Terribly!* **M**-melanoma, **C**-choriocarcinoma, **R**-renal cell carcinoma, **B**-bronchogenic, and **T**-thyroid

- · Transformation of an ischemic stroke
- · Trauma
- · Vascular malformation (See below)
- · Coumadin® (warfarin), Pradaxa® (dabigatran), Xarelto® (rivaroxaban), Eliquis® (apixaban), Lovenox® (enoxaparin), Heparin®, and/or other anticoagulants
- · Aspirin®, Plavix®, Aggrenox®, and/or other antiplatelets
- · Thrombocytopenia
- · Liver or Renal Disease

Hemorrhage by Anatomical Location

Putaminal Hemorrhage

The putamen is the **most common site of intracerebral hemorrhage**.

It is the **most common site where hypertensive hemorrhage occurs**.

It is associated with headache, hemiplegia, and eye deviation toward the lesion.

To remember that the putamen is the **#1** ICH location, think of this: "**Put 'em in there first.**"

Pontine Hemorrhage

Pontine hemorrhage causes **coma, quadriparesis**, and **pinpoint pupils**. The eyes do not move with doll's eyes maneuver.

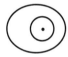 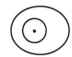

Cerebellar Hemorrhage

Cerebellar hemorrhage causes **headache, vomiting, gait ataxia**, and **dysarthria**.

It can cause **brainstem compression requiring surgery**. According to AHA guidelines for management of spontaneous ICH, "Patients with cerebellar hemorrhage >3cm in diameter who are neurologically deteriorating or who have brain stem compression and hydrocephalus from ventricular obstruction should have surgical removal of the hemorrhage as soon as possible.[5]

Ischemic cerebellar infarcts can also cause **mass effect** and surgery may be necessary.

Any cerebellar hemorrhages or infarcts that expand can cause herniation, so to prevent this catastrophe, patients may get a suboccipital craniectomy. This is different than a hemi-craniectomy surgery for malignant middle cerebral artery (MCA) infarcts or hemorrhages, which can also herniate if they expand. There have been a number of randomized clinical trials and meta-analyses that show that craniectomy in such cases saves lives, yet typically these are the sickest patients who survive with severe, longstanding neurologic deficits.

Thalamic Hemorrhage

Patients with thalamic hemorrhage have **contralateral hemisensory loss.**

They may have a fluent Thalamic Aphasia if the dominant hemisphere is involved.

Patients with Thalamic Aphasia want to take a **NAPP** – **N**eologism, **A**ttention fluctuation, **P**araphasia, and **P**erseveration.

Hemiparesis can be seen if the internal capsule is compressed.

Extension of the hemorrhage into the midbrain can result in a variety of eye findings such as impaired vertical gaze or skew deviation.

Cerebral Amyloid Angiopathy (CAA)

Pathophysiology

Cerebral Amyloid Angiopathy (CAA) results in deposition of amyloid β-protein (Aβ) in leptomeningeal and cortical capillaries (in the media and adventitia of small and medium vessels). This results in lobar hemorrhages, especially the frontal and parietal lobes. The term *Congophilic* is also used to describe the angiopathy because microscopic aggregations of amyloid are seen after applying the stain "Congo red" to brain tissue. This amyloid material is seen in the brain *only*; CAA is *NOT* related to other forms of Amyloidosis. An immune mechanism has also been proposed.

Epidemiology

There is a strong association between CAA and Alzheimer disease – 83% of Alzehimer's brains had CAA on autopsy.[6]

CAA may account for 50% of nontraumatic lobar ICH in 70-year-olds (20 cases per 100,000 people annually). CAA-related ICH risk increases with Alzheimer and Down syndromes.

CAA has been identified as occurring either sporadically (generally in elderly populations) or in familial forms.

---

[5] Stroke. 1999; 30: 905-915 doi: 10.1161/01.STR.30.

[6] Ellis RJ, Olichney JM, Thal LJ, Mirra SS, Morris JC, Beekly D, et al. Cerebral amyloid angiopathy in the brains of patients with Alzheimer's disease: the CERAD experience, Part XV. *Neurology.* Jun 1996;46(6):1592-6.

Genetics

Hereditary (familial) forms are usually associated with Aβ and "Abeta-related angiitis" yet other types are linked to certain genes:

> · "Icelandic type" associated with Cystatin C
>
> · "British type" associated with ITM2B

Build up of Aβ in the brain is thought to be related to *more Aβ production* instead of *less Aβ clearance*. Mutations in Amyloid Precursor Protein (APP), Presenilin-1 (PS1) and Presenilin-2 (PS2) genes cause APP to be cleaved into Aβ.

It's pretty silly (presenilin) that Presenilin 1 is on chromosome 14 and Presenilin 2 is on chromosome 1.

Subarachnoid Hemorrhage (SAH)

Diagnosis

Patients with SAH present with WHOL: "Worst Headache Of (my) Life".

The patient may also have vomiting, photophobia, or meningismus.

CT misses about 10% of SAH, so if one is highly suspicious of SAH, a **spinal tap should be performed if the CT is negative.**

Complications

Complications of SAH include **hydrocephalus, seizures, vasospasm, rebleeding**, and **hyponatremia**.

Nimodipine is used to prevent vasospasm, which usually occurs 5-14 days later. Vasospasm can lead to a disabling ischemic stroke in the territory of the vasospastic artery.

SAH is dangerous: 15% of SAH patients die immediately, 25% at 1 day, and 60% at 6 months.

To remember SAH fatality data, think of this: ~**24**% die at **24** hours, and **60**% die at **6** months.

Classification

Hunt and Hess System for Grading Aneurysmal Subarachnoid Hemorrhage (SAH)

Grade	Patient's symptoms/ signs
0	Asymptomatic
I	Mild headache, slight nuchal rigidity
II	More severe headache, nuchal rigidity. No neurologic deficit other than cranial nerve palsy.
III	Drowsiness/confusion and mild deficit
IV	Stupor, moderate to severe hemiparesis
V	Coma, decerebrate posturing

Etiology

Causes of subarachnoid hemorrhage (SAH):
- Amyloid angiopathy
- Anticoagulation
- Arteriovenous malformation
- Bleeding diatheses
- Drugs (i.e., cocaine)
- Mycotic (Infectious) aneurysm
- Saccular aneurysm
- Sickle cell disease
- Trauma
- Vasculitis

SAH is usually secondary to **saccular/berry aneurysms**.

Aneurysms

Aneurysms are classified as saccular, fusiform, or dissecting.

- **Saccular aneurysms** (also known as berry aneurysms) are the most common, accounting for 90% of all cerebral aneurysms. Usually they are located at the major branch points of large arteries.
- **Fusiform aneurysms** (also known as dolichoectatic or arteriosclerotic aneurysms) account for just 7% of all cerebral aneurysms. Typically, they are elongated outpouchings of proximal arteries.

Saccular aneurysms are situated in the anterior circulation in 90% of cases, whereas fusiform aneurysms predominantly occur in the vertebrobasilar system (posterior circulation).

sAccular aneurysms usually are located in the Anterior circulation, while Fusiform aneurysms form in the Fertebrobasilar system.

Anterior communicating artery-to-ACA aneurysms are the most common (35%), followed by **Posterior communicating artery-to-ICA aneurysms** (30-35%), then **MCA bifurcation aneurysms** (20%), then **aneurysms at the Basilar artery and other posterior circulation sites** (5%).

Mycotic (Infectious) **Aneurysms** are due to septic emboli, usually associated with bacterial endocarditis. Typically they are situated **peripherally** and comprise only 0.5% of all cerebral aneurysms.

Chart	sAccular (Berry)	Fusiform (Dolicho)	Mycotic (Infectious)
% of all aneurysms	90%	7%	0.5%
Location	**A**nterior	**F**ertebrobasilar (posterior)	Peripheral

A posterior communicating artery aneurysm can cause a CN III palsy due to compression.

Also, recall that CN III passes between the posterior cerebral and superior cerebellar arteries. Aneurysms at the junction of these arteries and the basilar artery may also compress CN III.

Recall from the Neuro-ophthalmology chapter:

The parasympathetic fibers are near the surface of the nerve, so compressive lesions tend to cause a dilated pupil prior to extraocular muscle weakness.

 Parasympathetic pupilloconstrictor fibers are along the periphery of CN III.

There may be a warning prior to a major subarachnoid hemorrhage. This is referred to as a **sentinel hemorrhage.**

 Conditions associated with aneurysms: POMPE FAN

       Autosomal dominant polycystic kidney disease (PCKD)

       Ehlers-Danlos type IV

       Marfan's syndrome

       Neurofibromatosis I

       Pompe disease[7]

       Pseudoxanthoma elasticum

       Osler-Weber-Rendu syndrome

       Fibromuscular dysplasia

---

[7] Please see the Metabolic Diseases chapter.

Subdural Hematoma

Subdural hematomas usually are due to **torn bridging veins**.

Blood is found between the dura and arachnoid. It does not cross suture lines.

 Think of this in the case of an **unresponsive alcoholic found in the street or a confused elderly person.**

Epidural Hematoma

Epidural hematomas are classically due to **tearing of the middle meningeal artery**.

Blood is found between the skull and dura. It may cross suture lines. *doesn't*

 A **lucid interval** may occur between the time of injury and neurological deterioration.

Cerebral Venous Thrombosis (CVT)

Risks for Cerebral Venous Thrombosis (CVT)

Risk factors for venous thrombosis include: My BODy ITCHeS

- **M**eningitis

- **B**ehçet disease (vasculitis associated with meningoencephalitis, oral ulcers, genital ulcers, and uveitis), **B**aby (Pregnancy and the post-partum period)
- **O**ral contraceptives
- **D**ehydration

- **I**nfection
- **T**rauma
- **C**ancer
- **H**ematologic (prothrombotic) conditions, **H**ypercoagulable states
- e
- **S**urgery, **S**ystemic disease

Factor V Leiden

Factor V Leiden is a mutation in Factor V that results in resistance to activated protein C.

This is the most common inheritable cause of venous thrombosis.

Sinus Thrombosis by Location

Cavernous Sinus Thrombosis (CST)

Cavernous sinus thrombosis presents with **PAP, PROPT, POP: Papilledema, Proptosis, and Painful ophthalmoplegia**.

Recall that the cavernous sinus contains CN III, IV, V1, V2, VI, postganglionic sympathetic fibers, and the internal carotid artery.

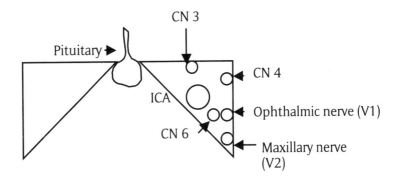

Recall that the rhino-orbital-cerebral form of Mucormycosis, which can be found in diabetics, can cause cavernous sinus thrombosis and hemorrhagic brain infarction.[8]

Transverse Sinus Thrombosis (TST)

Transverse sinus thrombosis is due to otitis, mastoiditis.

It can cause Gradenigo syndrome (CN VI palsy with facial pain due to CN V involvement).

Sagittal Sinus Thrombosis (SST)

The superior sagittal sinus receives blood from superficial veins and absorbs CSF through arachnoid villi.

---

[8] Please see the Infectious Diseases chapter for more details.

An **empty delta sign** is a filling defect in the sagittal sinus on a contrast enhanced scan indicating a sagittal sinus thrombosis.

Sagittal sinus thrombosis can present with paraparesis, seizures, or altered mental status.

Sagittal sinus thrombosis can cause bilateral parasagittal hemorrhagic infarction.

Since it can cause increased intracranial pressure, vomiting, and papilledema, it is in the differential for pseudotumor cerebri.

There is an increased risk of sagittal sinus thrombosis during pregnancy and in the post partum period.

Vascular Malformations

Types of Vascular Malformations

There are 4 types of vascular malformations:
- · Venous angiomas
- · Cavernous malformations
- · Capillary telangiectasias
- · Arteriovenous malformations (AVM)

The most common type is venous angiomas.

Venous Angiomas

Usually these have no neurologic complications.

Cavernous Malformations/Angioma

Cavernous malformations are Compact Collections of Calcific Channel-vessels without elastic tissue.

There's no normal parenchyma between these hyalinized vessels. Calcification, thrombus, or hemosiderin may be present inside the Cavernous malformations in multiple stages of evolution. This gives them a "Popcorn" appearance due to the extracellular methemoglobin.

80% of **C**avernous malformations are found supratentorially in the **C**erebral hemispheres, and frequently present with seizures.

Often near the ventricles, they are not seen well on arteriograms. They are seen better on MRI, particularly T2 and gradient echo sequences. They may be mistaken for small intracerebral hemorrhages on noncontrast head CT.

HOT TIP One familial form (CCM1) is due to a mutation in the KRIT1 gene, which has been mapped to 7q. It is autosomal dominant. These patients can also have retinal cavernous malformations.

Capillary Telangiectasias

Capillary telangiectasias are capillary-sized vessels that have normal brain tissue in between them.

They tend to be found in the **pons**.

Arteriovenous Malformation (AVM)

An AVM is a structure made of arteries and veins **without capillaries** in between; the parenchyma in the AVM is abnormal.

MNEMONIC With **abnormal parents** (parenchyma), **A** **V**ery **M**iserable child has **no pillars** (no capillaries) to admire.

Carotid-Cavernous Fistula

A carotid-cavernous fistula is a type of AVM.

The most common type is the direct type where there is direct flow from the ICA cavernous segment to the venous system.

Often these are due to trauma.

Patients may have **pulsatile proptosis, limited eye movement, vision loss, and a bruit**. The trigeminal nerve can also be affected.

Craniocervical Dissection

Dissection is when a tear in the intima allows blood to enter the arterial wall.

EXTRA-EXTRA-EXTRA, Read all about it!

The **extra-cranial** segment of the ICA and the **extra-cranial** vertebral arteries are the **extra-common** sites of dissection.

Carotid dissection can cause a painful Horner's syndrome.

COMMON CAROTID ARTERY (CCA) dissections involve all 3 signs of **Horner**'s Syndrome (**Hornblower PAM**): **P**tosis, **A**nhydrosis, and **M**iosis

PAM is a **COMMON** name, and **PAM** in traffic **COMMON**ly honks her **Horn**.

BUT in INTERNAL CAROTID ARTERY (ICA) dissections, only **M**iosis and **P**tosis may be seen, sparing facial sweat glands; in EXTERNAL CAROTID ARTERY (ECA) dissections, only **A**nhydrosis is seen **A**lone, sparing oculosympathetics.

Ann (**A**nhydrosis) is **A**lone **outside** (**EXTERNAL** Carotid Artery) where nobody can **see** her (**oculo**sympathetics spared).

Dissection of a vessel results in a **tapered appearance** on an angiogram.

Risk factors

Risk factors for dissection: **SCAM OF TIME** (think of the chiropractor – neck manipulation is sometimes viewed as both a **SCAM** and a waste **OF TIME**!)

Strangulation, **C**hiropractic manipulation, **A**ccidents (motor vehicle whiplash), **M**arfan syndrome, **O**ral contraceptive pill (OCP) use, **F**ibromuscular dysplasia, **T**rauma, **I**nfections (pharyngeal), **M**oyamoya, **E**hlers-Danlos syndrome.

Also: heavy lifting, complicated migraines, swinging a golf club or orchestral baton too violently, going on amusement park rides (like rollercoasters) and even having an elongated styloid process have all been associated with craniocervical dissection in the literature.

Complications

Complications of craniocervical dissection include aneurysm formation, artery-to-artery emboli, or ischemic stroke due to occlusion of the parent artery.

Delay in diagnosing a dissection is perilous because of the potential vowels **AEIOU**: **A**neurysm formation, **E**mbolism (artery-to-artery), or **I**schemic stroke due to **O**cclusion of **U**r artery!

Look out for an Ostrich[9] or a Puppy[10]

A patient with bilateral internal carotid artery dissections on axially-sliced MRA (Magnetic Resonance Angiography) fat-saturated sequences can give the appearance of the face of a puppy dog with the sclerae of the eyes represented by the internal carotid artery lumen irregularities from the dissections. This is given the neuroradiologic term "Puppy Sign". Additionally, bilateral vertebral artery dissection on such MRA sequences is given the neuroradiologic term "Ostrich Sign" due to the vertebral artery lumen irregularities and the surrounding structures resembling the eyes and face of an ostrich.

Cervicocephalic FMD

Fibromuscular dysplasia (FMD) is a non-atheromatous angiopathy that tends to affect women. It may be associated with aneurysms and is a risk factor for dissection.

Cervicocephalic FMD tends to affect the cervical carotid arteries. It is often bilateral.

On angiogram, a **string of beads** can be seen in FMD, due to medial fibroplasia.[11]

To remember that FMD is associated with a string of beads sign on an angiogram: If your honey is **FuMeD (fumed)**, you may want to get her a **string of beads**.

---

9 Rose DZ, Husain R. (Nov 2012) "'**Ostrich Sign**' Indicates Bilateral Vertebral Artery Dissection." *J Stroke Cerebrovasc Dis.*;21(8), p. 903.

10 Feddersen B, et al. (Oct 2007) "'**Puppy sign**' indicating bilateral dissection of internal carotid artery." *J Neurol Neurosurg Psychiatry*, 78, p. 1055

11 Medial fibroplasia is the most common histological finding in FMD, but others can be seen.

Stroke in the Young

CADASIL

CADASIL stands for Cerebral Autosomal Dominant Arteriopathy with Subcortical Infarcts and Leukoencephalopathy.

CADASIL presents with **migraine with Aura, subcortical stroke, psychiatric complaints, and/or progressive dementia.**

MRI shows small infarcts in the subcortical white matter with sparing of U fibers. Customarily, the external capsules and the anterior temporal lobes are affected; the external capsule lesions, when confluent and bilateral, give the appearance of closed parentheses "(" and ")" – a very classic neuroimaging finding for this disorder.

CADASIL is an **autosomal dominant** condition due to a mutation of the **Notch-3 gene** on **chromosome 19q.**

To remember that CADASIL is associated with Notch-3 gene mutations on chromosome **19** and closed **parentheses** on MRI, , remember: A CAD puts a Notch in his belt for every woman he smooches (**parentheses** – who is over age **19** – **parentheses**).

The **diagnosis** can be confirmed with a **skin biopsy.**

A notch in the skin (skin biopsy) helps to diagnose CADASIL, which is due to a Notch-3 mutation.

Eosinophilic inclusions are found in arterioles.

Electron microscopy demonstrates **granular osmophilic** material in the media.

Ehlers-Danlos Syndrome (also known as "Cutis hyperelastica")

Ehlers-Danlos syndrome is a connective tissue disorder due to deficiency of collagen.

There are many types, some of which are associated with **hypermobile joints and skin hyperelasticity.** Some types, such as type IV, are associated with neurovascular complications.

Clinical Features of ED-type IV

· Characteristic facial appearance: large eyes, small chin, thin nose/lips, lobeless ears

· Thin, pale, translucent skin – you can see veins on their chest and abdomen!

· **Dissections, aneurysms, arteriovenous fistulae, GI/GU rupture** and **cardiac defects**.

Some risk factors for dissection: Remember **SCAM OF TIME**.
Strangulation, **C**hiropractic manipulation, **A**ccidents (motor vehicle whiplash), **M**arfan syndrome, **O**ral contraceptive pill (OCP) use, **F**ibromuscular dysplasia, **T**rauma, **I**nfections (pharyngeal), **M**oyamoya, **E**hlers-Danlos syndrome.

Genetics of ED-type IV

Autosomal Dominant. Chromosome 2q. Defect in collagen type III.

Homocystinuria

Multiple enzyme deficiencies in methionine metabolism can cause homocystinuria including cystathionine synthase, methylenetetrahydrofolate reductase deficiency (MTHFR); methionine synthase reductase (MTRR); or methionine synthase (MS), which is also known as 5-methyltetrahydrofolate-homocysteine methyltransferase (MTR). Defective methylcobalamin synthesis is also associated with homocystinuria.[12]

Cystathionine beta-synthase deficiency is the most common genetic form of homocystinuria.

Patients with homocystinuria are **marfanoid** and have **mental retardation** and **down**ward **ectopia lentis**.

To remember that Marfan's is associated with **up**ward lens deviation and homocystinuria with **down**ward deviation:

· We look **up** to see Marfan's patients, who are really, really tall, so their lens dislocation is **upwards**.

· Vitamin treatment for the Homocysteinemic patient should **bring down their homocysteine level,** so their lens dislocation is **downwards**!

Stroke in patients with homocystinuria is because homocysteine causes injury to the endothelium and premature atherosclerosis.

To lower the risk of stroke in patients with homocystinuria, a combination of **folate, vitamin B6, and vitamin B12** is given.

---

[12] Please see the Metabolic Diseases chapter.

Marfan Syndrome

Marfan syndrome is an autosomal dominant connective tissue disease due to defects in synthesis of fibrillin.

Patients with Marfan syndrome have arachnodactyly, hyperextensible digits, long limbs, and joint laxity.

Cardiovascular defects, such as **dilatation of the aortic root, coarctation of the aorta**, and **mitral valve prolapse** are common. These put patients at **risk for thromboemboli**.

Patients also can have **saccular intracranial aneurysms** or **carotid dissection**.

Mitochondrial Encephalopathy, Lactic Acidosis, and Stroke-like episodes (MELAS)

MELAS is a multisystem disorder due to a mutation in mitochondrial DNA.

The most common mutation is in the gene ***MT-TL1***, which encodes **tRNA leucine**.

To remember the clinical and genetic features associated with MELAS, remember the phrase **"Me lass Lucy GIVES Out $10 at carnivals to children!"**

- **Me lass Lucy** = **MELAS-Leucine**,
- **GIVES Out**: **G**eneralized tonic-clonic seizures, **I**ntolerance to exercise, **V**omiting, **E**levated lactate in blood & CSF, **S**hort stature, **O**ccipital lobe involvement,
- **$10 at carnivals** = coenzyme Q**10** and **carn**itine = MELAS therapy!
- **to children** = MELAS presents in childhood.

MELAS presents in childhood with **headaches, vomiting, generalized tonic-clonic seizures**, and **stroke-like episodes** resulting in **transient hemiparesis or blindness**.

Patients may have **short stature, sensorineural deafness**, and **exercise intolerance**.

MRI shows multiple infarctions that do not fit a vascular distribution. Initially they are seen in the occipital lobes.

Labs show elevated blood and CSF lactate.

Muscle biopsy shows ragged-red fibers.

MELAS is treated with a cocktail that may include coenzyme Q10 and carnitine.

Moyamoya Disease

Epidemiology

Moyamoya disease is a non-atherosclerotic vasculopathy of intracranial vessels found primarily in Asians.

There are 2 peaks, the first around age 5 (more common), the second around age 30-40 (less common).

Pathophysiology

Patients have stenosis of both distal Internal Carotid Arteries (ICA) due to thickening of the intima with fibrous tissue. To make the diagnosis of moyamoya, neither vasculitis nor atherosclerosis may be present!

 Numerous collaterals cause a **"puff of smoke"** appearance on angiogram.

 Where there's **smoke**, there's **FIRE**!
Fibroplasia of the **I**ntima & **R**eduplication of the **E**lastica (**FIRE**) are thought to cause moyamoya.

Moyamoya syndrome (not Moyamoya disease) is associated with similar radiographic findings, but can be unilateral and due to numerous etiologies such as neurofibromatosis, sickle cell disease, and radiation.

Classic case is a 5-year-old girl blowing out her birthday cake candles and then having a TIA or stroke. Presumably the hyperventilation causes cerebral vascular constriction and further narrows her moyamoya-ravaged ICAs, causing neurologic deficit.

 Children typically present with strokes, whereas adults are more likely to develop ICH.

The natural history of untreated moyamoya disease is poor, 73% develop a major deficit or die 2 years after diagnosis. Medical treatment is with aspirin, surgical treatment includes either "***Direct***" or "***Indirect***" bypass:

> ***Direct***: connects the STA (Superficial Temporal Artery) to the MCA; may not work in children younger than 2 years of age
>
> ***Indirect***: an **EDAS** (**E**ncephalo**D**uro**A**rterio**S**ynangiosis - a synangiosis between a scalp artery and the dura) or an **EDAMS** (**E**ncephalo**D**uro**A**rterio**M**yo**S**ynangiosis - a synangiosis involving the temporalis muscle).

Hereditary Hemorrhagic Telangiectasia/ Osler-Weber-Rendu Disease

Osler-Weber-Rendu disease/ Hereditary hemorrhagic telangiectasia (HHT), which is autosomal dominant, occasionally presents with **ischemic stroke**.

Patients with HHT have skin angiomas and angiomas in the gastrointestinal and genitourinary tracts, nose, lung, and CNS.

Neurologic complications of HHT:

· Stroke.

· Brain abscess(es) due to pulmonary arteriovenous malformation.

· Subarachnoid hemorrhage can occur due to brain AVMs.

· Paraparesis may occur if a spinal AVM bleeds.[13]

Sickle Cell Disease

Infarction in patients with sickle cell disease occurs when the internal carotid or proximal anterior or middle cerebral arteries becomes occluded due to intimal and medial hyperplasia, which follows stasis and ischemia in the vasa vasorum. In severe cases, this can lead to Moyamoya syndrome.

Takayasu Arteritis

Takayasu arteritis is also known as "the pulseless disease".

Like temporal arteritis, this is a giant cell arteritis.

It involves the aorta and its major branches.

It is typically found in young Asian women.

Takayasu arteritis presents with **fever, weight loss, myalgia, and arthralgia**.

Later in the disease, **syncope, subclavian steal, stroke, limb claudication**, and **amaurosis fugax** are seen.

Takayasu arteritis is treated with **steroids.**

---

[13] For more information please see the Neurocutaneous Disorders chapter.

Systemic Lupus Erythematosus (SLE)

Stroke in patients with SLE may be due to endocarditis, an increased risk for thrombosis (due to antiphospholipid and anticardiolipin antibodies), vasculitis, or atherosclerosis secondary to hypertension.

Brain Perfusion

Cerebral Perfusion Pressure is equal to Mean Arterial Pressure minus IntraCranial Pressure.

CPP = MAP - ICP

Normal Cerebral Blood Flow (CBF) is approximately 50ml/100g/min in adults.

HyperPerfusion Syndrome (HPS)

 >100% increase in Cerebral Blood Flow (CBF) after a surgery or stenting procedure that opens the carotid artery compared to baseline.

- **May provoke ICH and/or seizures** after a Carotid EndArterectomy (CEA) or Carotid Artery Stenting (CAS)
    - ➢ Due to changes in previously low-flow, carotid vascular bed
    - ➢ *"exhausted micro-cerebro-vascular reactivity"*
    - ➢ Besides CBF, Cerebral Blood Perfusion (CBP) also rises s/p CEA or CAS
- *Hyperperfusion* after a CEA occurs in 9–14% of cases
    - ➢ The classic clinical **triad for HPS is seizures, ipsilateral headache, and focal neurological deficits.**

- Unknown; possibly lowering BP may help
- No definitive evidence favoring any particular antihypertensive drug or best ranges of BP
- Incidence of post-op stroke in HPS 10x higher compared to patients who did not experience HPS

Medical Therapies for Stroke

Medication	Mechanism
Heparin (unfractionated)	Augments the ability of antithrombin III to inactivate thrombin and activated factor X (factor Xa); used sparingly for carotid or vertebral dissection and/or severe intracranial stenosis that causes stuttering, stereotyped TIAs, otherwise little to no role in acute stroke therapy, even for patients with stroke due to Atrial Fibrillation because of risk of hemorrhagic transformation of recent infarction!
Lovenox (enoxaparin)	Low-molecular-weight heparin. Primarily used for patients with ischemic stroke due to cancer-related thrombophilia (hypercoagulability of malignancy) in therapeutic doses, and in for deep vein thrombosis prevention in prophylaxis doses.
Warfarin (Coumadin)	Inhibits synthesis of vitamin K-dependent clotting factors (II, VII, IX, X, protein C, and protein S). This Vitamin K Antagonist (**VKA**) has been approved/marketed since 1954. Side effects (besides bleeding) include purple toe syndrome, osteoporosis, fetal warfarin syndrome (teratogenic skeletal abnormalities), and interaction with >700 known meds and leafy-green, vitamin K-containing foods!
Aspirin "ASA"	Inhibits platelet aggregation by inactivating cyclooxygenase. The daily 81mg tablet ("baby aspirin") appears to be just as effective as larger doses (ie., 325mg and up).
Plavix (clopidogrel)	A pro-drug that inhibits platelet aggregation by preventing the binding of adenosine diphosphate (ADP) to its platelet receptor. Likely as effective as aspirin, but liver enzyme CYP2C19 interactions with PPIs and other medications have limited its use; also some minorities are found to be hypo-responders of clopidogrel metabolism.
Aggrenox (aspirin+ dipyridamole)	Combination pill (Aspirin inactivates cyclooxygenase, and dipyridamole inhibits platelet phosphodiesterase). It must be taken BID. One of the most common side effects of Aggrenox is headache. Aggrenox can cause an agonizing headache.
Pradaxa (dabigatran)	Oral Direct Thrombin Inhibitor (DTI), approved for anticoagulation in non-valvular Atrial Fibrillation; 150mg BID standard dose, and 75mg BID for renal patients. Dabigatran lowers stroke/systemic embolism risk vs. **warfarin**.[14] It does not require INR checks, has very few drug interactions, and its well-known side-effect is G.I./dyspepsia.
Xarelto (rivaroxaban), Eliquis (apixaban)	These newer medications are factor Xa inhibitors and also are used for stroke prevention in non-valvular A-Fib patients. Notice the **Xa** in their names! Like dabigitran, these oral anticoagulants also do not require INR checks and have very few drug interactions.
tissue Plasminogen Activator (tPA)	Activates plasminogen to form plasmin, which results in fibrinolysis of the clot. TPA is indicated for acute stroke patients presenting within three hours from symptom onset, or in select cases within <4.5 hours from symptom onset. The dose is 0.9 mg/kg (max 90mg), with 10% given I.V. Push over 1 minute, followed by a continuous infusion over 1 hour. Risk of any hemorrhage from tPA is about 11% overall, intracranial hemorrhage about 6%, and fatal hemorrhage about 3% according to the original NINDS-tPA trial.

---

[14] **RELY:** *NEJM* 361;12 1139-51 (2009).

The Unlucky 13 Contraindications to I.V. tPA

1. Spontaneously clearing neurological signs (dramatic improvement in Stroke Scale score)

2. Seizure at onset of symptoms

3. History of any previous ICH or brain tumor (excluding extraaxial meningioma)

4. Head trauma, MI, or prior ischemic stroke **in the previous 3 months**

5. GI or GU hemorrhage **in the previous 3 weeks**

6. Major surgery **in the previous 2 weeks**

7. Arterial puncture at a noncompressible site **in the previous 1 week**

8. Uncontrolled HTN at time of treatment: systolic BP>185 or diastolic>110mmHg

9. INR >1.7, or known bleeding diathesis

10. If receiving heparin in previous 48 hours, abnormal aPTT

11. Platelet count <100,000 mm3

12. Blood glucose <50 or >400 mg/dL

13. CT with infarction hypodensity >one-third of cerebral hemisphere

Surgical Therapies for Stroke

Carotid EndArterectomy (CEA)[15]

The Asymptomatic Carotid Atherosclerosis Study (ACAS) showed an absolute risk reduction of 5.9% and a relative risk reduction of 53% over 5 years in **asymptomatic** patients with 60-99% stenosis who underwent CEA.

The North American Symptomatic Carotid Endarterectomy Trial (NASCET) showed benefit of surgery in **symptomatic** patients with 50-99% stenosis as seen in the table below.

% stenosis	Ipsilateral stroke Medical arm	Ipsilateral stroke Surgical (CEA) arm	Absolute Risk Reduction
NASCET:			
70-99%	26.1% over 2 yrs	12.9% over 2 yrs	13.2%
50-69%	22.2% over 2 yrs	15.7% over 2 yrs	6.5%
ACAS:			
60-99%	11.0% over 5 yrs	5.1% over 5 yrs	5.9%

---

[15] **CREST**: *NEJM* 363 11-23 (2010). **NASCET**: *NEJM* 325:445 (1991). **ACAS**: *JAMA* 273: 1421 (1995).

For more information on stroke trials, go to this site: www.strokecenter.org. (Internet Stroke Center web site, Goldberg, MP [ed]).

The 9 major Complications of CEA

1. Post-op Cardiac events***
2. Post-op Stroke***
3. Hyperperfusion syndrome #
4. Cranial Nerve injury @
5. Re-stenosis @
6. Infection
7. Parotitis
8. Bleeding
9. Death***

@ = see below for more detail
# = see above for more detail
*** = really bad

Cranial Nerve Injury after CEA

· Nerves at risk for injury during CEA include:

➢ X Vagus nerve (Recurrent laryngeal)
   · Runs posterior and medially
➢ VII Facial nerve (mandibular branch)
   · Due to retraction; Recovers in 6 months
➢ IX Glossopharyngeal nerve
➢ XII Hypoglossal nerve
   · Runs along Anterior surface of JV near bifurcation
➢ V Branches of Trigeminal nerve

Re-stenosis after CEA

· Re-stenosis following CEA occurs in 3-10% at 5 years, and 20% of patients overall
· *Early* Re-stenosis (within 6 months) common when smooth muscle cells abundant in lesion; less likely when lesion rich in lymphocytes and macrophages
· *Late* Re-stenosis (years) results from progression of atherosclerotic disease

Carotid Artery Stenting (CAS)

Benefits:

- Percutaneous catheterization techniques (carotid angioplasty and stent placement) in practice for many years now
- Less invasive (can be done with local anesthesia and sedation)
- Can repair more cephalad stenosis that CEA can't reach
- Less likely to precipitate cardiac events, as per **CREST** (Carotid Revascularization Endarterectomy versus Stenting Trial)
  - MI rate = 1.1% for stenting vs. 2.3% for CEA

Risks:

And also as per the CREST trial, there were higher rates of stroke in patients undergoing catheterization/ stenting, presumably due to the guide wire flicking off atherosclerotic emboli junk to the brain during the procedure.

Transient Global Amnesia (TGA)

A patient with transient global amnesia is alert but confused, asking the same question over and over. He/she usually is oriented to self, but may not be oriented to time or place. This may last for hours.

The etiology of this is unclear. It may be a migraine variant. Presumably, TGA is not related to stroke or cerebral ischemia.

Stroke Quiz

(Answers on page 759)

1. Match the condition with its angiogram findings
    1) Fibromuscular dysplasia
    2) Carotid dissection
    3) Moyamoya disease

    A. Tapered vessel
    B. Puff of smoke
    C. String of beads

2. Match the lacunar syndrome to its anatomy.
    1) Pure hemiparesis
    2) Pure hemisensory loss

    A. Lesion of the posterior limb of the internal capsule.
    B. Lesion of the ventral posterior lateral nucleus of the thalamus.

3. The recurrent artery of Huebner is a branch of which artery?
    A. Internal carotid artery
    B. Anterior cerebral artery
    C. Middle cerebral artery
    D. Posterior cerebral artery

4. The anterior choroidal artery is a branch of which artery?
    A. Internal carotid artery
    B. Anterior cerebral artery
    C. Middle cerebral artery
    D. Posterior cerebral artery

5. The left vertebral artery arises from which artery?

      A. Subclavian

      B. Aorta

      C. Brachiocephalic

6. The right common carotid arises from which artery?

      A. Subclavian

      B. Aorta

      C. Brachiocephalic

7. Which of the following is NOT a major complication of CEA?

      A. Post-op MI

      B. Hyponatremia

      C. Hyperperfusion syndrome

      D. Cranial Nerve injury

      E. Re-stenosis

8. What is the 2-year recurrent ipsilateral stroke risk with an 80% internal carotid artery stenosis and a recent stroke treated medically with aspirin?

      A. 1%

      B. 4%

      C. 13%

      D. 26%

      E. 50%

9. Which of the following is an absolute contraindication for I.V. tPA?

      A. INR 1.4

      B. Diastolic Blood Pressure 120

      C. Major surgery 3 weeks ago

      D. Previous stroke a year ago

      E. Platelets 115,000

10. What is the rate of intracranial hemorrhage in ischemic stroke patients given IV tPA?

    A. 0.5%

    B. 6%

    C. 18%

    D. 33%

    E. 50%

11. What is the maximum number of hours since time of ischemic stroke onset that IV tPA can be given?

    A. 2

    B. 3

    C. 3-1/2

    D. 4-1/2

    E. 6

12. Which of the following is NOT a lacunar stroke territory?

    A. Putamen

    B. Thalamus

    C. Internal capsule

    D. Basal ganglia

    E. Occipital lobe

13. A patient comes to the ER with Worst Headache Of Life, but after reviewing the STAT CT Head, you see no hemorrhage. What's your next step?

    A. Order another CT Head in 2 hours

    B. Perform EEG to rule out seizures

    C. Perform Lumbar Puncture to look for xanthochromia

    D. Send the patient home because if CT Head is negative, it's not a cranial bleed

    F. Give stronger pain medicine until headache resolves

Chapter 16

Neurotoxins

Please also see the Neuro-oncology chapter for toxic effects of chemotherapeutic agents, the Neuromuscular Diseases chapter, and the Neurotransmitters chapter.

Arsenic

Acute Arsenic Poisoning

Following acute exposure, **GI distress** and circulatory collapse can occur. Patients have abdominal pain, nausea, vomiting, and diarrhea. **Altered mental status** can progress to **coma** and **seizures**. **Hemoglobinuria** can progress to **black urine**.

To remember that acute arsenic poisoning is associated with *GI disturbances*, remember that arsenic poisoning causes *diarrhea to* come out your *arse*, which can be an acute problem.

Chronic Arsenic Exposure

With chronic arsenic exposure, patients also can have *GI symptoms, but they are less severe.* Patients may complain of *pain in the soles of their feet.* An *axonal neuropathy* is common.

Arsenic causes an **a**xonal neuropathy.

Hyperkeratosis of the palms and soles and **Mees' lines** are also seen with chronic arsenic exposure.

Mees' lines (white transverse lines on the fingernails) appear 2-3 weeks after an acute exposure. They are also seen in thallium poisoning.

Carbon Monoxide

Carbon monoxide causes **bilateral necrosis of the globus pallidus**.

To remember clinical findings in carbon monoxide poisoning, use **PEPSI**, a **carbon**ated drink.

Pallidus necrosis, **p**yramidal signs

Extrapyramidal signs

Parkinsonism

Seizures possible and **s**ight impaired

Irritability

Ciguatera

Ciguatoxin is found in over 400 species of reef fish, and can cause **Ciguatera** – a foodborne illness with serious GI and neurologic effects, which include:

- · nausea, vomiting, and diarrhea, followed by
- · headaches, muscle aches, ataxia, numbness, hallucinations and "cold allodynia," in which on contact with **cold**, a patient will feel **burning** sensation.

The culprits are Dinoflagellates like *Gambierdiscus toxicus*, which adhere to coral, algae and seaweed, which are eaten by herbivorous fish, which are eaten by carnivorous fish (like barracudas, snapper, parrotfishes, and groupers), which are eaten by humans, who regret it later!

Ciguatoxin is quite heat-resistant, hence fish containing ciguatoxin cannot be detoxified by standard cooking measures. There is no known antidote, and treatment is supportive. Ciguatoxin lowers the threshold for opening voltage-gated sodium channels in synapses, causing unnecessary depolarization. Mannitol has been used for treatment, but with mixed results.

Ethylene Glycol

Ethylene glycol is found in antifreeze.

It breaks down into aldehydes and oxalic acid.

 Patients **look drunk initially** but don't smell like alcohol and have a **metabolic acidosis**.

 At first, patients who have ingested ethylene glycol look like they have had ethyl alcohol. 🍸

They develop **seizures** and **nonreactive pupils**, **lose their corneal reflexes**, and **become comatose** and **cyanotic**.

 Antifreeze produces **4 C's**: **c**orneal reflexes lost, **c**onvulsions, **c**oma, and **c**yanosis.

Lead

Children

Children develop lead poisoning from eating paint containing lead.

 Children exposed to lead develop **GI symptoms** and **altered mental status**.

Lead encephalopathy is associated with seizures and increased intracranial pressure.

 GI symptoms, such as vomiting, **may lead children** with lead poisoning **to the bathroom**.

Adults

Encephalopathy is seen less frequently in adults, who are more likely to develop **neuropathy**. A **motor** or **sensory** neuropathy can be seen.

 A motor neuropathy causing **wrist and finger drop** can be seen with lead exposure.

The wrist and fingers become heavy as lead and can't be lifted.

Other clues to suggest lead poisoning:

- **Microcytic anemia with basophilic stippling** of red cells
- **Blue line (lead line) along the gingival margin**
- **Lead lines** (transverse lines at the metaphysis of growing bones) **on x-rays**
- **Increase in urine coproporphyrin levels**

Mercury

Inorganic Mercury

Tremor and personality changes can be seen with inorganic mercury poisoning. Remember the phrase "**Mad as a Hatter**"? Hatters of old worked with mercury.

Inorganic mercury can cause **acrodynia**, which is seen predominantly **in children**.

Acrodynia is characterized by **pink extremities, tachycardia, sweating on the trunk, hypertension,** and **encephalopathy**.

If I was out of my head from inorganic mercury and did acrobatics, I'd be tachycardic, hypertensive, and diaphoretic, like someone with acrodynia.

Organic Mercury

Organic mercury causes **distal paresthesias** due to DRG (dorsal root ganglion) degeneration. **Ataxia, constriction of visual fields,** and **cortical vision loss** can also be seen.

To remember that mercury poisoning affects the DRG: **Mercury sounds like Merck**, which **makes drugs/DRuGs**.

If one had organic mercury (**Hg**) poisoning, one might have to **Hug** the walls when walking due to ataxia and poor vision.

Methanol

Methanol is metabolized by alcohol dehydrogenase to formic acid and formaldehyde, which results in **acidosis with an increased anion gap.**

Methanol toxicity can cause **vomiting, headache, seizures, coma,** and **cardiorespiratory failure.**

It causes *degeneration of retinal ganglion cells*, which causes **blindness**, and degeneration of the putamen, which results in **parkinsonism.**

Treatment is with **ethyl alcohol or fomepizole**, which compete with methanol for alcohol dehydrogenease, and **bicarbonate** for the acidosis.

Nitrous Oxide

Patients can have **paresthesias of the distal extremities, gait ataxia,** and **lower extremity weakness**. Nitrous oxide causes a **myeloneuropathy**.

Nitrous oxide use can look like B12 deficiency.

N_2O interferes with the conversion of homocysteine to methionine by inactivating methionine synthase, a B12-dependent enzyme. Therefore, **homocysteine levels are elevated when nitrous oxide is abused**.

It looks like you have *NO B12* when you *abuse N$_2$O (nitrous oxide)*.

In **B12 deficiency**, homocysteine and methylmalonic acid are elevated.
In **nitrous oxide abuse**, *only homocysteine* is elevated.

Normal:

$$Methylmalonyl\ CoA \xrightarrow[B12]{} succinyl\ CoA$$

$$Homocysteine \xrightarrow[B12]{methionine\ synthase} methionine$$

Nitrous oxide inhibits methionine synthase:

$$N_2O$$
$$\downarrow -$$
$$Homocysteine \xrightarrow[B12]{methionine\ synthase} methionine$$

Organophosphates

Organophosphates are found in pesticides for agriculture, residential landscaping, mosquito eradication and other public health programs.

Common ones include parathion, **malathion** (especially in the USA), fenitrothion, diazinon, chlorpyrifos, azinphos methyl, and phosmet. Uncommon yet deadly ones include **sarin** and **VX** nerve agent (which irreversibly inactivate acetylcholinesterase); these have been used for chemical terrorism.

Immediate Effect of Organophosphates

Organophosphates bind to acetylcholinesterase, causing an increase in acetylcholine at the receptor. This can cause a **cholinergic crisis.**

A cholinergic crisis is characterized by **miosis, increased salivation** and **secretions, diarrhea, cramps,** and **fasciculations**.

OP toxicity makes you say "**O**h, **P**oop" as you run to the bathroom in a **crisis**.

You want to douse yourself with <u>chlorine</u> during a <u>cholinergic</u> crisis due to diarrhea and other secretions. It's good that you are miotic, because you don't want to see yourself.

Organophosphate poisoning is treated with atropine and **pralidoxime (2-PAM)**. **Atropine** counteracts the muscarinic effects. Pralidoxime speeds up the reactivation of acetylcholinesterase.

Delayed Effect of Organophosphates

Organophosphates can cause a delayed symmetric sensorimotor polyneuropathy. This is an axonopathy that is thought to be due to inhibition of neuropathy target esterase (NTE).

Strychnine

Strychnine is an antagonist of glycine.

Strychnine can be found in **rat poison**.

It has been used as an **adulterant of cocaine**.

Clinical features include **apprehension, nausea, muscle twitching, extensor spasm, opisthotonus,** and **seizures. Strychnine** causes **severe muscle spasms** that can lead to **rhabdomyolysis** and **renal failure.**

Strychnine makes you **st**iff with spasms.

Remember the clinical features of strychnine poisoning by linking it to the word RAT and MOUSE or STRYCHNINE:

Rigidity, rhabdomyolysis, and renal failure

Apprehension

Twitching of muscles and tight jaw

Muscle spasms and pain

Opisthotonus

Upchuck, urine is dark

Seizure

Extensor spasm

Alternatively:

Seizures

Twitching of muscles

Rhabdomyolysis, respiratory arrest due to respiratory muscle spasm, rat poison

Yak (vomit)

Competitive antagonist of glycine

Hyperthermia

Nausea

Increased lactate

Neck spasm

Extensor spasm/opisthotonus

If I saw a mouse, I would become nauseated, have a spasm, and twitch everywhere, like someone exposed to mouse poison/strychnine.

Thallium

Thallium affects Na+/K+-ATPase.

It also can be found in rat poison.

Acutely, vomiting and diarrhea may be seen. Then severe dysesthesias are seen. Cardiac and respiratory failure can occur.

Patients develop *alopecia* and an *axonal neuropathy* (sensory and motor involvement). *Mee's lines* may be seen.

 Thallium poisoning is in the differential diagnosis of Guillain-Barré syndrome.

 Ironically, thallium has been used in cardiac stress tests, so you won't have to pull your hair out trying to remember thallium toxicity can cause heart failure and alopecia.

Toluene

Toluene is found in paint thinner, fuel, and glue.

It can cause **emotional lability; tremor; neuropathy; optic, cerebral, and cerebellar atrophy;** and **white matter changes**.

Remember the word TOLUENE to remember the signs and symptoms of toluene toxicity:

Tremor
Optic atrophy, **o**psoclonus, **o**cular dysmetria
Loss of hearing and smell
Upper motor neuron signs, **u**nsteady gait
Euphoria
Neuropathy
Emotional lability

or
GLUE

Glee
Loss of hearing and smell
Unsteadiness
Eye findings: optic atrophy

Neurotoxins Quiz

(Answers on page 761)

1. Match the symptoms with the toxin.

   1) Wrist drop
   2) Hyperkeratosis of palms and soles, axonal neuropathy, and Mees' lines
   3) Mees' lines, axonal neuropathy, and alopecia
   4) Coma, cyanosis, convulsions, and loss of corneal reflexes
   5) Nausea, opisthotonus, rigidity, and renal failure

   A) Arsenic
   B) Ethylene glycol
   C) Lead
   D) Strychnine
   E) Thallium

2. Which toxin can cause a Guillain-Barré type picture?

   A. Arsenic
   B. Ethylene glycol
   C. Inorganic mercury
   D. Strychnine

3. Acrodynia is due to which toxin?

   A. Arsenic
   B. Inorganic mercury
   C. Organic mercury
   D. Thallium

4. Eye findings are seen with which toxin?

   A. Ethylene glycol
   B. Organic mercury
   C. Methanol
   D. Toluene
   E. All of the above

5. Which of the following symptoms are NOT seen in Ciguatera?

     A. Nausea/vomiting

     B. Cyanosis

     C. Headaches

     D. Ataxia

     E. "Cold allodynia," in which on contact with *cold*, a patient will feel *burning* sensation

Chapter 17

Neurotransmitters

Acetylcholine (ACh)

Acetylcholine is the neurotransmitter at the synapse of motoneurons that innervate striated muscle.

Acetylcholine is also used in the motor neurons of cranial nerve nuclei.

In the autonomic nervous system, acetylcholine is the neurotransmitter for all:

- Preganglionic neurons
- Parasympathetic postganglionic neurons
- Sudomotor sympathetic postganglionic neurons.

Acetylcholine is used by interneurons in the striatum and in the reticular formation.

Cholinergic neurons are found in the basal nucleus of Meynert, septal nuclei, and the basal forebrain. They project to the cortex and amygdala. Some septal neurons send axons to the hippocampus through the fornix.

Acetylcholine is also found in the pedunculopontine nuclei. Its release from these neurons promotes wakefulness.[1]

Acetylcholine Synthesis

Acetylcholine is synthesized from acetyl CoA and choline by choline acetyl transferase.

Acetylcholine Metabolism

Acetylcholinesterase breaks down acetylcholine into acetate and choline.

---

[1] Please see the Neurophysiology chapter for more information.

Acetylcholine Receptors

There are 2 types of acetylcholine receptors:

1. Nicotinic
2. Muscarinic

Nicotinic Acetylcholine Receptors

Nicotinic acetylcholine receptors are located in:

- Skeletal muscle (at the neuromuscular junction)
- Brain
- Autonomic ganglia.

In the **central nervous system**, most of the nicotinic acetylcholine receptors are found in the **spinal cord** and **superior colliculus**.

Nicotinic acetylcholine receptors are **ligand-gated**.

To remember that nicotinic acetylcholine receptors are l̲igand-gated: **nicotine** has caused lots of **l̲itigation.**

Muscarinic Acetylcholine Receptors

Muscarinic acetylcholine receptors are **more prevalent in the brain than nicotinic receptors**.

They are located at all:

- Preganglionic synapses
- Postganglionic parasympathetic synapses
- Sudomotor sympathetic postganglionic synapses.

There are five types of muscarinic receptors, all of which are **linked to G proteins**.

To remember that m̲uscarinic acetylcholine receptors are *associated with* **sweat glands**, remember that there are **mus̲k-scented deodorants**.

To remember that muscarinic acetylcholine receptors are **linked to G proteins**: to become **mus̲cular** people eat a lot of **G̲ritty protein̲ bars**.

Atropine is a muscarinic receptor an̲tagonist.

Diseases associated with Acetylcholine

Alzheimer's Disease

 Alzheimer's disease is associated with loss of acetylcholine nuclei in the nucleus basalis of Meynert.

Cholinesterase inhibitors are used to treat Alzheimer's disease. Examples include:

· Donepezil (Aricept)

· Galantamine (Reminyl)

· Rivastigmine (Exelon)

Autosomal Dominant Nocturnal Frontal Lobe Epilepsy

Defects in nicotinic receptors have been found in autosomal dominant nocturnal frontal lobe epilepsy.[2]

Huntington Disease

In Huntington's disease, there is a *loss of acetylcholine-containing neurons* (and GABA-containing neurons) *in the* **striatum**.

Lambert-Eaton Syndrome

Lambert-Eaton syndrome is due to *antibodies against the presynaptic voltage-gated calcium channel*. This leads to a **reduction in acetylcholine release**.

---

[2] Please see the Epilepsy chapter for more information.

Myasthenia Gravis

 Myasthenia gravis (MG) is due to *antibodies to the acetylcholine receptor at the neuromuscular junction.*

Edrophonium (Tensilon) is an *acetylcholinesterase inhibitor* used to diagnose MG.

 MG is treated with acetylcholinesterase inhibitors, such as pyridostigmine (Mestinon).

 An overdose of Mestinon results in <u>cholinergic crisis</u>.

A **cholinergic crisis** is characterized by *miosis, increased salivation* and *secretions, diarrhea, cramps,* and *fasciculations.*

 You want to douse yourself with <u>chlor</u>ine during a <u>chol</u>inergic crisis due to diarrhea and other secretions. It's good that you are miotic, because you don't want to see yourself.

Toxins affecting Acetylcholine

Botulinum Toxin

 Botulinum toxin **prevents acetylcholine release**. There are 7 types of Botox subtoxins, each named alphabetically: **A,B,C,D,E,F and G**.

Subtypes **A**&**E** work by cleaving the protein **SNAP-25**.

 Think of turning off **A&E** network (channel **25**) in a **SNAP** since your show was cancelled.

Subtypes **B,D,F and G** work by cleaving **VAMP** (Vesicle Associated Membrane Protein).

 Think of a **BaD FanGed VAMP**ire.

Subtype **C** is perhaps the most **C**lever toxin: it **C**leaves **SNAP-25** and **syntaxin**!

 Subtype **C** **C**leaves a **C**ombo of proteins in a **SNAP**!

Clostridium toxins	Target proteins cleaved
Botulinum	
A	SNAP-25
B	VAMP (Synaptobrevin)
C	SNAP-25; Syntaxin
D	VAMP (Synaptobrevin)
E	SNAP-25
F	VAMP (Synaptobrevin)
G	VAMP (Synaptobrevin
Tetanus	VAMP (Synaptobrevin)

Bungarotoxin

 There are 2 types of bungarotoxins: α-bungarotoxin and β-bungarotoxin.

β-**bungarotoxin**, a toxin produced by sea snakes, causes **acetylcholine release**.

α-**bungarotoxin** <u>irreversibly</u> **blocks acetylcholine receptors**.

 β-**b**ungarotoxin acts **b**efore the synapse. **A**lpha-bungarotoxin acts **a**fter the synapse.

Latrotoxin

Latrotoxin, which is **black widow spider toxin**, **augments acetylcholine release**.

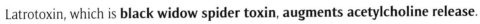

 Black widow spider toxin acts **b**efore the synapse.

Magnesium

 Hypermagnesemia results in **decreased** release of presynaptic acetylcholine at the neuromuscular junction. Magnesium competes with calcium for uptake at voltage-gated calcium channels.

Organophosphates

Organophosphates (which are found in pesticides) **bind to acetylcholinesterase**. This results in decreased acetylcholine breakdown in the synapse, which causes an **increase in acetylcholine at the receptor**. This can cause a **cholinergic crisis**. Common OP's include parathion and **malathion** (especially in the USA). Uncommon yet deadly ones include **sarin** and **VX** nerve agent (which irreversibly inactivate acetylcholinesterase); these have been used as chemical terrorism.

 A cholinergic crisis is characterized by **miosis, increased salivation** and **secretions, diarrhea, cramps,** and **fasciculations**.

OP toxicity makes you say "**O**h, **P**oop" as you run to the bathroom in a **crisis**.

Organophosphate poisoning is treated with **atropine** and **pralidoxime (2-PAM)**.
Atropine counteracts the **muscarinic** effects.
Pralidoxime speeds up the **reactivation of acetylcholinesterase**.

Plant Toxins

Deadly nightshade and jimson weed contain **atropine**.

Ingestion of these plant toxins results in confusion, tachycardia, and mydriasis.

Tick Paralysis

Tick paralysis is also thought to be due to **decreased acetylcholine release**.[3]

---

[3] Please see the Neuromuscular Diseases chapter for more information about this condition.

Dopamine

Dopamine is also known as **prolactin-inhibiting factor**.

Dopamine pathways:
- · Nigrostriatal
- · Tuberoinfundibular
- · Mesolimbic
- · Mesocortical

Dopamine Synthesis

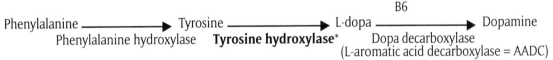

Phenylalanine ⟶ Tyrosine ⟶ L-dopa ⟶ Dopamine
Phenylalanine hydroxylase **Tyrosine hydroxylase*** Dopa decarboxylase
(L-aromatic acid decarboxylase = AADC)
B6

*The rate-limiting step is mediated by tyrosine hydroxylase.

Dopamine Metabolism

Dopamine breakdown

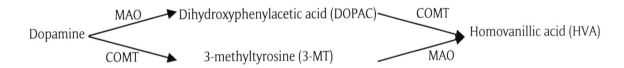

Dopamine
MAO ⟶ Dihydroxyphenylacetic acid (DOPAC) — COMT
COMT ⟶ 3-methyltyrosine (3-MT) — MAO
⟶ Homovanillic acid (HVA)

MAO = monoamine oxidase, COMT = catechol-O-methyltransferase

Dopamine Receptors

There are **5 types of dopamine receptors**.

D1 and D2 receptors are most prominent in the **striatum**.

D3-5 receptors are found in the **limbic system** and other pathways.

D1 versus D2:

D1 receptors are found in **striatonigral neurons** and are **excitatory**.

D2 receptors are found in **striatopallidal neurons** and are **inhibitory**.

Diseases associated with Dopamine

Tyrosine Hydroxylase Deficiency

Deficiency of tyrosine hydroxylase, the enzyme that mediates the rate-limiting step in dopamine synthesis, produces a form of **dopa-responsive dystonia**.[4]

Parkinson's Disease

D1 receptors are **decreased** in Parkinson's disease.

D2 receptors are **increased** in Parkinson's disease.

Neuroleptic Malignant Syndrome

Neuroleptic malignant syndrome (NMS) is due to **D2 receptor blockade**.[5]

GABA

GABA (γ-aminobutyric acid) is the major **inhibitory neurotransmitter** in the **CNS**. (Glycine is the major inhibitory neurotransmitter in the spinal cord.)

GABA is found in inhibitory interneurons.

Purkinje cells, Golgi cells, and basket cells in the cerebellum use GABA.

Neurons in the striatum projecting to the substantia nigra and globus pallidus use GABA. The projections from the globus pallidus to the thalamus and subthalamic nucleus also use GABA.[6]

GABA is also found in amacrine cells of the retina, granule cells of the olfactory bulb, and the hippocampus.

---

[4] Please see the Movement Disorders chapter for more information about dopa-responsive dystonia.

[5] Please see the Movement Disorders chapter for more information about NMS.

[6] Please see the Movement Disorders chapter for more information.

GABA Synthesis

GABA *is synthesized from* **glutamate by glutamic acid decarboxylase**, which *uses B6 as a cofactor*.

GABA Metabolism

GABA is *metabolized by* **GABA transaminase**, which uses *B6 as a cofactor*, into **succinic semialdehyde**.

Medications that Influence GABA Metabolism

Vigabatrin (Sabril) inhibits GABA-transaminase.

Tiagabine (Gabitril) blocks GABA reuptake.

GABA Receptors

There are **3 types of GABA receptors**:

       1. GABA A

       2. GABA B

       3. GABA C.

GABA **A** and GABA **C** receptors are responsible for **fast inhibitory neurotransmission**; they are *both ligand-gated chloride channels*.

GABA **B** receptors mediate **slow inhibitory neurotransmission**. They are *G protein-coupled*.

GABA A Receptors

GABA A receptors are **ligand-gated**.

The channel conducts **chloride** ions. Increased chloride conductance causes hyperpolarization of the neuronal cell membrane.

Barbiturates and benzodiazepines bind to GABA A receptors.

Benzodiazepines *increase the frequency of opening* of the channel.

Barbiturates *increase the time that the channel is open; they make it stay open longer.*

To remember that **ben**zodiazepines increase the frequency and <u>bar</u>biturates increase the time that the GABA A receptor is open, remember that **Ben** Affleck is photographed **frequently** and **bars** *stay open long into the night.*

Picrotoxin and bicuculline are antagonists to the GABA A receptor. They have been used to produce seizures in research animals.

GABA B Receptors

GABA B receptors are **metabotropic receptors** (which are associated with **G proteins**).

They mediate **slow inhibitory postsynaptic potentials**.

Activation of GABA B receptors results in opening of **potassium channels**, resulting in membrane hyperpolarization.

Baclofen is an **agonist** at the **GABA B receptor**.

Baclofen acts at the GABA **B** receptor.

GABA C Receptors

GABA **C** receptors are found in the **retina**.

GABA **C (see)** receptors are found in the **retina**.

Diseases associated with GABA

Angelman Syndrome

Children with Angelman syndrome may have epilepsy as a result of a **deletion** of the region of chromosome 15 that **codes for the β3 subunit of the GABA A receptor**.

Epilepsy

Defects in the GABA A receptor can cause:
- Generalized epilepsy with febrile seizures
- Autosomal dominant juvenile myoclonic epilepsy
- Childhood absence epilepsy and febrile seizures.

Huntington Disease

 Loss of GABAergic neurons in the striatum in Huntington disease leads to decreased inhibition of the substantia nigra.[7]

This leads to **increased dopamine production by nigrostriatal neurons**. As a result, **chorea is seen**.

Succinic Semialdehyde Dehydrogenase Deficiency

Succinic semialdehyde dehydrogenase (SSADH) deficiency, also known as Gamma-Hydroxybutyric Aciduria, is described in the Metabolic Diseases chapter.

Glutamate

 Glutamate is the **most common excitatory neurotransmitter**.

The **greatest concentrations of glutamate** are found in the:
- Dentate gyrus of the hippocampus
- Striatum
- Cortex.

Glutamate is the **neurotransmitter used by motor neurons of the cerebral cortex**.

Also, the **granule cells of the cerebellum** use glutamate.

Glutamate Synthesis

Glutaminase converts glutamine to glutamate.

Transaminase converts α-ketoglutarate to glutamate.

---

[7] See the Movement Disorders chapter for more information.

Glutamate Metabolism

 The primary mechanism of inactivation is reuptake.

Glutamate released from the nerve terminal is taken into glial cells and converted to glutamine.

Glutamate Receptors

Glutamate receptors include:
- NMDA
- AMPA
- Kainate
- Metabotropic.

NMDA (N-methyl-D-aspartate) Receptor

At rest, magnesium occupies the channel.

 For the channel to open, it must be depolarized, and 2 ligand sites must be occupied.

For instance, *glutamate and glycine both must bind while the channel is depolarized.*

When the membrane is **depolarized,**
- Calcium
- Sodium
- Potassium

………………flow through the channel.

Zinc <u>decreases</u> flow through the channel.

Phencyclidine and **ketamine <u>block</u>** NMDA receptors.

The **NMDA receptor** is important in **memory (long-term potentiation)** and has been implicated in **excitotoxicity**.

Memantine (Namenda), an NMDA receptor antagonist, has been used in patients with Alzheimer's disease.

AMPA (α-amino-3-hydroxy-5-methyl-4-isoxazole propionic acid) Receptor

 The AMPA receptor activates sodium channels.

The *GluR3 receptor is a subtype.*

Kainate Receptor

Domoic acid is an agonist for the kainate receptor.

Metabotropic Receptor

Metabotropic receptors are associated with G proteins.

Diseases associated with Glutamate

Anti-NMDA Receptor Encephalitis

Anti-NMDA Receptor Encephalitis is an autoimmune syndrome, often paraneoplastic in women with ovarian teratomas. Mean age of patients is 23 years old.

Patients may have preceding fever or other viral symptoms. Then they develop psychiatric symptoms such as **unusual behavior** and delusions/hallucinations. This is followed by movement disorders, for example orofacial **dyskinesias** and **choreoathetosis**. **Seizures** are also common. Patients become comatose, have **autonomic instability**, and have difficulty breathing.

It is treated with immunotherapy (steroids/IVIG/plasma exchange) and tumor removal if a tumor is present.

It is acute and potentially lethal. Autoantibodies are directed against NR1- and NR2-subunits of the glutamate NMDA Receptor. If diagnosed quickly and treated appropriately, full recovery is possible.

Amyotrophic Lateral Sclerosis (ALS)

Patients with *ALS* were found to have **elevated CSF glutamate levels**.

Therefore, **riluzole**, a *glutamate release inhibitor, is used to treat ALS.*

Parkinsonism-Dementia-ALS Complex of Guam

The **cycad plant**, which contains a chemical that activates NMDA receptors, is associated **with Parkinsonism-Dementia-ALS Complex of Guam**.[8]

Rasmussen's Encephalitis

Antibodies to the GluR3 receptor, an AMPA receptor subtype, have been found in patients with **Rasmussen's encephalitis.**

Toxins associated with Glutamate

Amnestic Shellfish Poisoning

Domoic acid, which is an *agonist for kainate receptors*, was found to be responsible for **amnestic shellfish poisoning.**[9]

Lathyrism

The **toxin in chickpeas** is an **AMPA receptor agonist** *in spinal neurons*. It causes **lathyrism**, which is characterized by **spastic paraplegia.**

---

[8] See the Neurodegenerative Diseases chapter.
[9] Salzman M, Madsen JM, Greenberg MI. Toxins: Bacterial and Marine Toxins. Clin Lab Med 2006;26:397-419.

Glycine

 Glycine is the **major inhibitory neurotransmitter in the spinal cord.**

It is the *neurotransmitter for* **Renshaw cells**, which inhibit alpha-motor neurons in the cord.

It is also found in the brainstem, particularly in the brainstem auditory pathways.

Glycine Synthesis

Serine is the precursor of glycine.

Glycine Metabolism

Glycine is inactivated by reuptake.

It is metabolized by the glycine-cleavage system, which mediates interconversion of glycine and serine.

Glycine Receptors

Like GABA, **glycine hyperpolarizes neurons by opening chloride channels.**

Also, glycine is a **ligand at NMDA receptors**, which are *excitatory*.

Diseases associated with Glycine

Nonketotic Hyperglycinemia

Nonketotic hyperglycinemia is an *autosomal recessive* condition due to a **defect in glycine cleavage.**

Neonates with nonketotic hyperglycinemia are **lethargic** and **hypotonic**. They have **multifocal myoclonus, hiccups**, and **apnea**.

EEG shows a *burst-suppression pattern*.

Diagnosis: **elevated CSF glycine** and **elevated CSF to plasma glycine ratio**.

Treatments for nonketotic hyperglycinemia include **sodium benzoate** and **dextromethorphan (NMDA receptor antagonist).**

Toxins associated with Glycine

Strychnine

Strychnine **inhibits the glycine receptor**.[10]

Tetanus

Tetanus toxin acts by **blocking release of glycine and GABA**.[11]

Norepinephrine (NE)

In the **CNS**, NE is found in **highest concentration in the locus ceruleus**.

It is the neurotransmitter **used by most postganglionic sympathetic neurons**.

 Remember that **sudomotor sympathetic postganglionic neurons** use **acetylcholine** instead.

Norepinephrine Synthesis

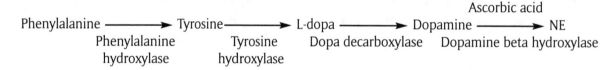

Phenylalanine ⟶ Tyrosine ⟶ L-dopa ⟶ Dopamine ⟶ NE

Phenylalanine hydroxylase   Tyrosine hydroxylase   Dopa decarboxylase   Ascorbic acid / Dopamine beta hydroxylase

Norepinephrine Metabolism

Norepinephrine inactivation is primarily through reuptake. This is blocked by amphetamines.

 Norepinephrine is metabolized by catechol-o-methyl transferase and monoamine oxidase.

In the *peripheral nervous system*, it is eventually degraded to **vanillylmandelic acid (VMA)**.

In the *central nervous system*, it is eventually degraded to **3-methoxy-4-hydroxy phenyl glycol (MHPG)**.

---

[10] Please see the Neurotoxins chapter.

[11] Please see the Infectious Diseases chapter for more information about tetanus.

Serotonin

Serotonin is found in the **raphe nuclei of the brainstem**.

Serotonin Synthesis

Serotonin is synthesized from tryptophan.

First, tryptophan hydroxylase converts tryptophan into 5-hydroxytryptophan. This is then converted into serotonin by aromatic acid decarboxylase (which uses B6 as a cofactor).

Serotonin Metabolism

The primary mechanism of inactivation of serotonin is reuptake.

Serotonin is broken down into **5-HIAA** (5-hydroxyindoleacetic acid) by monoamine oxidase A and aldehyde dehydrogenase.

Serotonin **can be converted to melatonin** in the **pineal gland**.

Conditions associated with Serotonin

Serotonin Syndrome

Serotonin syndrome is due to toxic levels of serotonin.

 First, **D**iarrhea is seen. This is followed by **R**estlessness. Then, **A**ltered **M**entation, autonomic **I**nstability, **R**igidity, and **T**emperature elevation are seen, similar to NMS.
Ser DR. -- AM I Rigid? MY TEMP Elevated?

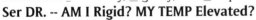 Unlike NMS, Serotonin Syndrome **may cause MYoclonus**.

In the final stages, serotonin syndrome can cause coma, status epilepticus, and cardiovascular collapse resulting in death.

Patients with Parkinson's disease who are taking MAO-B inhibitors, such as selegiline (Eldepryl) or rasagiline (Azilect), are at risk for Serotonin Syndrome, if they are placed on a SSRI.

Chapter 18

Triads

Neurology textbooks often state "Disease X is characterized by a triad: blah, blah, and blah." On the exam they may list these findings and expect you to recognize the disease.

Aicardi Syndrome

1) Agenesis of the corpus callosum

2) Infantile spasms

3) Chorioretinal lacunae

The first 3 letters of the name tell you what's in the triad:

Agenesis of the corpus callosum

Infantile spasms

Chorioretinal lacunae.

This is an X-linked **dominant** condition.

Bálint's Syndrome

Disconnection syndrome due to bilateral parietal-occipital damage.

1) Simultagnosia

2) Oculomotor-apraxia

3) Optic-ataxia

When you see **BAL** in **Bál**int's syndrome, think of base**Bál**l and the Boston Red **S.O.X.** who have difficulty getting 3 outs sometimes because of 3 visual deficits:

- **S**imultagnosia (they cannot perceive simultaneous objects -- only focusing on their huge salary and not the baseball),

- **O**culomotor-apra**X**ia (they cannot change to a new location of visual fixation -- the fielder cannot look over to see the baserunner), and

- **O**ptic-ata**X**ia (they cannot guide their hand toward an object using visual information -- the fielder is unable to tag the runner out!)

Behçet Disease

Type of vasculitis that can be associated with recurrent meningoencephalitis.

> 1) Oral ulcers
> 2) Genital ulcers
> 3) Uveitis

When you see Behçet, think Betcha It Hurts. These poor patients have oral and genital ulcers as well as uveitis.

Cushing's Triad

Signs of increased intracranial pressure.

> 1) Hypertension
> 2) Bradycardia
> 3) Irregular respirations

Dandy-Walker Syndrome

> 1) Agenesis of the cerebellar vermis
> 2) Cystic dilatation of the 4th ventricle
> 3) Enlarged posterior fossa with elevation of the tentorium

Foster Kennedy Syndrome

> 1) Ipsilateral anosmia
> 2) Ipsilateral optic atrophy
> 3) Contralateral papilledema

Classically associated with a mass, such as a meningioma, involving the olfactory groove or sphenoid ridge.

The mass compresses one optic nerve, causing optic atrophy, and increases intracranial pressure, resulting in papilledema of the contralateral eye.

Hutchinson Triad

Seen in congenital syphilis.

      1) Interstitial keratitis

      2) Notching of central incisors

      3) Nerve deafness

For more information, please see the Infectious Diseases chapter.

Gaucher's Disease Type 2

      1) Trismus

      2) Strabismus

      3) Opisthotonus

Isaac's Syndrome/Neuromyotonia

      1) Involuntary muscle twitching (fasciculations/myokymia)

      2) Muscle cramps/stiffness

      3) Myotonia

Lennox-Gastaut Syndrome

      1) EEG shows generalized slow spike and wave discharges at less than 2.5 Hz

      2) Developmental delay

      3) Specific seizure types: atonic, tonic, and atypical absence

Ménière's Disease

      1) Vertigo

      2) Tinnitus

      3) Hearing loss

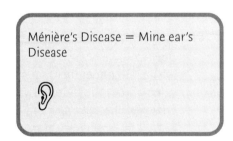

Ménière's Disease = Mine ear's Disease

MNEMONIC Ménière sounds like Mine ear. Remember: Mine ear is ringing and can't hear.

Miller-Fisher Variant of Guillain-Barré Syndrome

1) Ataxia

2) Ophthalmoparesis

3) Areflexia

 Associated with prior Campylobacter jejuni infection.

Associated with antibodies to the ganglioside GQ1b.

To remember that Miller-Fisher is associated with Campylobacter jejuni, remember that you go **fish**ing on a **camp**ing trip.

To remember that Miller-Fisher is associated with **A**taxia, **O**phthalmoparesis, and **A**reflexia and anti-**GQ**1b antibodies, remember this phrase: I bet Miller-Fisher was **A.O.A.** and perhaps **GQ** too when he wasn't **camp**ing..

Normal Pressure Hydrocephalus

1) Dementia

2) Ataxic gait

3) Urinary incontinence

"wet wacky wobbly"

Spasmus Nutans

1) Titubation / nodding of head

2) Nystagmus

3) Torticollis / neck in weird position

To remember that **sp**asmus nutans is associated with **T**itubation, **N**ystagmus, and **T**orticollis, remember the phrase: **I would spaz if I saw T.N.T. in my grandma's cellar!**
(supracellar glioma = grandma's super cellar)

Please see the Movement Disorders chapter for more information.

Susac's Syndrome

Microangiopathy involving the brain, retina, and cochlea.

     1) Branch retinal artery occlusions

     2) Encephalopathy

     3) Hearing loss

 Brain MRI findings may resemble Multiple Sclerosis.

Please see the Neuro-ophthalmology chapter for more information.

Tuberous Sclerosis

     1) Adenoma Sebaceum

     2) Mental retardation

     3) Epilepsy

Please see the Neurocutaneous Disorders chapter for the major and minor criteria used to diagnose Tuberous Sclerosis.

Wernicke Encephalopathy/Wernicke Disease

     1) Extraocular movement abnormalities

     2) Ataxia of gait

     3) Confusion   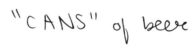

 Due to thiamine deficiency.

Observed mainly in alcoholics.

For more information, see the Behavioral Neurology chapter.

West Syndrome

     1) Infantile spasms

     2) Hypsarrhythmia

     3) Developmental delay

For more information, please see the Epilepsy chapter.

Whipple's Disease

1) Dementia

2) Supranuclear gaze palsy

3) Myoclonus

Patients also have systemic symptoms such as lymphadenopathy, steatorrhea, and weight loss.

For more information, please see the Infectious Diseases chapter.

Myoclonus, **Supra**nuclear gaze palsy, and **D**ementia can be remembered by **My Super Duodenum**.

Chapter 19

Reflexes, Signs and Other Phenomenon

Brudzinski Sign

 When the examiner flexes the patient's neck, the patient flexes the legs at the hip. This is a sign of meningeal irritation.

Ciliospinal Reflex

 When the neck is pinched, the ipsilateral pupil dilates if the sympathetic pathway is intact.

The pupil will not dilate if the patient has Horner's syndrome.

Collier Sign

 Bilateral upper eyelid retraction due to a dorsal midbrain lesion.

 This is seen as part of *Parinaud syndrome*.

Think of this as <u>Caller Sign</u>. *If someone is paranoid and has a persistent caller, his/her eyes will be bugging out/widened due to fear.* Likewise, if someone has Parinaud syndrome and Collier sign, his/her eyes seem to bug out because the eyelids are retracted.

Hoffman's Reflex

A reflex seen in patients with upper motor neuron lesions and in normal individuals with brisk deep tendon reflexes. If present on one side but not the other, it can confirm asymmetric reflexes.

When the patient's wrist is dorsiflexed, the examiner flicks the fingernail of the patient's middle finger. If the patient's thumb flexes and adducts, then Hoffman's reflex is present

Hoover's Sign

This refers to a test performed to determine if the patient is putting forth full effort during strength testing of the lower extremities.

When the patient is lying supine, the examiner puts his hand under one of the patient's legs and asks him/her to lift the other leg. Normally, if a patient is lifting the left leg and is giving full effort, he/she will push down on the examiner's hand with his/her right leg while lifting his/her left leg.

Hoover's sign is present if the patient does not push down with the normal leg when lifting the "weak" leg.

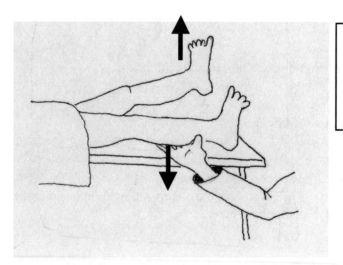

If a patient is putting forth full effort at lifting the left leg off the bed, the examiner will feel the right leg being pushed into the bed.

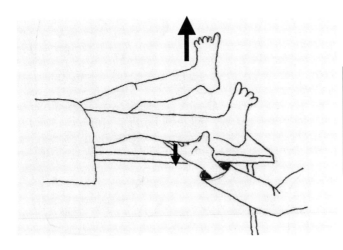

Hoover's Sign

The patient is not pushing down hard with the right leg while lifting the left leg.

Think of this as the Hover sign. **If someone is feigning weakness of the legs, both legs hover** (the leg being lifted and the leg on the bed). If the patient gave full effort, the leg on the bed would be actively pushing down.

Kernig Sign

When the examiner flexes the patient's leg at the hip and extends the leg at the knee, the patient complains of neck or back pain. *Like the Brudzinski sign, this is a sign of meningeal irritation.*

Lhermitte's Sign

A shock-like sensation travels down the back when the neck is flexed.

Classically, this is seen in **Multiple Sclerosis**. It can be seen with other **cervical lesions**.

Marcus Gunn Pupil

During the swinging flashlight test, the abnormal (Marcus Gunn) pupil appears to dilate when the light is pointed at it, rather than constricting. However it *does* react consensually when the normal pupil is illuminated. This is also known as **a relative afferent pupillary defect**.

An optic nerve lesion is one possible cause.

 If someone pointed a gun at your pupil, your eye would dilate wide open in horror and you'd ask the police to put out an **APB**.

Likewise, if someone has a Marcus Gunn pupil, the eye dilates when it's pointed at and there's an APD (**a**fferent **p**upillary **d**efect).

Myerson Sign

 The inability to stop blinking when tapped over the bridge of the nose or glabella.

This may be seen in Parkinson's disease.

Palmomental Reflex

Contraction of the ipsilateral mentalis muscle of the chin, when the palm is stroked. This can be seen in dementia but also in some normal individuals.

Phalen's Sign

When wrist flexion produces paresthesias in the median nerve distribution. It is used to help diagnose carpal tunnel syndrome.

Riddoch Phenomenon

When a person can see the examiner's fingers if they are moving but not if they are still.

 The examiner looks **rid**iculous wiggling his fingers but it is the only way to demonstrate **Rid**doch phenomenon.

Snout Reflex

 The patient's lips pucker in response to pressure/tapping. It is a primitive reflex and a frontal release sign.

Tinel's Sign

When tapping over the median nerve at the wrist elicits paresthesias in the median nerve distribution. It is used to help diagnose carpal tunnel syndrome.

Remember **Ph**alen's sign is when wrist flexion (**Phlexion)** produces paresthesias in the median nerve distribution, and **T**inel's sign is when **T**apping produces them.

Uhthoff's Phenomenon

Uhthoff's Phenomenon is the worsening of ANY neurologic symptoms from multiple sclerosis (MS) or other neurological demyelinating conditions when a person's body temperature rises.

Fever, saunas, hot tubs, sunbathing, and exercising heat up the body and slow down nerve conduction -- in a damaged optic nerve, for example provoking decreased acuity. When body temperature normalizes, so do symptoms.

Use the mnemonic **UHTHOFF** to remember the features off Uhthoff's phenomenon:

Under

Heat

The

Optic nerve

Fatigues

Fast

Chapter 20

X-Linked Diseases

This drawing was created by Dr. Anne Cross and redrawn by Jackie Brown, RN.

It was designed to help one remember X-linked diseases. It does not include all the X-linked diseases, but it covers quite a few.

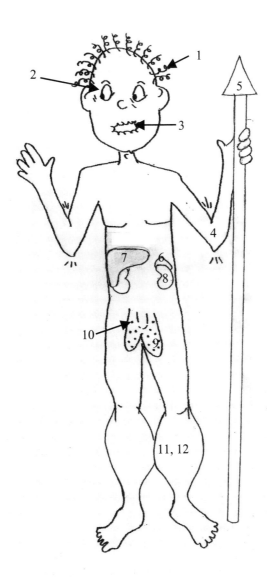

X-linked Diseases

1) Menkes' Kinky Hair Syndrome
2) Pelizaeus-Merzbacher disease
3) Lesch-Nyhan syndrome
4) Emery-Dreifuss muscular dystrophy
5) Hunter's syndrome
6) Adrenoleukodystrophy
7) Ornithine transcarbamylase deficiency
8) Lowe's (oculocerebrorenal) syndrome
9) Fragile X syndrome
10) Fabry's disease
11) Duchenne Muscular Dystrophy
12) Becker Muscular Dystrophy

Chapter 21

Psychiatry for Neurologists

Notes from the Authors

Although they say about 20% of the Neurology board exam (approximately 80 questions) covers Psychiatry, you may not be "in the mood" to memorize the entire *Diagnostic and Statistical Manual of Mental Disorders, Fourth Edition, Text Revision (DSM-IV-TR) or Fifth Edition (DSM-V, published in 2013)*. Don't fret -- this chapter contains key parts of most psychiatric conditions that Neurologists encounter, a few psychotically good mnemonics, and some sound advice:

First, review the bio-neuro-phenomenona[1] of psychiatric disorders – like the **genetics** of Schizophrenia, the **types** of Bulimia Nervosa, the **etiology** of Adjustment Disorder, and the **associated findings** of Pisa Syndrome.

Secondly, hit up the major diagnostic criteria for Depression, Mania, and Somatization Disorder. After all, we Non-psychiatrists shouldn't be giving out these diagnoses like free samples at Costco®.

Third, remember to look for obvious and not-so-obvious primary, secondary, and tertiary **Gain** in every patient. Conversion Disorder, Factitious Disorder, Munchausen's, and Malingering are not uncommon.

Fourth, don't skip mechanisms of action and side effects of psychopharmacological treatment. Reactions to meds are fair game!

Lastly but not leastly[2], take a peek at those pesky Neuro-Psych Tests (NPTs). A general overview of the NPTs highlighted below should suffice.

Now you'll be less nauseated when recalling details of Anorexia Nervosa and less stunned when facing a question on Electro-Convulsive Therapy – that's the psyche behind this chapter.

Multi-Axial System

To speak like a psychiatrist, you gotta know the fab 5 Axes below!!!!!

Axis I: Clinical disorders, including major mental disorders, and learning disorders, Substance Abuse Disorders *(examples: include Depression, Bipolar Disorder, ADHD, Autism Spectrum Disorders, Anorexia Nervosa, Bulimia Nervosa, Schizophrenia, and any of the anxiety disorders)*

---

[1] If that is actually a word in any language known to human or beast.
[2] Certainly not a word in any language known to humankind but perhaps one known to lesser mammals.

Axis II: Personality Disorders (see below)

Axis III: Medical conditions / physical disorders *(examples: Traumatic Brain Injury, Stroke, Epilepsy, Hypothyroidism, etc.)*

Axis IV: Psychosocial and environmental factors contributing to the disorder

Axis V: **G**lobal **A**ssessment of **F**unctioning (**GAF**) or **C**hildren's **G**lobal **A**ssessment **S**cale (**CGAS**, for children and teens) – measures psychologic, social, and occupational functioning, ranging from 1 (lowest level, with persistent danger to self and others) to 100 (highest level, asymptomatic, with many friends and positive qualities where "life's problems never out of hand"). *It is widely used in studies of treatment effectiveness.*

Neuro-Psychological Testing (NPT)

The hinterland between Neurology and Psychology is NPT. It helps with:

- *Hidden Diagnoses:* for example, depression may be difficult to diagnose in an articulate, well-compensated person but NPT can identify it;
- *Patient Safety:* NPT serves as a basis for increased supervision or reduced work responsibility (or even driver's license issues) in patients with dementia, cortical strokes, longstanding seizures, traumatic brain injury, and other neurologic disabilities that may affect personality, judgment, and daily living activities;
- *Follow-up Measurements:* serial NPT evaluations provide an established, objective baseline that can be contrasted annually or semi-annually to determine if a neuro-psychologic disease process is improving, deteriorating or stable.

There are many different categories of NPT. They include: Memory Testing, Dementia-specific Testing, Language Testing, Executive Function Testing, Intelligence Testing, Visuospatial Testing, and a combination of above.

Categories of NPT:

Memory Testing

3 types of testable memory are:

affected in TGA

1. Declarative or Explicit Memory:

Semantic Memory (for facts) and **Episodic Memory** (autobiographical details)

2. Non-Declarative or Implicit Memory:

- **Procedural Memory** (performance of skills) and **Priming** (memory facilitated by prior exposure to a stimulus)

- **Perceptual Learning** (pertaining to recall of visual, auditory, tactile, olfactory or taste senses-information, but in relation to experience and practice – such as moving chess pieces, playing piano, baking a cake, or discriminating X-ray images or even answering board review or RITE questions correctly in your case)

3. Working memory: short-term memory for information manipulation

Examples:
- California Verbal Learning Test
- Cambridge Prospective Memory Test (CAMPROMPT)
- Memory Assessment Scales (MAS)
- Rey Auditory Verbal Learning Test

Dementia-specific Testing

The four cognitive functions most often impaired by dementia are: Orientation, Language, Memory, and Problem solving,

OL' Miss Patsy (she was old and had dementia):
Orientation, **L**anguage, **M**emory, and **P**roblem **s**olving.

Certain NPTs evaluate presence of (and/or severity of) deficits in these 4 cognitive areas.

Examples:
- Clinical Dementia Rating; or
- **MCI** (**M**ild **C**ognitive **I**mpairment) Screen

Language Testing

Separate language functions can be selectively impaired, such as speech (expressing, understanding, naming and repeating), reading, and writing.

Examples:
- Boston Diagnostic Aphasia Examination
- Boston Naming Test
- **C**omprehensive **A**phasia **T**est (**CAT**)
- Lexical decision task
- Multilingual Aphasia Examination

Types of language difficulties:

Term	Definition
Adynamia	Difficulty with speech initiation
Agrammatism or Paragrammatism	Lack of (or misuse of) grammatical elements (such as articles, pronouns, prepositions, etc.)
Anomia	Lack of use of nouns
Circumlocution	"Dancing around the topic" – Cannot find a word so associated words or themes related to the missing word are used
Echolalia	Repeating others' words when not necessary
Palilalia	Repeating ones' own words when not necessary
Stereotypic speech	Repeating nonsensical syllables
Telegraphic speech	Condensed speech, in mostly nouns and verbs, like a telegram ("Water now!")
Logorrhea	"Diarrhea of the mouth" – Lengthy, incomprehensible speech
Neologisms	Invented words
Phonemic/Literal Paraphasia	An error of sound substitution (saying "hair" instead of "chair")
Semantic Paraphasia	An error of related-type substitution (saying "hammer" instead of "nail")
Remote Paraphasia	An error of **un**related-type substitution (saying "knee" instead of "apple")

Executive Function Testing

Executive Functions – localizing mostly to the **Dorso-Lateral Pre-Frontal Cortex (DLPFC), Orbito-Frontal Cortex (OFC)**, and **Cingulate Cortex** – include: planning, organizing, set-shifting, exhibiting selective attention, and controlling inhibitions. To be a successful CEO – Chief Executive Officer – you gotta do these things really well!

Examples:

· Continuous Performance Task (**CPT**)
· Controlled Oral Word Association Test (**COWAT**)
· Digit Vigilance Test
· Figural Fluency Test
· Halstead Category Test

· **Paced Auditory Serial Addition Test (PASAT)** ***
· **Wisconsin Card Sorting Task (WCST)** ***
· Symbol Digit Modalities Test

*** = these are particularly important executive function tests, used with some frequency

Lesions to the DLPFC, OFC and/or Cingulate each reveal separate dysfunctions:

*Lesions to the **Dorso-Lateral Pre-Frontal Cortex (DLPFC)** typically cause personality changes, and lack of ability to plan or to sequence actions or tasks. **DLPFC** is also involved in verbal and design fluency, organization skills, problem-solving, abstract thinking, shifting sets/topics, and creative reasoning.*

DLPFC – **D**rastic personality change, **L**ack of planning, **P**roblem-solving, verbal and design **F**luency, and **C**reative reasoning/abstract thinking.

*Lesions to the **Orbito-Frontal Cortex (OFC)** typically cause disinhibition, emotional lability (impulsiveness, jocularity, hypersexuality), and "acquired sociopathy" or "pseudopsychopathic disorder."*

lateral orbitofrontal → echopraxia

OFC – **O**h, **F**rank took his **C**lothes **OF**f!

*Lesions to the **Cingulate Cortex** typically cause akinetic mutism, apathy and abulia (if superior) or anterograde and retrograde amnesia and confabulation (if inferior mesial, or basal forebrain).*

Cing – **Cing** a **Confabulated** song or don't **Cing** at all (akinetic mute)

Intelligence Testing

Examples:
· Ammons Quick Test
· National Adult Reading Test
· Stanford-Binet Intelligence Scales
· **W**echsler **A**dult **I**ntelligence **S**cale (**WAIS**) ***
· **W**echsler Intelligence Scale for Children (WISC)

· **W**echsler Preschool and Primary Scale of Intelligence (WPPSI)

· **W**echsler Test of Adult Reading (WTAR)

*** = WAIS is the most famous and most commonly administered psychological test; it gets updated every decade*

This man who invented so many **intelligence** tests, David **"Wex"** Wechsler, must have been **intelligent** himself! Think he **Was cheer**ing on his test-takers? Or, if his students failed his test, did he make them wax his car and say, "**Wex** On, **Wex** Off!?"

Visuospatial Testing

Visuospatial NPT includes testing visual perception, construction and integration (mostly functions that involve the parietal lobe).

Examples:

· Clock Test

· Hooper **V**isual **O**rganisation **T**ask (**VOT**)

· Rey-Osterrieth Complex Figure

Combined NPT

Some batteries combine tests to assess many cognitive skills simultaneously. Such "megatests" evaluate all functions to find problem areas that need help.

Examples:

· **C**ognitive **F**unction **S**canner (**CFS**)

· Hooper Visual Organization Test

· **MMSE** (see below)

Mini-Mental Status Examination (MMSE)[3]

The MMSE (or Folstein exam) is the most commonly used, most referenced, most well-known, quickest mentation evaluation. There are 7 basic parts of the MMSE: **L**evel of Consciousness, **O**rientation, **C**oncentration/Calculation, **A**ttention, **M**emory, **L**anguage, and **T**hought process.

To remember the **7 various parts of the MMSE think** of the *MMSE Mnemonic:* **LOCAM-LT**[4] (or, if you want to use our interpretation of this mnemonic: **L**eave **O**ur **C**omrades **A**lone **M**ost **L**oathe **T**ests.)

---

[3] Folstein MF, Folstein SE, McHugh PR. "Mini-mental state." A practical method for grading the cognitive state of patients for the clinician. J Psychiatr Res. 1975;12(3):189-198.

[4] Baron, E. "Proposed LOCAM-LT Mnemonic for Mastering Examination of Mental Status and Cognitive Function." J Am Osteopath Assoc. 2010;110(9) 553-555.

Level Of Consciousness (LOC)

 There are 5 **fishy** LOC's: **HADOC**: **H**yperalert, **A**lert, **D**rowsy, **O**btunded, **C**omatose.

Orientation

A patient can be oriented to Person (self); Place (country, state, city, hospital, floor, room); and Time (year, month, date, day, time of day).

Concentration/Calculation

Spell W-O-R-L-D forward and backwards, or Subtract 7 from 100 (100-7=93), and then 7 from that (93-7=86), etc, continuing in that pattern for 5 total subtractions ("Serial 7's").

Attention

Is the patient attentive and focused or inattentive and distracted?

Memory (3 subtypes)

· *Immediate memory* – 3-item recall (apple, table, penny) or 7-digit recall.

· *Recent memory* – repeat/recall the same 3 items for immediate memory, after a minute distraction

· *Remote memory* – personal information (date of birth, place of birth, family members' birth order, historical events).

· *Eidetic "photographic" memory* – recall large amount of images, sounds and objects in an visualized sense

Language

· *Comprehension* – ask patient to perform 2- or 3-step commands, make purposeful movements, such as comb their hair or brush their teeth

· *Repetition* – repeat "no ifs, ands, or buts about it" or "it's a sunny day outside."

· *Naming* – name high-frequency, common objects (pen, finger, watch),
   then medium-frequency (thumb, necktie, button),
   then low-frequency (stethoscope, lapel, hammock).
(or, name as many *category items* in 1 minute; >12 words is normal):

· "S" words (sock, stove, sale, scare, etc...) screen for frontal dysfunction (Fronto-Temporal Dementia, FTD)

· Animal naming (cat, dog, lion, mouse, etc...) screens for temporoparietal dysfunction (Alzheimer Disease)

· **Reading** – read the sentence, "close your eyes," and to follow the instructions. (or, ask illiterate patients to describe events in a picture)

· **Writing/drawing** – write a random sentence, copy a diagram of intersecting pentagons, bisect a horizontal line, or insert missing numbers into a picture of a clock (screens for dementia and hemineglect syndromes)

· **Fluency** – listen for smoothness of speech and ability to construct and deliver full grammatically normal sentences

Thought Process

· **Abstraction** – discuss similarities and differences between various objects or settings—such as a tent vs a cabin or a river vs a lake (screens for psychosis, delusions, and tangential or pressured speech)

Somatoform Disorders

Somatization

Experiencing and communicating mental distress as physical symptoms

Somatoform Disorder

Physical symptoms that suggest but are not entirely explained by a general medical condition (or medication effect) which:

· causes impairment in social, occupational or physical functioning

· are unintentional (**unlike** Factitious Disorders and Malingering)

· mostly occur in unmarried, non-white, less educated women who live in rural areas.[5]

· *Lifetime Prevalence:* 0.13%

· **Somatization Disorder:** a subtype of Somato<u>form</u> Disorder where, over years, patient seeks medical attention for many physical symptoms with no evidence of organ pathology. Somatic complaints must start before age 30, involve pain in at least 4 different body areas, 2 or more GI problems, 1 sexual dysfunction, and 1 pseudo-neurologic condition, according to DSM-IV-TR. The most common complaints:

   ○ **S**exual problems (classically, "burning in sex organs") and/or **D**ysmenorrhea *

   ○ **E**xtremity pain

---

[5] According to survey of 20,000 Americans in the Somatization Disorder Epidemiological Catchment Area (ECA) Study.

○ **C**hoking (lump in throat = "globus" phenomenon) and shortness of breath (psychogenic dyspnea and/or hyperventilation)

○ **N**ausea/Vomiting

○ **A**mnesia

○ **T**rouble walking, hearing, seeing, or something neurologic-like

 Somatization **D**isorder **E**xperiences **C**hoking, **N**ausea, **A**nd other **T**roubles.

 If the patient does not complain of **S**exual problems and/or **D**ysmenorrhea, the diagnosis **S**omatization **D**isorder is less secure!

 All these symptoms do not all have to occur at the same time but rather typically occur in a chronic, fluctuating pattern. Patients may see dozens of doctors.

· **Somatization Syndrome:** as above but with fewer symptoms (total of 4 for men, 6 for women).

Body Dysmorphic Disorder (BDD)

· type of **Somatoform Disorder** excessively concerned with body image

· perceived defect of physical features

· causes impairment in social, occupational or physical functioning

· linked to Depression, Social Phobia, and Obsessive Compulsive Disorder (OCD)

· often a history of mental and physical abuse, emotional neglect

· discrepancy between "actual self" and "ideal self" (dissociation)

· **suicidal ideation rate of 80%!**

· symptom onset: adolescence (self-criticism of personal appearance starts in early adulthood)

· occurs equally among men and women

· **Incidence**: 1 – 2%

· cognitive behavioral therapy (CBT) and Selective Serotonin Reuptake Inhibitors (SSRIs)

Hypochondriasis

- type of **Somatoform** Disorder which fears having a serious disease
- hypersensitive to physical sensations, ruminate obsessively
- causes impairment in social, occupational or physical functioning
- concern must last at least <u>6 months</u>
- persists despite thorough medical evaluation and reassurance

- Identify, address underlying obsessional thinking or disease phobia; SSRIs like **P**axil (**P**aroxetine) are often chosen for **P**hobias

Differentiating **Hypochondriasis** from **Somatization Disorder** depends on the patient's focus – **Hypochondriacs** focus **less on the actual symptoms** and more on what the symptoms **signify**, and the **fear** of dying from them.

Conversion Disorder

- type of **Somatoform Disorder** where emotional stress unintentionally undergoes a **"conversion"** into neurological symptoms (like numbness, paralysis, aphasia, blindness, pseudoseizures, etc.)
- symptoms classically suggest a **neurologic** condition (like Stroke, Tourette's Syndrome, MS, Epilepsy, etc.) but thorough medical evaluation is unremarkable
- according to DSM-IV, Conversion Disorder diagnosis explicitly requires exclusion of deliberate feigning
- DSM-IV also requires clinician to identify preceding stressors or conflicts related to developing Conversion Disorder
- psychological factors / conflicts / stressors can precede the initiation or exacerbation of symptoms by years
- Pseudoseizures are now also called Psychogenic Non-Epileptic Seizures (PNES) or non-epileptic attack disorders, and may be seen in 20% of patients in epilepsy clinics. About 75% are women, with features during the "event" that can include tongue-tip-biting, eye-closing, pelvic thrusting, and moving the head side-to-side.
- Historically referred to as "hysteria".

CBT and SSRIs, but if hospitalized, symptoms may disappear within a week regardless

· **Recurrence:** 25% in 1 year

· **Prognosis:** better for patients with acute onset, clearly identifiable stress, and faster treatment

 Patients with **Conversion** Disorder will **religiously** have their mental stress undergo a **Conversion** into physical symptoms!

Factitious Disorder *(pseudologia fantastica, or mythomania)*

· intentional, false symptoms or gross exaggeration of minor symptoms

· **Gain** or motivation to assume the sick role and to receive care, often is initially unclear (see below on **type of Gain**)

· causes impairment in social, occupational or physical functioning

· if multiple hospitalizations, then diagnosis is **Munchausen's Syndrome**

· if multiple hospitalizations of a family member, friend, or surrogate, then diagnosis is **Munchausen's Syndrome by Proxy**

· when external incentives found (i.e., financial), diagnosis is **Malingering**

Patients with **Fact**itious Disorder got their **Facts** wrong!

Differentiating **Malingering** from **Somatization Disorder** depends on the degree of conscious voluntary control the person has over their *illness behavior*. The way everyone acts while assuming the "sick role" is different: some are stoic, others dramatic, some express verbal complaints, others reveal physical distress. Although both disorders display maladaptive attempts to be granted thc benefits of the sick role inappropriately, Malingering is a lot more deliberate and intentional.

Gain: Primary vs. Secondary vs. Tertiary

The type of Gain (1 vs. 2 vs. 3) is the psychological motivation for reporting symptoms

Primary Gain (1)

· *Internal Motivation* (illness helps the patient's psyche)

· example: feeling less guilty about missing work, when due to medical condition

Secondary Gain (2)

· *External Motivation* (symptom benefits the patient)

· example: reducing jail sentence by using the sick role

Tertiary Gain (3) – less well-studied

· *Third Party Motivation* (patient's illness benefits someone else)

· example: a relative, friend, or treating psychiatrist gets benefits/rewards from the victim's sickness

Remembering *Gains are as easy as 1-2-3!*

Primary (1): **P**atient's **P**syche **P**ampered and **P**andered

Secondary (2): **S**ymptom's **S**ympathy **S**ecured for **S**ufferer

Tertiary (3): **T**herapist's **T**rophy

Eating Disorders

Bulimia Nervosa

Bulimia is Greek for "ravenous hunger" and has strong genetic linkage in families. Twin studies estimate the heritability of syndromic Bulimia to be as high as 83%. Bulimics often have an affective disorder, such as Depression or General Anxiety Disorder (GAD).

There are two sub-types of Bulimia Nervosa, based on what happens after a binge:

· **Purging type** – primarily self-induce vomiting by gagging or taking emetics

· **Non-purging type** – primarily exercise or fast excessively to offset caloric intake; this subtype is more rare, representing <10% of cases

Bulimia: **R**eal **L**ife **R**egular **P**eople **B**inge

Recurrent episodes of binge eating (minimum of 2 required for diagnosis)

Lacks control during a binge (over-eating can be unstoppable once started)

Regular abuse of laxatives, diuretics, vomit-induction (with gastric acid from continuous self-emesis causing bad teeth), and/or rigorous exercise (watch for electrolyte imbalances!!)

Persistent over-concern with bodyweight (associated with distorted body image and depression)

Bodyweight higher than required for diagnosing Anorexia (weight loss of 15% of original body weight)

Anorexia Nervosa

Anorexic patients eat tiny amounts of food, despite hunger pains. The average anorexic patient's daily intake is 600 calories, but some self-impose total starvation.

Anorexia has the **highest mortality rate of any psychiatric disorder**. Anorexia is most prevalent among adolescent girls, with onset as early as age 9 to 12 years old.

Anorexia-→ FFFFAT, *there are Four F's in this FAT mnemonic*

Feels **FAT** (despite obvious skinniness)

Fears becoming **FAT** by weight-gain (and thus refuses to maintain normal body weight)

Factors for weight loss must be non-organic *(i.e., rule out hypothyroidism)*

Food always on mind

Amenorrhea

Tummy hurts (Epigastric discomfort and other peculiar symptoms are common)

Personality Disorders (Axis-II)

Personality Disorders are subdivided into 3 "clusters" – **A**, **B**, and **C**.

A, **B**, and **C**: **A**typical, **B**eastly, and **C**owardly/**C**lingy/**C**ompulsive
(or **A**, **B**, and **C**: *Weird*, *Wild*, and *Wacky*, respectively)

Cluster A

Atypical, or *Weird* (Odd Eccentrics): ***Paranoid, Schizoid and Schizotypal*** Personality Disorders

Paranoid Personality Disorder: **SUSPECT**

Suspicious

Unforgiving

Spouse infidelity Suspected

Perceives attacks (and reacts quickly)

Enemies of associates / friends

Confiding in others feared

Threats from normal events

Schizoid Personality Disorder: **NO FUN**

No close relations

Opposed to sex

"asteroid" off M another world

Flat / detached affect

Unresponsive to criticism / praise

No desire to participate in tasks / activities with others

Schizotypal Personality Disorder: **MAGIC**

Magical thinking

Anxiety in social situations, lacks friends

Goofy (odd) speech, behavior or appearance

Ideas of reference

Constricted, inappropriate affect

Rule out Psychotic Disorders and Pervasive Developmental Disorder (PDD) prior to making diagnosis of ***Schizotypal*** PD.

Cluster B

Beastly, or *Wild* (Dramatic, Erratic Extraverts): ***Antisocial, Borderline, Histrionic, and Narcissistic*** Personality Disorders

 Antisocial Personality Disorder: **CRIME**

    Cons others without remorse

    Reckless disregard for safety of self / others

    Ignores obligations, laws, rules, plans

    Mad, bad temper (irritable and aggressive)

    Everything is a lie

 Borderline Personality Disorder: **UNSTABLE**

    Unstable, intense relationships

    No control of anger / rage

    Suicidal, **S**elf-mutilating, **S**plitting behavior*

    Transient dissociative or paranoid states

    Abandonment

    Bad mood with marked reactivity

    Lack of identity

    Emptiness

 Splitting can occur in either ***Borderline*** or ***Narcissistic PD*** – Those with ***Borderline PD*** cannot integrate the good and bad images of both self and others (a *bad representation* dominates the *good representation*) whereas those with ***Narcissistic*** PD split via idealization and devaluation of others, due to "narcissistic rage and injury."

 Histrionic Personality Disorder: **O-PLEASE**

    Outward, physical appearance "made up" to draw attention to self

    Provocative / seductive behavior

    Love: relationships considered more intimate than reality

    Easily influenced

    Attention-seeker uncomfortable without the spotlight

    Speech impressionistic, vague, lacks detail

    Emotions exaggerated, shallow, shift rapidly, theatrical!

***Narcissistic* Personality Disorder: <u>SPECIAL-U</u>**

<u>S</u>elf-belief of <u>S</u>pecial <u>S</u>uccess and power, <u>S</u>plitting behavior*

<u>P</u>reoccupation with fantasies of unlimited brilliance, beauty, love

<u>E</u>nvious of <u>E</u>verybody

<u>C</u>onceited, high self-importance, entitled "VIP"

<u>I</u>nterpersonal exploitation

<u>A</u>rrogant

<u>L</u>acks empathy

<u>U</u>nable to recognize feelings/needs of others

Cluster C

<u>C</u>owardly/<u>C</u>lingy/<u>C</u>ompulsive, or *Wacky* (Anxious, Fearful Neurotics): *Avoidant* (<u>C</u>owardly), *Dependent* (<u>C</u>lingy), and *Obsessive-Compulsive* (<u>C</u>ompulsive) Personality Disorders (OCPD, not OCD)[6,7,8,9]

***Avoidant* Personality Disorder: <u>CRINGE</u>**

<u>C</u>ontemptuous self-image (viewed as an unappealing, inept, and/or inferior person)

<u>R</u>ejection (or criticism) preoccupies thoughts in social situations

<u>I</u>nhibition of <u>I</u>ntimate and/or new relationships

<u>N</u>eeds <u>N</u>umerous <u>N</u>ods of approval before engaging socially (certainty of being liked required before willing to get involved with others)

<u>G</u>ets around occupational activity with any interpersonal contact

<u>E</u>mbarrassment (potential) prevents new activity or taking risks

***Dependent* Personality Disorder: <u>DEPEND</u>**

<u>D</u>ependent upon constant companionship

<u>E</u>ncouragement <u>E</u>ssential (lacks self-confidence)

<u>P</u>owerless, helpless, <u>P</u>anic-<u>P</u>rone

<u>E</u>veryone <u>E</u>lse is responsible for <u>E</u>verything

<u>N</u>urturing <u>N</u>eeded (goes to excessive lengths to obtain)

<u>D</u>oesn't <u>D</u>isagree (for fear of losing support or approval)

---

[6] American Psychiatric Association (1994). Diagnostic and statistical manual of mental disorders (4th ed.). Washington, DC: Author.

[7] Benjamin, L. S. (1996). Interpersonal diagnosis and treatment of personality disorders (2nd ed.). New York: Guilford.

[8] Eysenck, H. J. (1987). The definition of personality disorders and the criteria appropriate for their descriptions. Journal of Personality Disorders, 1, 211 " 219.

[9] Pinkofsky, H. B. (1997). Mnemonics for DSM-IV personality disorders. Psychiatric Services, 48. 1197-1198.

Obsessive-Compulsive Personality Disorder (OCPD): <u>**SCRIMP**</u>

Stubbornness (rigidity)

Cannot discard worthless **C**rap, **C**annot **C**oncentrate on **C**olossal **C**oncerns, only on **C**rummy details

Rule-obsessed

Inflexible, scrupulous, overconscientious (on ethics, values, or morality, not accounted for by religion or culture); excludes friendships and leisure due to devotion to work

Miserly (toward self and others)

Perfectionistic to a fault – cannot complete tasks because compromised by perfectionism, and cannot delegate to others unless all guidelines followed

OCPD *(Axis II) is quite different from* ***OCD*** *(Axis I, below)*

Affective (Mood) Disorders

Depression, Dysthymia, and Mania (Bipolar I)

Depression

SIG: E CAPS

Suicidal thoughts

Interests decreased

Guilt

Energy decreased

Concentration impaired

Appetite disturbance

Psychomotor changes (agitation or retardation)

Sleep disturbance

Dysthymia

HE'S 2 SAD

Hopelessness

Energy decreased

Self-esteem decreased

2 years minimum of depressed mood most of the day, for more days than not

Sleep disturbance

Appetite disturbance

Decision-making, concentration impaired

Mania

HIDES

Hyperactive

Indiscreet

Distracted

Extravagant, grandiose

Speech Tangential with "Flight of Ideas" (loose associations rambling from one idea to an unrelated idea), and **S**leep deficit

Anxiety Disorders

Obsessive-Compulsive Disorder (OCD), Generalized Anxiety Disorder (GAD), Post-Traumatic Stress Disorder (PTSD), Neurasthenia, and *General Medical Condition-Anxiety Not Otherwise Specified (GMC-ANOS?)*

Obsessive-Compulsive Disorder (OCD)

OCD (Axis I) is different from **OCPD** (Axis II, above) in that it's more than just a personality thing, it's a real anxiety disorder – the obsession, which is routinely followed by its compulsion, results in alleviation of the anxiety

Generalized Anxiety Disorder (GAD)

Worry WARTS

> **Worry: Wor**n-out (low energy)
>
> **W**ound-up
>
> **A**rousal increased
>
> **R**estless, irritable
>
> **T**ense muscles
>
> **S**leepless, with decreased concentration (absentminded)

Post-Traumatic Stress Disorder (PTSD)

TRAUMAS

> **T**raumatic event occurred
>
> **R**e-experience / flashbacks
>
> **A**voidance of **A**ssociations to event
>
> **U**nable to function / **U**ninterested in **U**sual activities
>
> **M**onth or More of symptoms
>
> **A**rousal increased
>
> **S**ympathetic Surges

Neurasthenia ("Tired Nerves" or "Nervous Exhaustion")

FOG

> **F**atigue after mental effort
>
> **O**verlaps with Chronic Fatigue Syndrome, Depression, and anxiety disorders
>
> **G**eneral symptoms (dizziness, headaches, irritability and insomnia)

General Medical Condition-Anxiety Not Otherwise Specified

(**GMC-ANOS**: Diseases associated with anxiety)

 PATCHED – your shrink **PATCHED** up your **GMC-ANOS** when labs revealed you had a medical condition explaining your anxiety!

Pheochromocytoma (check urine catecholamines)

Arrhythmias (check EKG)

Temporal lobe epilepsy (check EEG)

Carcinoid (10% of carcinoids secrete excessive hormones, most notably serotonin, or 5-HT, so the most useful initial test is the 24-hour urine level of 5-hydroxyindoleacetic acid, or 5-HIAA – a serotonin breakdown product)

Hyperthyroidism (check TSH)

Ethanol withdrawal (check CAGE questionnaire, below)

Diabetes mellitus (check blood glucose and HbA1c %)

Panic Disorder

 The 5 components of Panic Disorder spell out the word **PANIC**:

Palpitation and **P**erspiration

Abdominal pain

Nausea/Vomiting

Increased awareness/anxiety about surroundings

Chest pain, **C**hills, and **C**hoking (lump in throat = "globus" phenomenon)

Phobia

 An anxiety disorder with extreme, irrational fear of simple things or social situations

SSRIs like Paxil (Paroxetine) are often Picked for Phobias

List of common (and some uncommon) phobias:

Ablutophobia – Fear of washing or bathing *(just like Bluto from Animal House!)*

Acrophobia – Fear of heights (just like an acrobat)

Agateophobia – Fear of insanity

Agoraphobia – Fear of open spaces or of being in crowded, public places like markets

Aichmophobia – Fear of needles or pointed objects

Allodoxaphobia – Fear of opinions

Androphobia – Fear of men (just like an android is a Robot-man)

Arachnophobia – Fear of spiders (like the infamous movie)

Athazagoraphobia – Fear of being forgotten or ignored or forgetting

Claustrophobia – Fear of confined spaces

Entomophobia – Fear of insects

Erotophobia – Fear of sexual love or sexual questions

Geliophobia – Fear of laughter

Gelotophobia – Fear of being laughed at

Genophobia – Fear of sex (becoming too genial, perhaps?)

Homophobia – Fear of sameness, monotony or of homosexuality

Hypnophobia – Fear of sleep or of being hypnotized

Iatrophobia – Fear of going to the doctor or of doctors

Ichthyophobia – Fear of fish

Neophobia – Fear of anything new (or fear of that guy from the Matrix)

Nosocomephobia – Fear of hospitals

Nosophobia – Fear of becoming ill

Numerophobia – Fear of numbers

Odontophobia – Fear of teeth or dental surgery

Ophidiophobia – Fear of snakes

Ornithophobia – Fear of birds

Pathophobia – Fear of disease

Parturiphobia – Fear of childbirth

Pedophobia – Fear of children

Philophobia – Fear of falling in love or being in love[10]

Phobophobia – Fear of phobias

Photophobia – Fear of light (frequently experienced in migraines)

Phonophobia – Fear of noises or voices (frequently experienced in migraines)

Psychophobia – Fear of mind

---

[10] Arguably normal variant in the male half of the species !

Radiophobia – Fear of radiation, x-rays

Ranidaphobia – Fear of frogs

Scotophobia – Fear of darkness

Sinistrophobia – Fear of lefties

Somniphobia – Fear of sleep

Verminophobia – Fear of germs

Xenophobia – Fear of strangers or foreigners

Zoophobia – Fear of animals

Adjustment Disorder

A stronger-than-expected **Behavioral** and **Emotional** response to an identifiable *"life stressor"* such as financial or marital troubles, death of a loved one, or job problem.

Behavioral signs include: fighting; shunning family or friends; ignoring bills, deadlines, chores, or homework; performing poorly in school or work; truancy; vandalism; general recklessness; or theft

Emotional signs include: sadness, crying, nervousness, insomnia, difficulty concentrating, and suicidal ideations

Adjustment Disorder does not meet criteria for Anxiety Disorder, PTSD, or Acute Stress Disorder – Anxiety Disorder lacks the presence of a stressor, and PTSD and Acute Stress Disorder are associated with a more intense stressor than the typical "life stressors".

Adjustment Disorder may be **acute** (< 6 months) or **chronic** (> 6 months) but symptoms cannot last > 6 months after the stressor (or its consequences) has ended. The difference between Adjustment Disorder and Major Depressive Disorder is that the latter is **caused by an outside stressor** which, when removed, or constructively adapted to, typically **resolves**.

Incidence: 5-21% among adult psychiatric consultations (women diagnosed twice as often as men, but girls and boys receive diagnosis with equal frequency.

To **adjust** to *"life stressors"* and not develop Adjustment Disorder, you must **BE** all that you can **BE** (**Behavioral** and **Emotional** responses).

Substance <u>Dependence</u> versus Substance <u>Abuse</u>

Substance Dependence

ADDICT

Activities **A**bandoned

Dependence is physical: *tolerance* versus *withdrawal*

Duration of substance use more than intended

Intrapersonal and **I**nternal consequences

Can't **C**ontrol use or **C**ut back

Time-consumed

Tolerance (the capacity to endure or become less responsive to a substance with repeated use or exposure) and *withdrawal* (painful physical and psychological symptoms that follow discontinuing a substance) are *neither necessary nor sufficient to develop an addiction,* but together contribute to physical **Dependence**.

Substance Abuse

COLD turkey

Consequences, personal or social

Obligations Omitted at work, school, or home

Legal problems

Danger

Alcohol Abuse – **the 4-question CAGE** questionnaire is popular:

1. Have you ever felt you should **C**ut back on your drinking?

2. Have people **A**nnoyed you by criticizing your drinking?

3. Have you ever felt **G**uilty about your drinking?

4. Have you ever had an **E**ye-opener? It's a drink first thing in the morning to steady your nerves or eliminate a hangover...

Behavioral Problems of Alcoholism –the 5 **D**'s to self-**D**estruction

> **D**omineering
>
> **D**ependency
>
> **D**eception
>
> **D**emanding
>
> **D**enial

How to deal with a denier of harsh realities? (**DENY**)

> **D**on't always confront them **D**irectly
>
> **E**GO might hold the key to a deeper knowledge
>
> **N**O! might **N**ot be a possibility, so beware!
>
> **Y** is this happening? – A good question to ask! The dynamics of Denial may include Neuro-psychiatric, Family-legal-situational, Personality-embellishment-lie, and/or Chemical-dependency-addiction-medication-mismanagement.

Delirium (acute confusional state) and Encephalopathy

- Acute/subacute onset, fluctuating attention, with disorganized behavior and psychotic features such as hallucinations or delusions
- Arousal affected (hyperactive, hypoactive, or mixed)
- Altered sleep-wake cycle
- Etiology usually extracranial – such as infection (UTI, pneumonia) or medication-related (especially CNS depressants such as opioids, anticholinergics, benzodiazepines, and barbiturates)
- **Delirium** overlaps with **Encephalopathy** but **Delirium** may involve **agitation**.
- Both can be easily confused with Dementia, Depression, and Psychosis because of multiple symptom overlap
- most common disorder in hospitalized adults
  - 20% overall
  - 40% in elderly patients
  - 80% in ICU patients
- Life-threatening causes of Delirium/Encephalopathy:

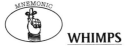

WHIMPS

Wernicke's encephalopathy, **W**ithdrawal of medication or drugs

Hypertensive emergency, cerebral **H**ypoperfusion, **H**ypoxia, **H**ypoglycemia (always check a fingerstick glucose in delirious patients!), **H**yperthermia or **H**ypothermia

Infection (especially meningitis)

Metabolic derangement (sodium, magnesium, calcium, urea, ammonia, glycine) and **M**itochondrial encephalopathy

Poisons and toxins

Status epilepticus, **S**troke, and **S**pongiform disorders

Schizophrenia

- characterized by a breakdown of thought processes and by emotional instability along with separation from realism, resulting in a withdrawal into self
- most commonly manifests as auditory hallucinations, paranoid or bizarre delusions, or disorganized speech and thinking
- symptoms divided into Positive and Negative (below)
- causes impairment in social, occupational or physical functioning
- occurs as frequently in men as in women, but much **earlier in men**
    ○ age of peak onset: 18-24 years in men and 24-35 years in women
- *Prevalence:* 0.3–0.7%
- *Risk:* if 1st-degree relative = 6.5%; if monozygotic twin = > 40%
- *Genetic link (candidate genes):* NOTCH4, histone protein loci, zinc finger protein 804A; Glycine transporter 1 inhibition

Positive Symptoms:

Symptoms present in Schizophrenics but absent in normal people

- Bizarre ideation
- Hyperactivity
- Delusions / Hallucination

Negative Symptoms:

Symptoms Absent in Schizophrenics but present in normal people

 The 4 **A**'s for negative (**A**bsent) symptoms of schizophrenia

Affect flattening:
Affect on emotional stability making person unresponsive

Alogia:
Poverty of speech. Schizophrenics have very little to share or say.

Avolition:
Lack of motivation. The person is not goal/objective oriented.

Anhedonia:
Inability to experience pleasure

For diagnosis, Schizophrenia requires at least 2 or more of the following:

· **C**atatonia or grossly disorganized behavior (like dressing inappropriately, or crying frequently)
· Any of the four negative **A**'s Above
· **S**peech Disorganized (derailment, incoherence)
· **H**allucinations / Delusions *

* = if delusions are bizarre, or if hallucinations are a voice of "running commentary," or if 2 or more voices are chatting with each other, then only 1 criterion is needed!

 Schizophrenics can't get a job and are strapped for **CASH!**

Prognosis of schizophrenia

A better overall prognosis in schizophrenia has been linked to six factors:

 POSITIVE-MOOD F.R.O.G.

Positive (rather than negative) symptoms

Mood symptoms

Female

Rapid (rather than insidious) symptom onset

Older age of first episode

Good pre-illness function

Schizophreniform Disorder

 Same criteria as Schizophrenia, but duration is different – Schizophreniform Disorder must be shorter than 6 months (yet still longer than 1 month).

 Unlike Schizophrenia, in which prodromal symptoms may develop over several years, Schizophreniform Disorder requires a rapid period from the onset of prodromal symptoms to the point of developing the diagnostic symptoms

Schizoaffective Disorder

Schizoaffective Disorder patients have features of Schizophrenia and a mood disorder but do not fully meet the criteria for either diagnosis alone.

If a patient simultaneously meets criteria for Schizophrenia and Major Depressive Disorder or Mania (plus psychosis for at least 2 weeks without a mood disorder) then the diagnosis is secure.

Men with Schizoaffective Disorder can show traits of **Antisocial Personality Disorder.**

Prognosis: Schizoaffective Disorder patients may fare better than Schizophrenics.

Schizo-**A**ffective **D**isorder patients have **Schizo**phrenia and are **SAD** (have a mood disorder).

Brief Psychotic Disorder

· A brief episode of psychosis, non re-occurring, of sudden onset
· symptoms can include delusions, hallucinations, disorganized speech or catatonic behavior (not better accounted for by Schizophrenia, Schizoaffective Disorder, Delusional Disorder or Mania / Bipolar Disorder, or due to medication or drug toxicity or side effect or general medical illness)
· *Duration:* usually at least 1 day, no more than 1 month
  ○ eventual return to *full* baseline functioning
· stressor may or may not be apparent
· *Incidence:* uncommon in the United States, but 10 times more common in developing countries, twice as often in women than men
· *Age of onset:* late 30s and early 40s

---

11 Macdonald, JM (1963). "The threat to kill". Am J Psychiatry 120: 125–130.

Triad of Sociopathy (Macdonald triad)[11]

· 3 characteristics, if present together, may be associated with violent tendency:

- ○ CRUELTY to ANIMALS
  - · Vulnerable animals = rehearsal for killing humans (yikes!)
- ○ FIRESETTING
  - · Releases aggression, due to extensive childhood humiliation
- ○ ENURESIS
  - · unintentional bed-wetting during sleep, persistent after age 5

 Sociopaths can't stand the food in the **CAFÉ** and will get angry! They'll **burn** the **CAFÉ** down, **urinate** on it, and then go eat at **MacDonald's**.

Grief Reaction (the 5 "Kubler-Ross" Stages)

There are 5 normal stages we all typically go through when grieving:

 "**D**eath **A**lways **B**rings **D**ifficult **A**cceptance"

1. **D**enial
2. **A**nger
3. **B**argaining
4. **D**epression
5. **A**cceptance (last stage)

Dissociative Disorders

Dissociative disorders are thought to primarily be caused by psychological trauma and result in disruptions of one's **A**wareness, **I**dentity, **M**emory, and/or **P**erception.

Am **I** **M**ultiple **P**eople?

· Dissociation is a pathologic and involuntary defense mechanism to a trauma

· *Lifetime Prevalence:* 10% in the general population, 46% in psychiatric inpatients

· In the DSM-IV, there are 5 types of Dissociative Disorders:

Depersonalization Disorder: detachment from self (or surroundings), felt as dreamlike imaginary, unnatural, unreal, or "outside" oneself. Subject knows that this feeling is not a reality and maintains awareness.

Dissociative Amnesia: ("Psychogenic Amnesia"): extreme memory loss due to emotional trauma; have *retrograde amnesia* (cannot retrieve stored memories prior to onset of amnesia) <u>without</u> *anterograde amnesia* (cannot form new memories)

Dissociative Fugue: ("Psychogenic Fugue" or "Fugue State"): unplanned physical desertion, travel, or wandering, away from familiar surroundings and with reversible amnesia for personal identity. The duration of a fugue can last hours to days, rarely months or years. Afterwards, there is often no recollection of the fugue or the original stressor (Dissociative Amnesia, above).

> Fugues cannot be due to alternate etiologies like Delirium, Dementia, Bipolar Disorder, Depression, or any other general medical condition, use of psychotropic substances, or to physical trauma.

Dissociative Identity Disorder: ("Multiple Personality Disorder" or "Split Personality"): the interchange of two or more distinct personality states (one may be the host) that recurrently take control of behavior. When the alternate personality takes over, severe amnesia can result. It is the least common Dissociative Disorder, (1% of all cases)! Significant physical and sexual abuse as a child is usually noted.

Dissociative Disorder Not Otherwise Specified: any pathological dissociation not covered by any of the above. It is the most commonly diagnosed Dissociative Disorder (40% of all cases)! An example is "prison psychosis" whereby prison inmates try to dissociate for jail time leniency.

Psychopharmacology

Anti-depressants, Anti-psychotics, Anxiolytics, Sedative-Hypnotics and Mood-Stabilizers

Anti-depressants

8 classes (don't get depressed, they're easy!)

1. Selective Serotonin Reuptake Inhibitors (SSRIs)
- Current standard 1st-line treatment for Depression
- Increases the amount of available Serotonin (5-hydroxytryptamine, or 5-HT) in the synapse by preventing reuptake of serotonin by the presynaptic neuron
- Side-effects – usually fewer than other anti-depressants:
  - weight gain, decreased libido, drowsiness, dry mouth, anxiety

· 33% efficacious in 1st week of treatment, but usually takes 2-6 weeks to work
· *Examples:*
  ○ Citalopram (Celexa®, Cipramil®)
  ○ **Escitalopram (Lexapro®**, Cipralex®, Seroplex®, Lexamil®)
    · The most prescribed anti-depressant in the USA
  ○ Fluoxetine (Prozac®, Sarafem®, Symbyax®)
  ○ Fluvoxamine (Luvox®)
  ○ Paroxetine (Paxil®, Aropax®)
  ○ Sertraline (Zoloft®)
  ○ Vilazodone (Viibryd®)

2. Serotonin-Norepinephrine Reuptake Inhibitors (SNRIs)

· Work on both Norepinephrine and Serotonin
· *Side-effects* – Similar to SSRIs, but with more "activating" alertness, concentration
· withdrawal syndrome on discontinuation (must taper dose when discontinuing!)
· *Examples:*
  ○ Desvenlafaxine (Pristiq®)
  ○ Duloxetine (Cymbalta®)
    · FDA-approved for "neuropathic pain"
  ○ Milnacipran (Ixel®)
    · FDA-approved for Fibromyalgia
  ○ **Venlafaxine (Effexor®)**
    · The first and most commonly used SNRI
    · At low doses (<150mg), it works only on Serotonin
    · At moderate doses (150-300mg), it works on Serotonin and Norepinephrine
    · At high doses (>300mg), it works on Serotonin, Norepinephrine and Dopamine

    · **S**ven did **SeND** the **fax** about how **Effe**ctive this drug is at highest doses, working on three neurotransmitters -- **S**erotonin, **N**orepinephrine and **D**opamine!!!

3. Norepinephrine Reuptake Inhibitors (NRIs)

· Works on Norepinephrine
· *Side-effects* – palpitations / tachycardia, anxiety, nervousness, and more "activating" alertness, concentration symptoms
· withdrawal syndrome on discontinuation (must taper dose when discontinuing!)

· *Examples:*

    ○ Atomoxetine (Strattera®)

    ○ Mazindol (Mazanor, Sanorex®)

    ○ Reboxetine (Edronax®)

    ○ Viloxazine (Vivalan®)

4. Norepinephrine-Dopamine Reuptake Inhibitors (NDRIs)

· inhibit reuptake of Dopamine and Norepinephrine

· *Side-effects* – differ from SSRIs: lowers seizure threshold, and does not cause weight gain or sexual dysfunction

· helps with smoking cessation and other reward disinhibitions

    ○ antagonist at Nicotinic Acetylcholine Receptor

· *Example:*

    ○ Bupropion (Wellbutrin®, Zyban®)

5. Tricyclic Anti-depressants (TCAs)

· Less selectively block the reuptake of Norepinephrine and Serotonin

· used less commonly now due to more selective, safer options

· *Side-effects* – dry mouth, constipation, urinary retention, blurred vision, dizziness, confusion, drowsiness, sexual dysfunction, palpitations / tachycardia, and fatal arrhythmias in very high doses (pill-ingestion suicide not uncommon with TCAs)

· Very effective, especially for severe depression or those intolerant to SSRI side-effects

· *Examples:*

    ○ Amitriptyline (Elavil®, Endep®)

      · Also commonly used in migraine prophylaxis

    ○ Clomipramine (Anafranil®)

    ○ Desipramine (Norpramin®) ← *less anti-cholinergic side effects*

    ○ Doxepin (Adapin®, Sinequan®)

    ○ Imipramine (Tofranil®)

    ○ Nortriptyline (Pamelor®, Aventyl®, Noritren®) ←

    ○ Protriptyline (Vivactil®)

    ○ Trimipramine (Surmontil®)

6. Noradrenergic and Specific Serotonergic Anti-depressants (NaSSAs) or "Tetracyclics"

· Also work on both Norepinephrine and Serotonin; block presynaptic 1-adrenergic and 2-adrenergic, and 5-HT2A, 5-HT2C, and 5-HT3, receptors and enhance 5-HT1A-mediated transmission

· *Side-effects* – Similar to SSRIs, with more weight gain / appetite issues

· *Examples:*

    ○ Mirtazapine (Remeron®, Avanza®, Zispin®)

    ○ Esmirtazapine

    ○ Mianserin (Bolvidon®, Norval®, Tolvon®)

    ○ Setiptiline (Tecipul®)

7. Monoamine Oxidase Inhibitor (MAOIs)

· block enzyme **monoamine oxidase**, which breaks down Dopamine, Serotonin, and Norepinephrine.

· as effective as TCAs, but used less frequently because of **fatal interactions** between MAOIs and **tyramine**-containing foods, like wine, cheese, and meat

· Hypertensive crisis or Serotonin Syndrome can develop

·   When **Tyra** gets **M**ad **A**t **O**nly **I**, then the reaction is an explosion – **WE** go **BAM**!

    ○ **W**ine and cheese

    ○ **E**ggplant

    ○ **B**eans – broad, green, fava and soy

    ○ **A**vocado

    ○ **M**eats – pickled, smoked, or processed (and liver)

· Also, **fatal interactions** can occur between MAOIs and medications, such as meperidine, tramadol, and dextromethorphan!!!

· *Examples of MAOIs:*

    ○ Isocarboxazid (Marplan®)

    ○ Moclobemide (Aurorix®, Manerix®)

    ○ Phenelzine (Nardil®)

    ○ Selegiline (Eldepryl®)

        · transdermal patch (Emsam) bypasses stomach, less likely to induce tyramine-crisis

8. Herbal / Supplemental Anti-depressants

· *Examples:*

    ○ St. John's Wort – most widely-used and well-studied

    ○ Saffron (Crocus sativus L.) – presumably as effective as imipramine or fluoxetine

    ○ Pineapple sage (Salvia elegans) – from Mexican traditional medicine, possibly works by modulating Dopamine

    ○ Omega-3

Anti-depressant Discontinuation Syndrome

FINISH

Flu-like symptoms

Insomnia

Nausea

Imbalance

Sensory disturbances

Hyperarousal

Anti-psychotics

3 classes (don't get psychotic, they're easy!)

· Most Anti-psychotics block the brain's D2 Dopamine receptors

· Excess Dopamine in the mesolimbic pathway has been linked to psychosis

· Potency of the Anti-psychotic depends on its ability to cling to the D2Rs, and are listed below as "H" for high, "M" for medium, and "L" for low potency

o potency does not equal efficacy

1. **First-Generation Anti-psychotics "Typicals"**

· *Side-effects* – Tardive Dyskinesia, EPS, Akathesia and prolongation of the QT interval

Butyrophenones

Haloperidol (Haldol®) - H

Droperidol (Droleptan®) - H   -dol

Phenothiazines

Chlorpromazine (Thorazine®) - L

Fluphenazine (Prolixin®) - H   -azine

Perphenazine (Trilafon®) - M

Prochlorperazine (Compazine®) - L

Thioridazine (Mellaril®) - L

Promethazine (Phenergan®) - L

Pimozide (Orap®)

Cyamemazine (Tercian®)

Thioxanthenes

Chlorprothixene (Cloxan®)

Clopenthixol (Sordinol®)

Flupenthixol (Depixol®)

Thiothixene (Navane®) - H

Zuclopenthixol (Cisordinol®)

2. Second-Generation Anti-psychotics "Atypicals"

· lower likelihood of Tardive Dyskinesia, EPS, and Akathesia than the Typicals

Clozapine (Clozaril®) – *risk of* **agranulocytosis**, *check CBC*

Granny's **2nd Cloz**et is full of **C**lean **B**eautiful **C**lothes

Olanzapine (Zyprexa®) – for Bipolar

Risperidone (Risperdal®) – for Tourette syndrome (off-label) *to make them risper (whisper)*

Quetiapine (Seroquel®) – for Bipolar, Schizophrenia

Ziprasidone (Geodon®) – for Bipolar, *risk of prolonged* **QT interval**

Paliperidone (Invega®) – derivative of Risperidone

Iloperidone (Fanapt®)

Lurasidone (Latuda®)

3. Third-Generation Anti-psychotic (TGAs)

Aripiprazole (Abilify®)

· Abilify is the 1st TGA on the market

· for Bipolar Disorder, Depression, Schizophrenia, and Autism (reduces aggression, irritability, quick-changing moods, and self-injury)

Abilify has the **ability** to improve the **BADS** (**B**ipolar, **A**utism, **D**epression, **S**chizophrenia)

Order of Appearance of Side-Effects of Anti-psychotics

The order of appearance of the 7 major side effects of Anti-psychotics can be remembered by this

"**D**oes **A**nyone **R**eally **T**hink **A**bout **P**sychotic **R**abbits?"

1. **D**ystonias
2. **A**kinesia
3. **R**igidity
4. **T**remors
5. **A**kathisia
6. **P**isa Syndrome
7. **R**abbit Syndrome

Pisa Syndrome "Pleurothotonus"

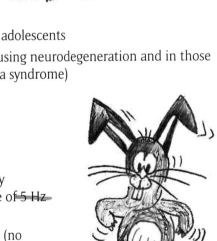

· A dystonia characterized by twisting of the thorax (Pleurothotonus), neck and head to one side

· Tonic trunk flexion eventually causes the body to lean (like the Leaning Tower of Pisa, in Italy)

· Primarily due to longstanding overuse of neuroleptics but also seen in anticholinergic medication and Anti-depressant overuse

· Reported mostly in elderly demented women and in adolescents

· it has also been seen in those with other diseases causing neurodegeneration and in those who are not receiving any medication (idiopathic Pisa syndrome)

Rabbit Syndrome

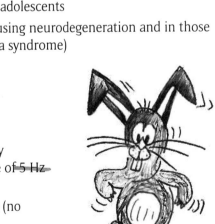

· Extrapyramidal side effect syndrome characterized by involuntary, fine, rhythmic, perioral tremors at a rate of 5 Hz – just like a cute, gnawing bunny rabbit!

· Mouth masticatory motions occur in a vertical plane (no tongue involvement)

· *Incidence:* 2 – 4% in reported studies

· Seen typically after years of high-potency Anti-psychotics (Haloperidol, Fluphenazine, and Pimozide) but also can occur with Thioridazine, Clozapine, Olanzapine, Aripiprazole, and Risperidone

· ~~Anticholinergics~~ (or use an Atypical Anti-psychotic with high anti-cholinergic properties)

Anxiolytics, Sedative-Hypnotics, and Mood-Stabilizers

· Mostly are ~~Barbiturates~~ and ~~Benzodiazepines~~

  o both act at ~~GABA (A)~~ receptors

· **Benzodiazepines** increase the **frequency** of opening of the GABA channel

· **Barbiturates** increase the duration of time the GABA channel is **open**

Ben Affleck is photographed with **frequency** and **bars** stay **open** long into the night

Benzodiazepines

· short-term relief of severe and/or disabling **anxiety** and Panic Disorder (at moderate doses); **sedative-hypnotic** at higher doses; also for Status Epilepticus

· *Side-effects* – amnesia, impairs motor skills, relaxes skeletal muscle, **withdrawal** and/or **rebound** (if abruptly discontinued after 2 weeks); **tolerance** and **dependence** (if used for months)

· *Examples* (and half-lives):

Generic name	Trade name	Half-life
Alprazolam	(Xanax®)	9 - 20
Chlordiazepoxide	(Librium®)	24 - 100
Clonazepam	(Klonopin®, Rivotril®)	19 - 60
Diazepam	(Valium®)	30 - 200
Etizolam	(Etilaam®)	8 - 24
Lorazepam	(Ativan®)	8 - 24
Oxazepam	(Serax®)	3 - 25
Midazolam	(Versed®)	1 - 4
Temazepam	(Restoril®)	3 - 25
Triazolam	(Halcion®)	1.5 - 5

Barbiturates

· anxiolytic effect linked to the sedation they cause

· abuse and addiction is high

· rarely prescribed anymore

· obsolete for treating anxiety but valuable for the short-term treatment of severe insomnia, though only after benzodiazepines or non-benzodiazepines have failed

· *Examples:*

　○ Amobarbital (Amytal®) – intermediate-acting "truth serum" which decreases inhibitions (caught off-guard when questioned); also used in the Wada Test

　○ Pentobarbital (Nembutal®) – for seizures and pre-op sedation

　○ Phenobarbital (Luminal®) – for anxiety and seizures, especially in children; risk: Hyperactivity, cognitive disturbances, Dupuytren's Contractures

　○ Secobarbital (Seconal®) – for short surgical procedures, also abused under nickname "Red Devils"

　○ Thiopental (Pentothal®) – ultra-short acting

Azapirones

· 5-HT_{1A} receptor agonists

· 　　　　　anxiety disorders, and add-on for Depression, but less effective than benzodiazepines in benzodiazepine-treated patients

· *Side-effect*s – less cognitive impairment, sedation and dependence than benzodiazepines

· *Examples:*

　○ Buspirone (Buspar®)

　○ Tandospirone (Sediel®)

　○ Gepirone (Ariza®)

Anticonvulsants / Anti-Epileptic Drugs (AEDs)

· Many AEDs are also mood stabilizers

· *Examples:*

rapid cycling bipolar & AIDS - mania

    ○ Valproic acid (Depakene®), Divalproex Sodium (Depakote®), Sodium Valproate (Depacon®), risk: liver or bone marrow toxicity

    ○ Lamotrigine (Lamictal®) – risk: Stevens–Johnson syndrome

    ○ Carbamazepine (Tegretol®) – risk: leukocytopenia

    ○ Oxcarbazepine (Trileptal®) – risk: hyponatremia

Lithium

· mood stabilizer, strong use in Bipolar

· drug monitoring required

· lithium level therapeutic range: 0.6-1.2mEq/L

· *Side-effects* –

↑level c̄ captopril (ACE), thiazides, NSAIDS, CCBs, Flagyl

LITHIUM:

    Leukocytosis

    Insipidus, Diabetes

    Tremor, Teratogenicity (first Trimester), Thyroid disturbance

    Heaviness (weight gain)

    Intestinal disturbance (nausea, vomiting, diarrhea)

    Ugliness (acne breakouts)

    Major EKG changes (T-wave flattening, prolonged QT interval, ventricular tachycardia and ventricular fibrillation)

Non-Benzodiazepine "Z-drug" Sedatives

· Examples:

    ○ Eszopiclone (Lunesta®)

    ○ Zaleplon (Sonata®)

    ○ Zolpidem (Ambien®)

Electro-Convulsive Therapy – what a <u>SHOCK</u>, it's still in use

- ECT induces a clonic seizure therapeutically for at least *15 seconds*
- The **Hippocampus** is implicated in the mechanism of action (? "reboot" or "jumpstart" the brain's center of memory and mood, boosts neurotransmission in its dense synaptic connections)
- *Indications:* Often used if unresponsive to other interventions (medication and psychotherapy), or intolerant of Anti-depressant medication side effects, or prior good response to ECT, or in relapse prevention, but can consider ECT for Schizophrenia, Schizoaffective or Schizophreniform Disorder, after failing Anti-psychotics. ECT may also work for quick, definitive response to psychosis, suicide ideation, manic delirium, or catatonia.
- 70% of ECT patients are women (women are at twice the risk of depression)
- Older and more wealthy patients are also more likely to receive ECT

SHOCK

Seizure (clonic) induced therapeutically for at least ***15 seconds***

Hippocampus implicated in ECT mechanism of action

Often used if unresponsive to other interventions (medication and psychotherapy), **O**r intolerant of Anti-depressant side effects, **O**r prior good response to ECT, **O**r in relapse prevention

Consider after unsuccessful treatment with Anti-psychotic medication for Schizophrenia, Schizoaffective or Schizophreniform Disorder.

Key for quick, definitive response to psychosis, suicide ideation, manic delirium, or catatonia

New from DSM-V

Some of the items below were not in DSM-IV-TR but have wiggled onto DSM-V:

Compulsive Hoarding (Packratting or Pathological Collecting)

Excessive acquisition of objects that fill up the home or workplace and collectively become an impediment to social, occupational, behavioral, or other areas of functioning

For diagnosis, a patient must be living in a **DUMP**:

Difficulty **D**iscarding possessions, regardless of actual value

Urge to save **U**nnecessary stuff

Many **M**essy areas (home or workplace) completely cluttered, making intended use impossible

Psychiatric/Neurologic or **P**re-morbid Medical conditions mustn't cause the hoarding (e.g., brain injury, stroke, obsessions from OCD, Major Depressive Disorder, delusions from Schizophrenia, cognitive deficits from Dementia, etc.)

Dermatillomania (Skin Picking Disorder or Neurotic/Psychogenic excoriation)

· characterized by repeated urges to pick at one's own skin, causing tissue damage.
· symptoms should cause clinically significant distress in social, occupational, or other areas of functioning.

Skin pickers are quite **PICKY**:

Picking Preceded by tension, anxiety, or stress of a **P**erceived skin defect

Impulse Control Disorder with **I**magined "Irregularities" felt on the skin -- typically the face, but can include arms, legs, fingers/toes, scalp, gums, lips, back, and chest

Complications include infection at the site of picking, epidural abscess, sepsis, disfigurement, and even tissue damage requiring skin grafts as needed

Knowledge of the harm/complications, but compulsion to engage in the negative behavior regardless

Yale–Brown Obsessive Compulsive Scale gives a score ranging from 0 (subclinical) to 40 (severe/extreme disease)

To be diagnosed with **Dermatillomania**, the patient must first **scratch out** other medical conditions causing **itching/picking** by asking for **HELP**:

        Hodgkin's Disease

        Eczema

        Liver Disease, **L**upus

        Psoriasis, **P**olycythemia

 Treatment: SSRIs and/or opioid antagonists

Trichotillomania

- self-induced pulling of and recurrent loss of hair.
- Patients may have increasing sense of tension before pulling out their hair and gratification/relief as hairpulling occurs
- Complications include:
  - infection,
  - permanent alopecia,
  - carpal tunnel syndrome,
  - trichophagia (eating the hair just pulled out) which can lead to a trichobezoar (or a "hair ball" for the cat lovers out there – meow!) and even Rapunzel Syndrome (below)

Rapunzel Syndrome

- occurs when the "tail" of a trichobezoar extends from the stomach down into the intestines
- on abdominal imaging, it looks like the character Rapunzel "letting down her hair" from the Brothers Grimm fairy tale
- can cause gastrointestinal obstruction
- can be fatal if misdiagnosed
- often requires urgent surgery because the GI tract is unable to digest human hair

Hypnosis (neuro-hypnotism or "nervous sleep")[12,13]

Hypnotherapy is a type of psychotherapy that employs innovative, unique, and fresh thoughts, feelings, behaviors and attitudes to help form unconscious change in a patient being hypnotized. Optimal candidates for hypnosis typically have heightened suggestibility to this concept and responsiveness to new ideas; this hypnotizability may be determined by a "Hypnotic Induction Profile" (HIP).

To induce hypnosis, you gotta be a **HIPSTER**:

Heightened/intense focus on a specific thought or memory

Induced by **I**nstructions and role-enactment to reach **I**nner Core of one's being

Psychological state resembling sleep but with quazi-awareness "other than the ordinary conscious state"

Suggestibility (hypnotizability)

Trance-state **T**echnique of...

Eye-fixation, or **E**ye-roll, along with ...

Reclining posture and **R**elaxation of muscles

· Patients with DID and PTSD may have the highest hypnotizability.

· For more on Hypnotherapy and delving into patients' Inner Core and own motivations (or if you just want to get HIP and learn about latest techniques in neuropsychotherapy), check out this book: "The Still, Soft Voice: Breaking Through to the Inner Core" by Clifford K. Brickman (Kempner Books: 2010). An interesting read to say the least!

Recommended Reading

Caplan J, Stern T. Mnemonics in a mnutshell: 32 aids to psychiatric diagnosis. *Curr Psychiatr.* 2008;7:27-33.

This is a great resource for psychiatry mnemonics, some of which are included in this chapter.

---

[12] "The Still, Soft Voice: Breaking Through to the Inner Core" by Clifford K. Brickman (Kempner Books: 2010).

[13] Spiegel, D.; Loewenstein, R. et al. (2011). Dissociative Disorders in DSM-5. *Depression and Anxiety* 28 (9): 824–852.

Psychiatry for Neurologists Quiz

(Answers on page 763)

1. Which of the following is NOT part of the SIG-E-CAPS Major Depressive Disorder screening symptoms?

    A. Sleep disturbance

    B. Appetite disturbance

    C. Pressured speech

    D. Concentration disturbance

2. Which of the following is NOT part of the MacDonald Triad of Sociopathy?

    A. Animal Cruelty

    B. Running Amok

    C. Firesetting

    D. Bedwetting

3. A 24-year-old woman who was otherwise previously healthy, was just diagnosed with schizophrenia. Symptoms were mostly hyperactivity and hallucinations, and onset was quick. Which of the following is NOT a good prognostic indicator?

    A. her gender

    B. the speed of the onset of her symptoms

    C. the positive symptom complex

    D. her age of onset of illness

    E. her pre-morbid functionality

4. Which of the following interact with Monoamine Oxidase Inhibitor medications?

    A. Avocado

    B. Beans

    C. Cheese

    D. Dextromethorphan

    E. all of the above

5. Link the phobia with its definition. An answer may be used only once.

    1) Geliophobia   A. fear of heights

    2) Agoraphobia   B. fear of love or falling in love

    3) Philiophobia   C. fear of open spaces, markets

    4) Acrophobia   D. fear of laughter

6. Match the Mood Stabilizer medication with its side effect.

    1) Valproic acid   A. Hyponatremia

    2) Oxcarbazepine   B. elevated liver function tests

    3) Lamotrigine   C. Leukocytosis and Ugliness

    4) Lithium   D. Stevens-Johnson Syndrome

    5) Alprazolam   E. Amnesia

7. After a fall and TBI, your cousin Milty now is emotionally labile, hypersexual, and exhibits sociopathic behavior. This dysfunction is due to damage in his:

    A. Orbito-Frontal Cortex (OFC)

    B. Dorso-Lateral Pre-Frontal Cortex (DLPFC)

    C. Cingulate gyrus

    D. Mesial Temporal lobe

    E. None of the above, he was like that even before the TBI

Quiz
Answers

Neuroanatomy Quiz Answers

1. A

    CN I has no relay through the thalamus.

2. B.

    The flocculonodular lobe is responsible for vestibular function.

3. D

Purkinje cells carry output from the cerebellum.

4. A

    The Triangle of Mollaret connects the dentate nucleus, the red nucleus, and inferior olive.

5. A

    The anterior nucleus of the thalamus receives information from the mamillary bodies and sends information to the cingulate gyrus.

6. C

    The dentatorubrothalamic tract goes through the ventral lateral thalamus

7. 1. A
    2. B
    3. B
    4. A
    5. B
    6. A

CN V (Trigeminal nerve)	CN VII (Facial nerve)
Muscles of mastication	Muscles of facial expression
Anterior belly of the digastric	Posterior belly of the digastric
Tensor tympani	Stapedius
Mylohyoid	Stylohyoid
Sensation to the anterior 2/3 of the tongue	Taste to the anterior 2/3 of the tongue

MNEMONIC

The stylohyoid is innervated by cranial nerve seven, which exits the skull through the stylomastoid foramen.

8.   B

Macules in the utricle and saccule detect linear acceleration.

The semicircular canals detect angular acceleration.

Behavioral Neurology Quiz Answers

1. 1. B
    2. C
    3. A
    4. D

2. 1. C
    2. A
    3. D
    4. B
    5. E

3. 1. D
    2. B
    3. A
    4. C

4. B
    A patient with an IQ of 45 has moderate mental retardation "Intellectual Disability".

Epilepsy
Quiz Answers

1. 1) D
   2) C
   3) B
   4) A

2. 1) A
   2) A
   3) C
   4) C

3. 1) A
   2) D
   3) C
   4) B

4. C
   Carbamazepine even induces its own metabolism (autoinduction).

5. A
   Levetiracetam (Keppra), vigabatrin (Sabril), pregabalin (Lyrica), and gabapentin (Neurontin) are relatively free of drug interactions.

Infectious Diseases
Quiz Answers

1. G
    Variant CJD has a longer clinical course than sporadic CJD.

2. 1) B
    Coccidiodes is found in the Southwest.

    2) A
    Histoplasma is found in the Ohio and Mississippi River Valleys.

3. 1) B
    New variant CJD is due to the agent that causes mad cow disease.

    2) C
    Trichinosis is due to eating undercooked pork.

    3) A
    Cryptococcus is found in pigeon droppings.

    4) D
    Bartonella henselae causes cat scratch disease.

4. D
    Neurosarcoidosis and TB both tend to cause basal meningitis, which can result in
    cranial neuropathies.

5. E
    Diabetic patients are at increased risk for infection with *Mucoraceae*, which causes mucormycosis.

6. D
    Tetanus does not produce a Guillain-Barré Syndrome-like picture.
    Botulism, Diphtheria, Rabies, and West Nile Virus can produce a Guillain-Barré Syndrome-
    type picture.

7. 1) D
    Naegleria fowleri causes hemorrhagic meningoencephalitis after swimming in a fresh water lake.

    2) G
    Tropheryma whippelii can cause supranuclear palsy, myoclonus, and dementia.

    3) A
    Cryptococcus causes soap bubbles in the parenchyma.

    4) C
    Mycobacterium leprae prefers the peripheral nerves due to cooler temperatures there.

    5) B
    Group B Streptococcus is the most common cause of neonatal bacterial meningitis.

    6) E
    Neisseria meningitidis is the most common cause of meningitis in children.

    7) F
    Streptococcus pneumoniae is the most common cause of meningitis in adults

Metabolic Diseases
Quiz Answers

1.   E
Farber's disease, which is due to ceramidase deficiency, is associated with a cherry-red spot.

Other diseases that cause a cherry-red spot are:
    Sandhoff disease
    Sialidosis
    Tay Sachs disease

Abetalipoproteinemia is associated with retinitis pigmentosa.
Canavan disease causes optic atrophy.
Cerebrotendinous xanthomatosis causes cataracts.
Fabry's disease causes corneal deposits.

2.   1) A
Canavan disease is due to aspartoacylase deficiency.

    2) D
Gamma-hydroxybutyric acidemia is also known as succinic acid dehydrogenase deficiency.

    3) C
Gaucher's disease is due to glucocerebrosidase deficiency.

    4) B
Krabbe disease is due to galactocerebrosidase deficiency.

3.   1) C
Glutaric acidemia type II causes a sweaty foot odor.

    2) C
Isovaleric acidemia also causes a sweaty foot odor.

    3) A
Maple syrup urine disease conveniently causes a maple syrup odor.

    4) B
Phenylketonuria causes a musty odor.

4.   1) C
Some patients with ethylmalonic-adipicaciduria, which is a form of glutaric acidemia type II, respond to riboflavin.

2) D
Some patients with maple syrup urine disease respond to thiamine.

3) A
Some patients with methylmalonic acidemia respond to B12.

5.   D

6.   B
The ABCD1 gene encodes for an ATP-binding cassette protein. Mutations in this gene on Xq28 cause adrenoleukodystrophy.
Mutations in the sulfatase-modifying factor-1 (SUMF1) gene cause multiple sulfatase deficiency.
Mutations in the PLP1 gene cause Pelizaeus-Merzbacher disease.

7.   A

8.   1) B

2) B

3) B

4) B

5) A

6) A

Gray Matter	White Matter
Sandhoff disease	Alexander disease
Tay-Sachs disease	Canavan disease
	Krabbe disease
	Pelizaeus-Merzbacher disease

Movement Disorders Quiz Answers

1.   **1) A**
DRPLA is an autosomal dominant ataxia due to an expansion of a CAG repeat in *ATN1*, the gene encoding atrophin-1, on chromosome 12.

2) C
Friedreich's ataxia is due to an expanded GAA repeat in the *FXN* gene on chromosome 9q, which encodes frataxin.

3) A
Huntington disease is due to an expanded CAG triplet repeat in the *HD* gene on chromosome 4p16.3, which encodes huntingtin.

4) A
SCA 3, which is the most common autosomal dominantly inherited ataxia in the US, is due to an expanded CAG repeat in the *ATXN3* gene on chromosome 14q24.3-q31.

5) B
SCA 8 is due to a CTG repeat.

2.   **D**
Vitamin E deficiency causes a phenotype similar to Friedreich's ataxia.

3.   **1) A**
In glutaric acidemia type 1, the MRI shows **frontotemporal atrophy** with prominent Sylvian fissures. This results in a **bat wing** appearance.

2) C
The eye of the tiger sign is seen in pantothenate kinase-associated neurodegeneration (PKAN).

3) D
Face of the giant panda is seen in Wilson's disease.

4) B
MSA is associated with the **hot-cross bun sign** on MRI due to pontine atrophy.

4.   B
Astrocytic tufts are found in progressive supranuclear palsy. Astrocytic plaques are found in CBGD.

CBGD is associated with **alien limb phenomenon**, cortical sensory loss, impaired balance, dystonia, dysphasia, and dysarthria.

Remember that ABCD can be used to remember the pathologic findings of CBGD:

Astrocytic plaques, which are astrocytic lesions that are immunoreactive for tau.

Ballooned neurons, which are swollen neurons, are seen. There are also seen in Pick's disease.

Cortical atrophy, especially of the parietal and frontal lobes and Coiled bodies of tau in oligodendrocytes.

Degeneration of the substantia nigra and striatum.

5.   1) C
Patients with abetalipoproteinemia (Bassen-Kornzweig syndrome) may have retinitis pigmentosa.

2) C
Retinitis pigmentosa may also be seen in ataxia with isolated vitamin E deficiency (AVED).

3) C
Retinitis pigmentosa is part of HARP syndrome. HARP syndrome is characterized by hypobetalipoproteinemia, acanthocytosis, retinitis pigmentosa, and pallidal degeneration.

4) B
Pendular eye movements are seen in Pelizaeus-Merzbacher disease.

5) E
Supranuclear gaze palsy can be seen in Whipple's disease.

6)   A, D
Kayser-Fleischer rings and sunflower cataracts are associated with Wilson's disease.

Neurocutaneous Disorders Quiz Answers

1.   1)C
   2)B
   3)B
   4)B
   5)A
   6)B
   7)B
   8)D

2.   1)E
   2)D
   3)A
   4)D
   5)B
   6)C

3.   1)B
   2)A
   3)E
   4)D
   5)C
   6)F

4.   1)C
   2)D
   3)E
   4)A
   5)A
   6)D
   7)B
   8)B and E
   9)D

10)D
11)D

Neurodegenerative Diseases Quiz Answers

1. E
   NARP is not associated with ragged red fibers.

2. B
   Astrocytic tufts are found in PSP.

   The following are found in Alzheimer's disease:
   Amyloid deposition
   Granulovacuolar degeneration
   Hirano bodies
   Neuritic plaques
   Neurofibrillary tangles.

3. D
   MSA is an alpha-synucleinopathy.

   Tauopathies include:
   Alzheimer's disease
   CBGD
   FTDP-17
   Pick's disease
   PSP

4. D

 Knife-edge gyri are associated with Pick's disease.

Neuromuscular Diseases
Quiz Answers

1. C
    The supinator is innervated by the posterior interosseous branch of the radial nerve.

 I think The Supinator is a radical name, and the supinator is innervated by the radial nerve.

2. A
    The anconeus is spared in a radial neuropathy at the spiral groove.

3. A
    The obturator and femoral nerves innervate the pectineus muscle.

4. B
    The obturator and sciatic nerves innervate the adductor magnus.

5. 1) A
    2) C
    3) B

    The inferior gluteal nerve innervates hip extensors.
    The obturator nerve innervates thigh adductors.
    The superior gluteal nerve innervates thigh abductors.

6. A
    The accessory peroneal nerve usually innervates the extensor digitorum brevis.

7. B
    Myokymia is found in radiation plexopathy.

8. E
    OPMD is due to a **GCG repeat expansion in the gene encoding PAPB2** (poly-A binding protein-2) on 14q11.

9. E
    Muscle biopsy shows **rimmed vacuoles** and fiber size variation in patients with OPMD.

10. D

Tomaculous neuropathy is another name for hereditary neuropathy with liability to pressure palsies (HNPP).

11. A

Anti-GM1 antibodies are found in multifocal motor neuropathy with conduction block.

12. 1) A

Bunina bodies and axonal spheroids are found in ALS.

2) D

Increased central nuclei are found in myotonic dystrophy (DM1).

3) B

Onion bulbs are seen in CMT1A.

4) E

Ragged red fibers are seen in zidovudine (AZT) myopathy.

5) C

Rimmed vacuoles are found in inclusion body myositis (IBM).

Neuro-Oncology Quiz Answers

1.   E

     Recall that Etoposide, Vincristine, Cisplatin, and Taxol EViCT cancer but leave you numb due to peripheral neuropathy.

2.   A

     Anti-Tr antibody is associated with Hodgkin's disease. It causes cerebellar degeneration.

3.   A

     Metaplastic meningiomas are grade I. Clear cell, choroid, rhabdoid, and papillary meningiomas are aggressive.

4.   1) E
     2) B
     3) D
     4) C
     5) A

Neuro-Ophthalmology Quiz Answers

1.   1) A
      2) D
      3) B
      4) C

2.   1) A
      2) B
      3) F
      4) C
      5) D

3.   A

      The optic nerve exits the skull through the optic canal.

      The oculomotor, trochlear, and abducens nerves exit through the superior orbital fissure.

4.   1) C
      2) D
      3) B
      4) A

5.   1) B

      Bitemporal hemianopia is due to an optic chiasm lesion.

      2) A

      Pie in the sky visual field defects are due to temporal lobe lesions.

      3) C

      Pie on the floor defects are due to parietal lobe lesions.

MNEMONIC
To remember that pie in the sky defects are due to temporal lobe lesions and pie on the floor defects are due to lesions in the parietal lobe:

Temporal lobe lesions make me tickled 'cuz pie is in the sky, and parietal lobe lesions make me pout 'cuz pie is on the floor.

Neuropathology Quiz Answers

1.　1) D
　　2) B
　　3) A
　　4) C

2.　1) A
　　2) D
　　3) B
　　4) C
　　5) E

3.　Multiple System Atrophy is a synucleinopathy, not a tauopathy. Other synucleinopathies are Parkinson's disease and dementia with Lewy bodies.

　　The tauopathies are: Alzheimer's disease, corticobasal ganglionic degeneration, Frontotemporal dementia with Parkinsonism, Pick's disease, and progressive supranuclear palsy.

4.　A

　　Alzheimer type I astrocytes are associated with Wilson's disease and hyperammonemia.

Neurophysiology Quiz Answers

1. 1) C
    Triphasic waves with anterior to posterior lag are seen in encephalopathy, for example hepatic encephalopathy.

    2) D
    Burst-suppression is seen in severe anoxic injury.

    3) A
    High amplitude generalized periodic sharp wave complexes every 4 to 15 seconds are found in SSPE.

    4) B
    Generalized periodic sharp wave complexes that occur every 0.5- 1.6 seconds are found in sporadic CJD.

2. 1) B
    Mu is attenuated by movement or thoughts of movement of the contralateral body.

    2) C
    Posterior slow waves of youth are characterized by delta activity with overriding alpha frequencies.

    3) D
    Wicket spikes are 6-11 Hz activity in the temporal region during drowsiness or light sleep in adults.

    4) A
    Lambda waves are positive sharp transients in the occipital area seen during visual scanning.

3. C
    The abductor pollicis longus is innervated by the posterior interosseous nerve.

4. D
    Narcolepsy has been associated with low CSF levels of orexin/hypocretin.

Pediatric Neurology Quiz Answers

1. B
When you are given a case of a neonate with hiccups, seizures, and a burst-suppression pattern on the EEG you should think of nonketotic hyperglycinemia.

2. D
A neonate with high output congestive heart failure and a cranial bruit may have a vein of Galen malformation.

3. 1) B
Mutations in the ubiquitin-protein ligase E3A (UBE3A) gene (15q11-13) can cause Angelman syndrome. Other mutations that cause Angelman syndrome include: deletion of maternally derived 15q11-13, duplication of paternal chromosome 15 (uniparental disomy), and mutation in the imprinting center (15q11-13).

2) C
Rett syndrome is due to a mutation in MECP2, which maps to Xq28. Mutations in the CDKL5 (cyclin-dependent kinase-like 5) gene, which is also known as STK9, have been found to cause an early-onset form of Rett syndrome that is associated with seizures.

3) A
Familial Hemiplegic Migraine-1 (FHM1) is due to a mutation in the *CACNA1A* gene on 19p13.

Recall that mutations in this gene also cause spinocerebellar ataxia-6 (SCA 6) and episodic ataxia-2 (EA2).

4) D
Periventricular nodular heterotopia is due to a mutation in the FIL-1 gene.

4. C
Pregnant women should take folate to prevent neural tube defects.

5. C
Cobblestone lissencephaly is associated with congenital muscular dystrophy. Examples of congenital muscular dystrophy include muscle-eye-brain disease, Fukuyama CMD, and Walker-Warburg CMD.

6.   1) B
Miller-Dieker syndrome is due to a deletion that includes the LIS1 gene, which encodes PAFAH1B1. The deletion also includes the 14-3-3 gene.

2) B
Isolated lissencephaly may be due to mutations in LIS1 on 17p13.3. It is also caused by DCX mutations on Xq22.3-23. Recall that males with DCX mutations have lissencephaly, and females have subcortical band heterotopia. To make things even more confusing, subcortical band heterotopia can also occur with LIS1 mutations.

3) C
Lissencephaly with agenesis of the corpus callosum is seen with ARX mutations on Xp22.13.

4) A
Lissencephaly with cerebellar hypoplasia is due to a mutation in the gene that encodes reelin at 7q22.

7.   1) C
Dandy-Walker syndrome is associated with PHACES syndrome. PHACES syndrome is characterized by **P**osterior fossa malformations, **H**emangiomas, **A**rterial anomalies, **C**oarctation of the aorta and other cardiac defects, **E**ye abnormalities, and **S**ternal clefting or **S**upraumbilical raphe.

2) A
Both DiGeorge's syndrome and velocardiofacial syndrome are CATCH syndromes. CATCH stands for **C**ardiac **A**bnormality, **T**-cell deficit, **C**lefting, and **H**ypocalcemia.

3) B
MASA syndrome (**M**ental retardation, **A**phasia, **S**huffling gait, and **A**dducted thumbs) is due to a mutation in the L1CAM gene and one of the syndromes included in CRASH syndrome.

4) A

Recommended Reading

Clark GD. Genetics of human brain malformations. Continuum Lifelong Learning Neurol 2005;11(2):143-160.

Stroke
Quiz Answers

1.   1. C
A string of beads is seen in fibromuscular dysplasia.

2. A
Carotid dissection is associated with a tapered vessel.

3. B
A "puff of smoke" is seen in patients with moyamoya disease.

2.   1) A
Pure hemiparesis can result from a lesion of the posterior limb of the internal capsule.

2) B
Pure hemisensory loss can result from a lesion of the ventral posterior lateral nucleus of the thalamus.

3.   B
The recurrent artery of Huebner is a branch of the anterior cerebral artery. It supplies the head of the caudate, anterior putamen, part of the outer segment of the globus pallidus, and the anterior limb of the internal capsule.

4.   A
The anterior choroidal artery is a branch of the internal carotid artery.

5.   A
The left vertebral artery arises from the left subclavian artery.

6.   C
The right common carotid arises from the brachiocephalic artery.

7.   B
All of the above except for hyponatremia are serious CEA complications.

8.   D

In the NASCET trial, the two year recurrent stroke risk with 70-99% stenosis was 26% in the medical arm, compared to 13% for patients undergoing CEA (surgery).

9.   B

Some of the 13 exclusion criterion include prothrombin time > 15 sec (INR>1.7), BP > 185/110, major surgery within 14 days, previous infarct within 3 months, and platelets < 100,000. Some experts say if you can get the BP to goal or below it quickly enough with minimal use of antihypertensives in the ER, then tPA can be given.

10.   B

The rate is 6.4%, per the NINDS trial.

11.   D

The I.V. limit is 4-1/2 hours now, no longer just 3 hours, per the ECASS-3 trial.

12.   E

13.   C

Lumbar puncture is the next step after CTH is negative if you suspect SAH.

Neurotoxins Quiz Answers

1. 1) C
    2) A
    3) E
    4) B
    5) D

1) Wrist drop	Lead
2) Hyperkeratosis of palms and soles, axonal neuropathy, and Mees' lines	Arsenic
3) Mees' lines, axonal neuropathy, and alopecia	Thallium
4) Coma, cyanosis, convulsions, and loss of corneal reflexes	Ethylene glycol
5) Nausea, opisthotonus, rigidity, and renal failure	Strychnine

2. A

    Arsenic can cause a Guillain-Barré type picture. Thallium and lead poisoning are also in the differential diagnosis of Guillain-Barré syndrome.

3. B

    Acrodynia is due to inorganic mercury poisoning.

4. E

    Ethylene glycol can cause nonreactive pupils and loss of corneal reflexes.
    Organic mercury can cause visual field constriction and cortical vision loss.
    Methanol can cause blindness due to damage to retinal ganglion cells.
    Toluene can cause optic atrophy, opsoclonus, and ocular dysmetria.

5. B

Psychiatry for Neurologists
Quiz Answers

1. C

2. B

3. D
    The POSITIVE MOOD F.R.O.G confers a good prognosis in schizophrenia. Early age of onset is a poor prognostic indicator.

4. E

5. 1) D
    2) C
    3) B
    4) A

6. 1) B
    2) A
    3) D
    4) C
    5) E

7. A

References

ACAS: *JAMA* 273: 1421 (1995)

AFFIRM Investigators. A randomized, placebo-controlled trial of natalizumab for relapsing multiple sclerosis. N Engl J Med. 2006 Mar 2;354(9):899-910.

Amar AP, Aryan HE, Meltzer HS, Levy ML. Neonatal subgaleal hematoma causing brain compression: report of two cases and review of the literature. Neurosurgery 2003;52:1470-1474.

Amato AA (ed). Muscle diseases. Continuum Lifelong Learning in Neurol 2006;12(3):33-168.

American Psychiatric Association (1994). Diagnostic and statistical manual of mental disorders (4th ed.). Washington, DC: Author.

Armstrong MJ, Miyaskaki JM. Evidence-based guideline: Pharmacologic treatment of chorea in Huntington disease. Neurology 2012;79:597-603.

Asher D. Transmissible spongiform encephalopathies: slow infections of the nervous system. In Long SS, Pickering LK, Prober CG, eds. Principles and practice of pediatric infectious diseases, 2nd edition. Philadelphia: Churchill Livingstone, 2003;316-319.

Baron, E. "Proposed LOCAM-LT Mnemonic for Mastering Examination of Mental Status and Cognitive Function." J Am Osteopath Assoc. 2010;110(9) 553-555.

Bartelson JD, Fish A, Edlund W. AAN pocket guidelines: summaries of AAN clinical practice guidelines. 2003 edition.

Baumann C, Bassetti C. Hypocretins (orexins) and sleep-wake disorders. Lancet Neurol 2005;4:673-82.

Benjamin, L. S. (1996). Interpersonal diagnosis and treatment of personality disorders (2nd ed.). New York: Guilford.

Berciano J, Boesch S, Pérez-Ramos JM, Wenning GK. Olivopontocerebellar atrophy: toward a better nosological definition. Movement Disorders 2006;21:1607-1610.

Berg AT, Berkovic SF, Brodie MJ, et al. Revised terminology and concepts for organization of seizures and epilepsies: report of the ILAE Commission on Classification and Terminology, 2005–2009. *Epilepsia* 2010;51:676–685.

Berman SA, Arshad S, Kari K, et al. Olivopontocerebellar atrophy. Emedicine October 18, 2006.

Bidichandani SI, Delatycki MB, Ashizawa T. (Updated August 25, 2006). Friedreich ataxia. In: GeneReviews at GeneTests: Medical Genetics Information Resource (database online). Copyright, University of Washington, Seattle. 1997-2007.
Available at **http://www.genetests.org**.

Bird TD. (Updated October 27, 2006). Hereditary ataxia overview. In: GeneReviews at GeneTests: Medical Genetics Information Resource (database online). Copyright, University of Washington, Seattle. 1997-2007. Available at **http://www.genetests.org**.

Blumenfeld, H. Neuroanatomy through clinical cases. Sunderland: Sinauer Associates, Inc., 2002.

Bobustuc GC, Gilbert MR. Whipple disease. Emedicine April 11, 2006.

Bonne G, Leturcq F, Récan-Budiartha D, Yaou RB. (Updated April 26, 2007). Emery-Dreifuss muscular dystrophy. In: GeneReviews at GeneTests: Medical Genetics Information Resource (database online). Copyright, University of Washington, Seattle. 1997-2007. Available at **http://www.genetests.org**.

Bradley WG, Daroff RB, Fenichel GM, Jankovic J. Neurology in clinical practice: principles of diagnosis and management, 4th edition. Philadelphia: Elsevier, Inc., 2004.

Brazis PW, Masdeu JC, Biller J. Localization in clinical neurology, 4th edition. Philadelphia: Lippincott Williams & Wilkins, 2001.

Britton WJ. Leprosy. In Cohen J, Powderly WG, eds. Infectious diseases, 2nd edition. Edinburgh: Mosby, 2004;1507-1514.

Bucurescu G, Suleman A. Neurosarcoidosis. Emedicine November 7, 2006.

Cardoso F, Seppi K, Mair K, et al. Seminar on choreas. Lancet Neurol 2006;5:589-602.

Carrera E, Bogousslavsky J. The thalamus and behavior: effects of anatomically distinct strokes. Neurology 2006;66:1817-1823.

Chaturvedi S, Bruno A, Feasby T, et al. Carotid endarterectomy – an evidence-based review: report of the Therapeutics and Technology Assessment Subcommittee of the American Academy of Neurology. Neurology 2005;65:794-801.

Chenevix-Trench G, Spurdle A, Gatei M, et al. Dominant negative ATM mutations in breast cancer families. J Natl Cancer Inst 2002;94:205-215.

Chesson AL, Wise M, Davila D, et al. Practice parameters for the treatment of restless leg syndrome and periodic limb movement disorder. Sleep 1999;22:961-968.

Clark GD. Genetics of human brain malformations. Continuum Lifelong Learning Neurol 2005;11(2):143-160.

Cohen ME, Duffner PK. Weiner and Levitt's Pediatric Neurology, 4th edition. Philadelphia: Lippincott Williams & Wilkins, 2003.

Comella CL, Shannon KM (eds). Movement disorders. Continuum Lifelong Learning in Neurol 2004;10(3):15-188.

Conroy JA. Progressive myoclonic epilepsies. J Child Neurol 2002;17:S80-S84.

Crawford P. Best practice guidelines for the management of women with epilepsy. Epilepsia 2005;46(Suppl 9):117-124.

CREST: *NEJM* 363 11-23 (2010).

Cross JH. Neurocutaneous syndromes and epilepsy- issues in diagnosis and management. Epilepsia 2005; 46:17-23.

Delgado-Escueta AV, Perez-Gosiengfiao KB, Bai D, et al. Recent developments in the quest for myoclonic epilepsy genes. Epilepsia 2003;44(Suppl 11):13-26.

Ebersole JS and Pedley TA. Current practice of clinical electroencephalography, 3rd edition. Philadelphia: Lippincott Williams & Wilkins, 2003.

Ellis RJ, Olichney JM, Thal LJ, Mirra SS, Morris JC, Beekly D, et al. Cerebral amyloid angiopathy in the brains of patients with Alzheimer's disease: the CERAD experience, Part XV. *Neurology*. Jun 1996;46(6):1592-6.

Ellison D, Love S, Chimelli L, et al. Neuropathology. Barcelona: Harcourt Publishers Limited, 2000.

España RA, Scammell TE. Sleep neurobiology for the clinician. Sleep 2004;27:811-820.

Eysenck, H. J. (1987). The definition of personality disorders and the criteria appropriate for their descriptions. Journal of Personality Disorders, 1, 211 " 219.

Faught E. Pharmacokinetic considerations in prescribing antiepileptic drugs. Epilepsia 2001;42(Suppl. 4):19-23.

Feddersen B, et al. (Oct 2007) "**Puppy sign'** indicating bilateral dissection of internal carotid artery." *J Neurol Neurosurg Psychiatry*, 78, p. 1055.

Fenichel GM. Clinical pediatric neurology: a signs and symptoms approach, 5th edition. Philadelphia: Elsevier, Inc., 2005.

Filiano J. Neurometabolic diseases in the newborn. Clin Perinatol 2006;33:411-479.

Fisch BJ. Fisch and Spehlmann's EEG primer: basic principles of digital and analog EEG, 3rd edition. Amsterdam: Elsevier, 1999.

Fix JD. High-yield Neuroanatomy, 2nd edition. Philadelphia: Lippincott William & Wilkins, 2000.

Fluharty AL. (Updated May 30, 2006). Arylsulfatase A deficiency. In: GeneReviews at GeneTests: Medical Genetics Information Resource (database online). Copyright, University of Washington, Seattle. 1997-2007. Available at **http://www.genetests.org**.

Folstein MF, Folstein SE, McHugh PR. "Mini-mental state." A practical method for grading the cognitive state of patients for the clinician. J Psychiatr Res. 1975;12(3):189-198.

Franz D, Glauser T. Tuberous sclerosis. Emedicine February 14, 2007.

Fuller GN, Goodman JC. Practical review of neuropathology. Philadelphia: Lippincott Williams & Wilkins, 2001.

Gallagher RC, Van Hove JL, Scharer G, et al. Folinic acid–responsive seizures are identical to pyridoxine-dependent epilepsy. Ann Neurol 2009;65:550–556.

Gatti RA. (Updated February 15, 2005). Ataxia-telangiectasia. In: GeneReviews at GeneTests: Medical Genetics Information Resource (database online). Copyright, University of Washington, Seattle. 1997-2007. Available at **http://www.genetests.org.**

George AL. Inherited channelopathies associated with epilepsy. Epilepsy Currents 2004;4:65-70.

Geyer HL, Bressman SB. The diagnosis of dystonia. Lancet Neurol 2006;5:780-790.

Geyer JD, Keating JM, Potts DC, Carney PR. Neurology for the boards, 3rd edition. Philadelphia: Lippincott Williams & Wilkins, 2006.

Gilman S, Low PA, Quinn N, et al. Consensus statement on the diagnosis of multiple system atrophy. Journal of the Neurological Sciences 1999;163:94-98.

Goetz CG. Textbook of clinical neurology, 2nd edition. Philadelphia: Saunders, 2003.

Goldberg S. Clinical neuroanatomy made ridiculously simple. Miami: Med Master Inc, 1997.

Grossman RI, Yousem DM. Neuroradiology: the requisites, 2nd edition. Philadelphia: Mosby, 2003;331-409.

The Guarantors of Brain. Aids to the examination of the peripheral nervous system, 4th edition. London: W.B. Saunders, 2000.

Hankey GJ and Wardlaw JM. Clinical neurology. London: Manson Publishing Ltd, 2002.

Headache classification committee of the IHS. Classification and diagnostic criteria for headache disorders, cranial neuralgias and facial pain. *Cephalalgia* 1988 8: 1-96.

Headache Classification Subcommittee of the International Headache Society (2004). "The Classification of Headache Disorders, 2nd Edition". *Cephalalgia* (Oxford, England, UK: Blackwell Publishing) 24 (Supplement 1).

Holmes GL, Moshé SL, Jones, Jr HR. Clinical neurophysiology of infancy, childhood, and adolescence. Philadelphia: Elsevier, Inc, 2006.

Hyland, K. The lumbar puncture for diagnosis of pediatric neurotransmitter diseases. Ann Neurol 2003;54(Suppl 6):S13-S17.

Hyland K, Shoffner J, Heales SJ. Cerebral folate deficiency. J Inherit Metab Dis 2010;33:563-570.

J Neurol Neurosurg Psychiatry 2004;75:1135–1140.

Kabbani H, Raghuveer TS. Craniosynostosis. American Family Physician 2004;69:2863-2870.

Kaler SG. (Updated July 13, 2005). ATP7A-related copper transport disorders. In: GeneReviews at GeneTests: Medical Genetics Information Resource (database online). Copyright, University of Washington, Seattle. 1997-2007. Available at **http://www.genetests.org**.

Kaye EM. Update on genetic disorders affecting white matter. Pediatr Neurol 2001;24:11-24.

Kullmann DM. Genetics of epilepsy. J Neurol Neurosurg Psychiatry 2002;73:32-35.

La Spada AR. (Updated December 28, 2006). Spinal and bulbar muscular Atrophy. In: GeneReviews at GeneTests: Medical Genetics Information Resource (database online). Copyright, University of Washington, Seattle. 1997-2007. Available at **http://www.genetests.org**.

Lee AG, Brazis PW. Systemic infections of neuro-ophthalmic significance. Ophthalmol Clin N Am 2004;17:397-425.

Leppik IE. Classification of the myoclonic epilepsies. Epilepsia 2003;44(Suppl 11):2-6.

Levin KH, Lüders HO. Comprehensive clinical neurophysiology. Philadelphia: W.B.Saunders Company, 2000.

Libman RB, Wirkowski E, Alvir J, Rao TH. Conditions that mimic stroke in the emergency department. Implications for acute stroke trials. Arch Neurol 1995 Nov;52(11):1119-22.

Lion-François L, Cheillan D, Pitelet G, et al. High frequency of creatine deficiency syndromes in patients with unexplained mental retardation. Neurology 2006;67:1713-1714.

Lisko JH, Fish F. Klippel-Trenaunay-Weber syndrome. E medicine October 5, 2006.

Littner MR, Kushida C, Anderson WM, et al. Practice parameters for the dopaminergic treatment of restless legs syndrome and periodic limb movement disorder. Sleep 2004;27:557-559.

Louis DN, Ohgaki H, et al. The 2007 WHO Classification of Tumours of the Central Nervous System. Acta Neuropathol 2007;114:97-109.

Louis DN, Ohgaki H, Wiestler OD, Cavenee WK. (eds). WHO Classification of Tumours of the Central Nervous System, 4th edition. Lyon: International Agency for Research on Cancer, 2007.

Lublin FD, Tullman M (eds). Multiple Sclerosis. Continuum Lifelong Learning in Neurol 2004;10(6):120-172.

Lucchinetti CF, Parisi J, Bruck W. The pathology of multiple sclerosis. Neurol Clin 2005; 23:77-105.

Macdonald, JM (1963). "The threat to kill". Am J Psychiatry 120: 125–130.

Mahapatra RK, Edwards MJ, Schott JM, Bhatia KP. Corticobasal degeneration. Lancet Neurol 2004;3:736-743.

Mandava P, Kent T. Metabolic disease and stroke: Fabry disease. Emedicine January 5, 2006.

Marcus S. Toxicity, lead. Emedicine October 25, 2005.

Marra CM (ed). Infectious diseases. Continuum Lifelong Learning in Neurol 2006;12(2):13-94,111-132.

McArther JC, Brew BJ. Neurological complications of HIV infection. Lancet Neurol 2005;4:543-555.

McGovern MM, Desnick RJ. Lipidoses. In: Behrman RE, Kliegman RM, Jenson HB, eds. Nelson textbook of pediatrics,16th edition. Philadelphia: W.B. Saunders Company, 2000;398-405.

Mena-Segovia J, Bolam JP, Magill PJ. Pedunculopontine nucleus and basal ganglia: distant relatives or part of the same family? Trends in Neurosciences 2004;27:585-588.

Menkes JH, Sarnat HB. Child neurology, 6th edition. Philadelphia: Lippincott Williams & Wilkins, 2000.

Mills PB, Struys E, Jakobs C, et al. Mutation in antiquitin in individuals with pyridoxine-dependent seizures. Nat Med 2006;12:307-309.

Mitchell JJ, Scriver CR. (Updated July 19, 2005). Phenylalanine hydroxylase deficiency. In: GeneReviews at GeneTests: Medical Genetics Information Resource (database online). Copyright, University of Washington, Seattle. 1997-2007.
Available at **http://www.genetests.org**.

Mochida GH, Walsh CA. Genetic basis of developmental malformations of the cerebral cortex. Arch Neurol 2004;61:637-640.

Morita M, Al-Chalabi A, Andersen PM, et al. A locus on chromosome 9p confers susceptibility to ALS and frontotemporal dementia. Neurology 2006;66:839-844.

Moschella SL. An update on the diagnosis and treatment of leprosy. J Am Acad Dermatol 2004;51:417-426.

NASCET: *NEJM* 325:445 (1991).

Neary D, Snowden J, Mann D. Frontotemporal dementia. Lancet Neurol 2005;4:771-780.

Oliver SCN, Bennett JL. Genetic disorders and the optic nerve: a clinical survey. Ophthalmol Clin N Am 2004;17:435-445.

Online Mendelian Inheritance in Man, OMIM (TM). McKusick-Nathans Institute for Genetic Medicine, Johns Hopkins University (Baltimore, MD) and National Center for Biotechnology Information, National Library of Medicine (Bethesda, MD). World Wide Web URL: **http://www.ncbi.nlm.nih.gov/omim/**

Optic Neuritis Study Group. The clinical profile of optic neuritis. Experience of the Optic Neuritis Treatment Trial. *Arch Ophthalmol.* Dec 1991;109(12):1673-8.

Ottman R. Analysis of genetically complex epilepsies. Epilepsia 2005;46(Suppl 10):7-14.

Pahapill PA, Lozano AM. The pedunculopontine nucleus and Parkinson's disease. Brain 2000;123:1767-1783.

Pankratz ND, Wojcieszek J, Foroud T. (Updated February 5, 2007). Parkinson disease overview. In: GeneReviews at GeneTests: Medical Genetics Information Resource (database online). Copyright, University of Washington, Seattle. 1997-2007.
Available at **http://www.genetests.org**.

Patterson M. (Updated February 13, 2006). Niemann-Pick disease type C. In: GeneReviews at GeneTests: Medical Genetics Information Resource (database online). Copyright, University of Washington, Seattle. 1997-2007.
Available at **http://www.genetests.org**.

Paulson H. (Updated September 30, 2003). Spinocerebellar ataxia type 3. In: GeneReviews at GeneTests: Medical Genetics Information Resource (database online). Copyright, University of Washington, Seattle. 1997-2007.
Available at **http://www.genetests.org**.

Paulson HL (ed). Neurogenetics. Continuum Lifelong Learning in Neurol 2005;11(2):59-160.

Pearl PL, Hartka TR, Cabalza JL, Gibson KM. (Updated July 25, 2006). Succinic semialdehyde dehydrogenase deficiency. In: GeneReviews at GeneTests: Medical Genetics Information Resource (database online). Copyright, University of Washington, Seattle. 1997-2007.
Available at **http://www.genetests.org**.

Pestronk A (website author). Neuromuscular disease center. Washington University, St.Louis, Mo. World Wide Web URL: **www.neuro.wustl.edu/neuromuscular/**

Petersen RC (ed). Dementia. Continuum Lifelong Learning in Neurol 2004;10(1):29-134.

Picker JD, Levy HL. (Updated March 29, 2006). Homocystinuria caused by cystathionine beta-synthase deficiency. In: GeneReviews at GeneTests: Medical Genetics

Information Resource (database online). Copyright, University of Washington, Seattle. 1997-2007.
Available at **http://www.genetests.org**.

Pinkofsky, H. B. (1997). Mnemonics for DSM-IV personality disorders. Psychiatric Services, 48. 1197-1198.

Plecko B, Paul K, Paschke E, et al. Biochemical and molecular characterization of 18 patients with pyridoxine-dependent epilepsy and mutations of the antiquitin (ALDH7A1) gene. Hum Mutat 2007;28:19-26.

Pons R, Ford B, Chiriboga CA, et al. Aromatic L-amino acid decarboxylase deficiency: clinical features, treatment, and prognosis. Neurology 2004;62:1058-1065.

Preston DC, Shapiro BE. Electromyography and neuromuscular disorders. Newton: Butterworth-Heinemann, 1998.

Prineas JW. Pathology of multiple sclerosis. In Cook SD ed. Handbook of multiple sclerosis, 3rd edition. New York: Marcel Dekker, Inc, 2001;289-324.

Pryse-Phillips W. Companion to clinical neurology, 2nd edition. New York: Oxford University Press, 2003.

Ramaekers VT, Blau N. Cerebral folate deficiency. Dev Med Child Neurol 2004;46:843-851.

Ramaekers VT, Rothenberg SP, Sequeira JN, et al. Autoantibodies to folate receptors in the cerebral folate deficiency syndrome. N Engl J Med 2005;352:1985-1991.

RELY: *NEJM* 361;12 1139-51 (2009).

Rengachary DA. The Washington manual neurology survival guide. Philadelphia: Lippincott Williams & Wilkins, 2004.

Rezvani I. Defects in metabolism of amino acids. In: Behrman RE, Kliegman RM, Jenson HB, eds. Nelson Textbook of Pediatrics, 16th edition. Philadelphia: W.B. Saunders Company, 2000;344-377.

Rho JM, Sankar R. The Pharmacologic basis of antiepileptic drug action. Epilepsia 1999;40:1471-1483.

Rho JM, Sankar R, Cavazos JE. Epilepsy: scientific foundations of clinical practice. New York: Marcel Dekker, Inc., 2004.

Rice GPA, Hartung H, Calabresi. Anti-α4 integrin therapy for multiple sclerosis: mechanisms and rationale. Neurology 2005;64:1336-1342.

Ringholz GM, Appel SH, Bradshaw M, et al. Prevalence and patterns of cognitive impairment in sporadic ALS. Neurology 2005;65:586-590.

Rolak LA. Neurology secrets, 3rd edition. Philadelphia: Hanley and Belfus, Inc, 2001.

Rose DZ, Husain R. (Nov 2012) "'**Ostrich Sign**' Indicates Bilateral Vertebral Artery Dissection." *J Stroke Cerebrovasc Dis.*;21(8), p. 903.

Sadock BJ and Sadock VA. Kaplan and Sadock's pocket handbook of clinical psychiatry, 3rd edition. Philadelphia: Lippincott William & Wilkins, 2001.

Salzman M, Madsen JM, Greenberg MI. Toxins: bacterial and marine toxins. Clin Lab Med 2006;26:397-419.

Sandbrink F. Motor Unit Recruitment in EMG. Emedicine November 7, 2005.

Saul RA, Tarleton JC. (Updated March 15, 2007). FMR1-related disorders. In: GeneReviews at GeneTests: Medical Genetics Information Resource (database online). Copyright, University of Washington, Seattle. 1997-2007. Available at **http://www.genetests.org**.

Schapira AHV. Etiology of Parkinson's disease. Neurology 2006;66:S10-S23.

Schiff D (ed). Neuro-oncology. Continuum Lifelong Learning in Neurol 2005;11(5):13-29,69-92,116-160.

Schöls L, Bauer P, Schmidt T, et al. Autosomal dominant cerebellar ataxias: clinical features, genetics, and pathogenesis. Lancet Neurol 2004; 3:291-304.

Schuelke M. (Updated May 20, 2005). Ataxia with vitamin E deficiency. In: GeneReviews at GeneTests: Medical Genetics Information Resource (database online). Copyright, University of Washington, Seattle. 1997-2007. Available at **http://www.genetests.org**.

Seashore MR. (Updated December 27, 2006). The organic acidemias: an overview. In: GeneReviews at GeneTests: Medical Genetics Information Resource (database online).

Copyright, University of Washington, Seattle. 1997-2007. Available at **http://www.genetests.org**.

SENTINEL Investigators. Natalizumab plus interferon beta-1a for relapsing multiple sclerosis. N Engl J Med. 2006 Mar;354(9):911-23.

Shahwan A, Farrell M, Delanty N. Progressive myoclonic epilepsies: a review of genetic and therwapeutic aspects. Lancet Neurol 2005;4:239-248.

Sheen VL, Walsh CA. Developmental genetic malformations of the cerebral cortex. Current Neurology and Neuroscience Reports 2003;3:433-441.

Sheth RD, Iskandar BJ. Craniosynostosis. Emedicine January 9, 2007.

Siegel GJ, Agranoff BW, Albers RW, et al. Basic neurochemistry: Molecular, cellular, and medical aspects, 6th edition. Philadelphia: Lippincott-Raven Publishers, 1999.

Silver NA, Stobart K. Osler-Weber-Rendu. Emedicine March 21, 2003.

Simon JH. Update on multiple sclerosis. Radiol Clin N Am 2006;44:79-100.

Snell RS. Clinical Neuroanatomy: a review with questions and explanations, 3rd edition. Philadelphia: Lippincott Williams & Wilkins, 2001.

Sparks SE, Krasnewich DM. (Updated August 15, 2005). Congenital disorder of glycosylation type Ia. In: GeneReviews at GeneTests: Medical Genetics Information Resource (database online). Copyright, University of Washington, Seattle. 1997-2007. Available at **http://www.genetests.org**.

Sparks SE, Kransnewich DM. (Updated August 15, 2005). Congenital disorders of glycosylation overview. In: GeneReviews at GeneTests: Medical Genetics Information Resource (database online). Copyright, University of Washington, Seattle. 1997-2007. Available at **http://www.genetests.org**.

Spiegel, D.; Loewenstein, R. et al. (2011). Dissociative Disorders in DSM-5. *Depression and Anxiety* 28 (9). 824–852.

Spillantini MG, Goedert M. The alpha-synucleinopathies: Parkinson's disease, Dementia with Lewy Bodies, and Multiple System Atrophy. Ann N Y Acad of Sci 2000;920:16-27.

Stanley C. Disorders of mitochondrial fatty acid oxidation. In: Behrman RE, Kliegman RM, Jenson HB, eds. Nelson Textbook of Pediatrics: 16th edition. Philadelphia: W.B. Saunders Company, 2000;377-380.

Strauss KA, Puffenberger EG, Morton DH. (Updated January 30, 2006). Maple syrup urine disease. In: GeneReviews at GeneTests: Medical Genetics Information Resource (database online). Copyright, University of Washington, Seattle. 1997-2007. Available at http://www.genetests.org.

Stroke. 1999; 30: 905-915 doi: 10.1161/01.STR.30.

Suls A, Mullen SA, Weber YG, et al. Early-onset absence epilepsy caused by mutations in the glucose transporter GLUT1.

Summar ML. (Updated August 11, 2005). Urea cycle disorders overview. In: GeneReviews at GeneTests: Medical Genetics Information Resource (database online). Copyright, University of Washington, Seattle. 1997-2007. Available at http://www.genetests.org.

Swaiman KF, Ashwal S, Ferriero DM. Pediatric neurology: principles and practice, 4th edition. Philadelphia: Mosby, Inc., 2006.

Swoboda KJ, Hyland D. Diagnosis and treatment of neurotransmitter-related disorders. Neurol Clin N Am 2002; 20:1143-1161.

Swoboda KJ, Saul JP, McKenna CE, et al. Aromatic L-amino acid decarboxylase deficiency: overview of clinical features and outcomes. Ann Neurol 2003;54(Suppl 6):S49-S55.

Tabrize SJ, Collinge J. Transmissible spongiform encephalopathies of humans and animals. In Cohen J, Powderly WG, eds. Infectious diseases, 2nd edition. Edinburgh: Mosby, 2004;297-306.

"The Still, Soft Voice: Breaking Through to the Inner Core" by Clifford K. Brickman (Kempner Books: 2010)

Tomsak RL, Levine MR. Handbook of neuro-ophthalmology and orbital disease: diagnosis and treatment, 2nd edition. Philadelphia: Butterworth Heinemann, 2004.

Tran T, Kaufmann LM. The child's eye in systemic diseases. Pediatr Clin N Am 2003;50:241-258.

Trenkwalder C, Paulus W, Walters AS. The restless leg syndrome. Lancet Neurol 2005;4:465-475.

Tsuji S. (Updated December 22, 2006). DRPLA. In: GeneReviews at GeneTests: Medical Genetics Information Resource (database online). Copyright, University of Washington, Seattle. 1997-2007. Available at http://www.genetests.org.

Tyler KL. Prions and prion diseases of the central nervous system (transmissible neurodegenerative diseases). In: Mandell GL, Bennett JE, and Dolin R, eds. Principles and practice of infectious diseases, 6th edition. Philadelphia: Churchill Livingstone, 2005;2219-2222.

Venditti CP. (Updated January 18, 2007). Methylmalonic acidemia. In: GeneReviews at GeneTests: Medical Genetics Information Resource (database online). Copyright, University of Washington, Seattle. 1997-2007. Available at http://www.genetests.org.

Vetrugno R, D'Angelo R, Montagna P. Periodic limb movements in sleep and periodic limb movement disorder. Neurol Sci 2007;28:S9-S14.

Victor M, Ropper AH, eds. Principles of neurology, 7th edition. New York: McGraw-Hill, 2001.

Volpe J. Neurology of the newborn, 4th edition. Philadelphia: W.B. Saunders Company, 2001.

Weiner HL, Levitt LP, Rae-Grant A. Neurology, 6th edition. Philadelphia: Lippincott Williams & Wilkins, 1999.

Wenning GK, Colosimo C, Geser F, Poewe W. Multiple system atrophy. Lancet Neurol 2004;3:93-103.

Wingerchuk DM, Lennon VA, Pittock SJ, et al. Revised diagnostic criteria for neuromyelitis optica. Neurology 2006;66:1485-1489.

Wenning GK, Colosimo C, Geser F, Poewe W. Multiple system atrophy. Lancet Neurol 2004; 3:93-103.

Wyllie E, Gupta A, Lachhwani D. The treatment of epilepsy: principles and practice, 4th edition. Philadelphia: Lippincott Williams & Wilkins, 2006

Yoshida M. Cellular tau pathology and immunohistochemical study of tau isoforms in sporadic tauopathies. Neuropathology 2006;26:457-470.

Yen KG. Mucormycosis. E-medicine December 20, 2004.

Zesiewicz TA, Elble RJ, Louis ED, Gronseth GS, Ondo WG, Dewey RB Jr, Okun MS, Sullivan KL, Weiner WJ. Evidence-based guideline update: Treatment of essential tremor: Report of the Quality Standards Subcommittee of the American Academy of Neurology. Neurology. 2011 Nov 8;77(19):1752-5.

Zucconi M, Ferri R, Allen R, et al. The official World Association of Sleep Medicine (WASM) standards for recording and scoring periodic leg movements in sleep (PLMS) and wakefulness (PLMW) developed in collaboration with a task force from the International Restless Legs Syndrome Study Group (IRLSSG). Sleep Medicine 2006;7:175-183.

Index